21.00

SENSATION AND PERCEPTION

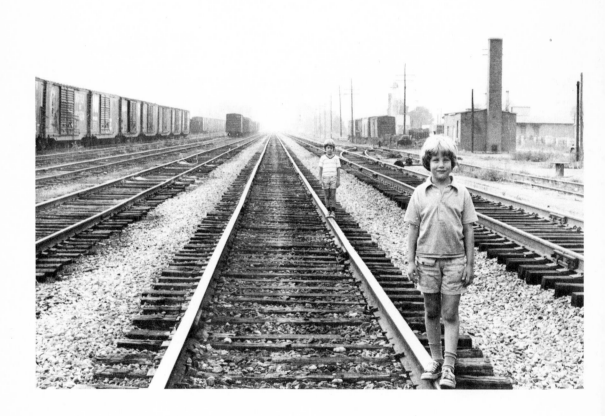

SENSATION AND PERCEPTION:
An Integrated Approach

Harvey Richard Schiffman
RUTGERS, THE STATE UNIVERSITY

JOHN WILEY & SONS, INC.   NEW YORK   LONDON   SYDNEY   TORONTO

Library of Congress Cataloging in Publication Data:

Schiffman, Harvey Richard, 1934–
   Sensation and perception.

   Bibliography: p.
   Includes index.
   1. Senses and sensation. 2. Perception. I. Title.

BF233.S44   152.1   76-185
ISBN 0-471-76091-9

Printed in the United States of America

10 9 8 7 6 5

To Jan and Noah

Preface

This book has two primary objectives. The first is to present the main principles of one of the oldest branches of experimental psychology, sensation and perception, within a biological context, organized around an evolutionary theme. Accordingly the reader will encounter many instances of specialized anatomy, physiological mechanism and behavior with adaptive consequences. The second primary objective is to present an integrated approach to the areas that are usually subsumed under the separate rubrics of sensation and perception. This book attempts to cover the fundamental concepts and principles of sense-receptor anatomy and mechanisms (sensation) that are presumed to underlie those cognitive processes that are usually labeled perceptual in nature, as well as to deal with the general topics of perception. Indeed, in the face of much research a clear or firm distinction between sensation and perception is impossible to maintain and as indicated in the first chapter such a distinction is not herein made.

Although the book should meet the needs, in terms of scope of coverage, of the upper-level undergraduate or beginning graduate course in sensation and perception, hopefully the inclusion of a glossary of technical terms will enable a more general readership. Moreover it is anticipated that this book will be of use to researchers and educators from many diverse areas of science, specialists who wish to acquaint themselves with the core of knowledge of sensation and perception or those who must consider the nature of sensation and perception within the framework of their own disciplines.

The orientation in bringing material together was that this book should be neither a handbook of methodologies nor an encyclopedic survey or inventory of the enormous number of hypotheses, theories, and accepted facts of sensation and perception. Rather an attempt has been made for a broad and balanced coverage of the theories, principles, and findings. Nonetheless the sophisticated reader may notice a neglect or omission of some topics. This is in the nature of a compromise between depth and scope. Fortunately there are numerous sources dealing with restricted topics for the interested reader.

The twenty chapters of this book were written so that each could be read at a single sitting (with the possible exceptions of Chapters 14 and 16). A departure from the usual topics of sensation and perception is the inclusion of a chapter on time perception (Chapter 20), an area of psychological inquiry that has recently been revitalized in the research literature and one that I feel bears a reading.

I have drawn heavily for both inspiration

and fact from a vast number of sources and their influence is obvious throughout the book. Although I cannot identify them all here some require special acknowledgement.

J. J. Gibson, *The Senses Considered as Perceptual Systems,* Boston: Houghton Mifflin, 1966.

Sir Stewart Duke-Elder, *Systems of Opthalmology. Volume I, The Eye in Evolution.* 1958, C. V. Mosby: St. Louis.

G. Walls, *The Vertebrate Eye and Its Adaptive Radiation.* Cranbrook Institute of Science, 1942; reprinted, 1963, New York: Hafner Press.

F. A. Geldard for his continuing contribution to human sensation: *The Human Senses. (second ed.)* 1972, New York: John Wiley.

I take this opportunity to acknowledge a special debt of gratitude to my teachers who at various times and places in my education instilled and nurtured an interest in sensation and perception. They are Marshall Curatolo and R. D. Walk, S. F. Fillenbaum, my teacher and a friend, H. F. Crovitz, who doubly served as my mentor and as a critical and humorous reader of this book when it was in manuscript form. A special thanks is owed to Harold Schiffman, who, at least at one time spoke to me more of the science of psychology than of the laws of chance.

The reviewers made many constructive criticisms and their careful reading expertly served to detect a number of errors and weaknesses. I hereby acknowledge my debt to William Stebbins, Herbert Crovitz, E. N. Pugh, and George Mandler. Though these psychologists have helped make this a better book, I bear complete responsibility for any remaining inaccuracies.

A special recognition is due to Jack Thompson, a friend and former graduate student who carefully read all portions of the manuscript at least once and helped in numerous ways to bring the manuscript to a published version. Also my thanks are due Douglas Bobko and other students who read and commented on portions of the manuscript and to those students who were exposed to much of the materials of this book in my undergraduate and graduate courses in sensation and perception.

I am especially grateful to Jack Burton, Psychology Editor and his staff at John Wiley & Sons, for their generous support and encouragement in all stages of the preparation of the manuscript. I am also indebted to the production staff and Illustration Department of John Wiley.

Finally and most significantly I must acknowledge my debt to Marjorie Faye Weiss Schiffman, who read, reread, and commented on the many drafts of the entire manuscript and helped in many diverse ways to bring it to a final form. Her encouragement and assistance has been considerable and important: however, she never typed a word.

H. R. Schiffman
New Brunswick, New Jersey
September 1975

Contents

SENSATION AND PERCEPTION

1 *Introduction*

In the chapters that follow is a presentation of the methods, principles, and findings concerning sensation and perception. Many meanings and distinctions have been attached to the terms sensation and perception, but it must be stressed at the outset that the distinction between the two is of greater historical relevance than of contemporary taxonomic utility. Traditionally, *sensations* refer to certain immediate and direct qualitative experiences—qualities or attributes such as "hard," "warm," "red," and so on—produced by simple isolated physical stimuli. Moreover, the study of sensations is primarily associated with structure, physiology, and general sense-receptor activity. The study of *perception,* on the other hand, generally refers to psychological processes whereby meaning, past experience, or memory and judgment are involved. Perceptions are associated with the organization and integration of sensory attributes, that is, the awareness of "things" and "events" rather than mere attributes or qualities.

The emphasis of our exposition will reflect the vast body of research literature on both structural and functional features of the receptor mechanisms as well as those "higher" processes that are perceptual in nature. Hence, although these terms will be part of our vocabulary we will generally avoid a clear sensation-perception distinction. (We would be remiss indeed to omit noting that there exist important controversies regarding definition and the proper subject matter of this domain of experimental psychology; see for example Gibson, J. J., 1963, 1966; Hebb, 1972, p. 217, 234–239; and Corso, 1967, p. 187; for a historical discussion see Boring, 1942, pp. 4–19).

Stated quite generally, sensation and perception refer to the study of a complex chain of interdependent processes: actuation of selectively tuned sensory receptors by energy changes in the physical environment resulting in an extraction of information and/or some form of potentially measurable behavior on the part of the receiving organism. We can thus identify a train of biological activity: stimulation from the external environment, impinging on sense receptors, which in turn produce neural activity, terminating in the behavioral phenomena of sensation and/or perception.

STIMULATION

The necessary information for effective stimulation of the sentient organism lies within the energy that emanates from the environment. A variety of forms of energy with particular biological utility can be identified: mechanical (including pressure and vibratory force), thermal, chemical, and electromagnetic (including photic energy). Each of these forms of energy acts on sense organs uniquely suited to their reception.

SENSORY RECEPTORS

Although our primary focus will be on human sensation and perception, our presentation will be organized around a functional, evolutionary theme. The assumption is made herein, for example, that the sense-receptor structures and mechanisms of a given species are shaped by natural selection to meet the informational needs required for survival. That is to say, random variations lead to the creation of adaptive sensory structures and functions that provide the form and level of sensory input adequate for the survival of each species of animal. Accordingly, we will encounter many instances of infrahuman specialized anatomy, physiology, and behavior with adaptive consequences.

All forms of life must interact with their external surroundings to extract information and to perform some form of energy exchange. For a one-celled animal such as the amoeba, the simplest of protozoa, environmental information is received without specialized receptors. Most of the amoeba's external surface is responsive to gravity, light, heat, and pressure. However, for most multicellular animals the demands of interacting with their habitat have led to the evolution of specialized receptor cells and units. All such receptor cells share in common the function of generating neural activity in response to stimulation, that is, of transducing or converting the energy of the incident stimulus from the environment into neural form.

Aggregations of such receptor units form sense organs of diverse structures and functions that are differentially sensitive to various forms of energy changes in the environment of the organism. Thus, receptive portions of the eyes are specialized to receive and react neurally to electromagnetic or radiant energy, the taste buds to react to chemical molecules in the mouth, the inner regions of the ear set to receive airborne vibrations, the skin surface to respond to thermal changes and to mechanical deformations, and so on. However, mechanical energy properly applied as pressure can produce effects on hearing and vision; similarly, because of the bioelectric basis of living tissue, electrical energy has the unusual property of actuating all sensory units.

In general, specialized sense receptors have evolved to perform the survival tasks of a species through selective response to particular forms of energy—energy that provides the species with information about its habitat. Indeed, sense-receptor structures and mechanisms can be studied in terms of their function in the behavior of the species, that is, by examining the relationship of a species' behavioral requirements for survival in its unique habitat to its sensory equipment. For example, the highly developed and specialized acoustic anatomy of the bat can be understood when this species is viewed in an ecological context. Bats are most active at night and often live in environments so dark that photoreceptor or light-sensitive mechanisms would be nearly useless. As an adaptive consequence, they have evolved sensory structures and behavioral capacities uniquely suited to locomotion in a lightless environment. Thus, their peculiar auditory structures and their extended range of sound emissions and receptions can be studied in terms of the bat's remarkable ability to locate and catch prey on the wing, and to navigate and avoid obstacles in the complete absence of light.

Sensory structures may also reflect a decrease in the functional demands of an organism's adaptation to its environment, as indicated by this unusual example:

The tunicate sea squirt in its larval form swims freely about, guided by its eyes and

ears, finding food and avoiding predators.
Reaching adulthood, it loses its tail and
attaches itself to a rock. For about two years,
it sits on the rock, vegetating. Its eyes, its
ears, and then its brain—all degenerate and
become useless. (Alpern, Lawrence, &
Wolsk, 1967, P. 1)

But in general, the outcome of the specialization of sensory structures is an increase in the potential information that can be extracted from the environment. As the range of functional demands increases, there is a need for greater sensitivity to energy and the capacity to make finer sensory discriminations. This is provided by the development of more specialized sensory mechanisms.

PLAN OF THE BOOK

Most meaningful sensory interactions between an organism and its environment are not restricted to a single sensory input. Hence, a study of the relationship of the total organism to its environment must generally take into account the biology and the ongoing activity of more than an isolated sense modality. However, there are vast differences in the nature of the effective physical energies, in the physiologies and functionings, and in the experimental methodologies required for studying the different sensory modalities. In order to make clear the detailed activity of the various sense modalities we will deal with each sense modality separately. Because more research has been performed on the visual modality it will be dealt with more extensively than the others.

CLASSIFICATION OF MODALITIES

The basis of organizing and classifying the sense modalities is not a simple matter and as is the case for most matters of definition, it is not universally agreed on. Some attempts at a taxonomy are made on the basis of specific morphological differences or distinct sensory qualities (e.g., Geldard, 1972), or are based on the nature of the energy to which receptors selectively respond (e.g., Corso, 1967; Christman, 1971). In contrast, J. J. Gibson (1966) has argued for a more functional organization. He has questioned the traditional study of a sense organ as a passive receiver of imposed stimulation; rather, he has stressed the information-gathering aspects of the senses. To this end he proposes a classification based on "modes of activity" and on the kinds of information picked up by the active organisms. Accordingly, his inventory is organized with respect to the organism's behavior—"smelling," "looking," and so on—accomplished by *perceptual systems* and the sorts of external information so obtained, rather than with respect to specialized receptor structures. His classification, shown in Table 1.1, corresponds to an extent with the usual sensory categories of vision, audition, touch, taste, and smell, but there are important differences. For example, his notion of a *haptic* system conceptually includes inputs from the skin, joints, and muscles. Another difference from the usual categorization is that taste (gustation) and smell (olfaction), usually treated as distinct sense modalities, are grouped into a unitary chemical-receiving system.

Functionally, Gibson's classification is a useful one and we will encompass aspects of it in the pages to follow. However, before discussing their processes and mechanisms we must introduce some of the methods for studying sensation and perception.

Table 1.1
THE PERCEPTUAL SYSTEMS[a]

System	Mode of Attention	Receptive Units	Sense
Basic orienting	General orientation	Mechano-receptors and gravity-receptors	Vestib-ular organs
Auditory	Listening	Mechano-receptors	Ear
Haptic	Touching	Mechano-receptors and possibly thermo-receptors	Skin, joints, and muscles
Taste-Smell	Smelling	Chemo-receptors	Nose
	Tasting	Chemo- and mechano-receptors	Mouth
Visual	Looking	Photo-receptors	Eyes

[a] Source: Gibson, 1966, p. 50; revised by Buss, 1973, p. 159.

Activity of the Organ	Stimuli Available	External Information Obtained
Body equilibrium	Forces of gravity and acceleration	Direction of gravity, being pushed
Orienting to sounds	Vibration in the air	Nature and location of vibratory events
Exploration of many kinds	Deformations of tissues Configurations of joints Stretching of muscle fibers	Contact with the earth Mechanical encounters Object shapes Material states; solidity or viscosity Heat or cold
Sniffing	Chemical composition of the medium	Nature of odors
Savoring	Chemical composition of ingested objects	Nutritive and biochemical values
Accommodation Pupillary adjustment Fixation, convergence Exploration	Light	Information about objects animals, motions, events, and places

Psychophysics 2

Virtually every living species has evolved some means of extracting information from its habitat for its survival—information such as the location and identification of food, water, prey, predators, and mates. Many facts on this characteristic have been gathered by ethologists, who observe behavior directly in natural, nonlaboratory situations. However, for certain requirements it is also necessary to resort to the experimental controls imposed by laboratory conditions of testing in order to investigate the dimensions and bounds of stimulus reception, that is, of sensation and perception.

Accordingly, it is the purpose of this chapter to introduce some of the general issues and quantitative methods employed for this task of measurement. The area of inquiry in which psychologists study the link between variation in specified characteristics of environmental stimulation (physical dimension) and the attributes and magnitude of subjective experience (psychological dimension) is called *psychophysics,* and the methodologies used to describe a lawful relationship between the physical and psychological dimensions are termed *psychophysical methods.* The problems of psychophysics are among the oldest of psychology, and historically they have often been tied to such philosophical issues as the

nature and meaning of subjective experience and the mind-body relationship. (For a historical perspective see Boring, 1942.)

As we noted in the preceding chapter, the physical dimensions of stimulation have been reasonably well identified and measured; as well as varying along an intensity dimension they take a variety of forms: photic, electrical, vibratory and mechanical, thermal and chemical. It is the determination of how these dimensions relate to subjective experience that accounts for an extensive experimental approach to quantification in psychology. In the course of much philosophical and scientific inquiry, a body of methods and facts has been gathered concerning the psychophysical problem. It must be stated that the issues of psychophysics define a distinct area of psychological inquiry with its unique set of problems and theoretical issues. However, our major objective will be well served by limiting the scope of this chapter to a general introduction to some of the main issues of psychophysics. We will focus on two of the most important: threshold measurement and the determination of the function relating the amount of physical energy to the perceived (or judged) magnitude of the resulting sensation. Although our focus will be on human judgment, note should be taken of the existence of a burgeoning literature on animal psychophysics (e.g., Stebbins, 1970).

DETECTION AND THE ABSOLUTE THRESHOLD

In the course of studying the relation of certain features of the stimulus to attributes of experience, an important and specific experimental question arises. What is the minimal amount of stimulus energy required for the detection of a stimulus? That is, how intense must the stimulus be in order for a viewer to reliably distinguish its presence from its absence. Clearly, no organism is responsive to *all* portions of the possible range of physical energies. Rather, the potential stimulus must be of sufficient or minimal intensity (and duration) to cause a certain degree of neural activation in order for it to be sensed.

The minimum magnitude values of the stimulus necessary for detection are generally known as *absolute threshold* values or *absolute limen* (Latin for threshold) values. Traditionally, these values define an approximation of the lower limit of the organism's absolute sensitivity. If the magnitude of the stimulus is too weak, not pro-

ducing a detection response, the stimulus magnitude is said to be *subthreshold* or *subliminal:* in contrast, above threshold values of the stimulus are termed *suprathreshold* or *supraliminal*. Some threshold values, not to be taken too seriously in their present form, are shown in Table 2.1. More detailed and precise values for most sensory modalities will be given in subsequent chapters. Quite obviously, the minimal detectable stimulus is not absolutely fixed and varies in the extreme with the modality investigated, with conditions of testing, and with a number of observer and experimenter factors.

There is a traditional set of procedures used to determine the threshold. One of the simplest procedures is called the *method of limits* or *the method of minimal change*. For example, to determine the absolute threshold for the detection of a light we might start with a light sufficiently intense to be perceived by a subject and then systematically reduce its intensity in small graded steps with a light dimmer until the subject reports that the light is no longer detectable. We then record that intensity level and then show the light at a still dimmer setting but now gradually increasing its intensity level until the subject reports that it is just perceptible. After a number of *descending* and *ascending* series of trials, we compute an average based on the energy levels at

Table 2.1
SOME APPROXIMATE DETECTION THRESHOLD VALUES[a]

Sense modality	Detection threshold
Light	A candle flame seen at 30 miles on a dark clear night (ca. 10 quanta).
Sound	The tick of a watch under quiet conditions at twenty feet (ca. 0.0002 dynes/cm^2).
Taste	One teaspoon of sugar in 2 gallons of water.
Smell	One drop of perfume diffused into the entire volume of a 3 room apartment.
Touch	The wing of a bee falling on your cheek from a distance of 1 cm.

[a] Source: Galanter, *New Directions in Psychology,* 1962, p. 97, Holt, Rinehart & Winston.

which the stimulus just becomes undetectable and just becomes perceptible. This serves as the statistical measure of the threshold for that subject under the general experimental conditions of testing. (As we will note in a subsequent chapter, the detectability of a light is very much a matter of the general conditions of lighting and the prior light exposure of the subject; indeed, the role of the present and prior conditions of stimulation apply to all sensory modalities.)

Another often employed technique of determining the absolute threshold, called the *method of constant stimuli*, requires a series of forced choice trials. In this case a fixed number of stimuli of different intensities are singly presented many times in random order. Upon each presentation the subject makes a detection response—either, "yes" he detects it, or "no" he does not. Then the percentage of the time that each stimulus is detected is computed and that stimulus value yielding a detection response 50% of the time serves as the measure of the absolute threshold.

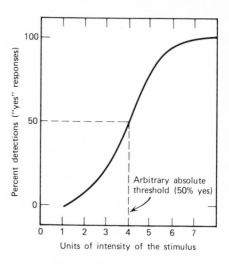

Fig. 2.1b *An empirical threshold function. By convention the absolute threshold is defined as the intensity at which the stimulus is detected on 50% of the trials. (From Psychology: Man in Perspective, by A. Buss, Wiley, New York, 1973, p. 153. Reprinted by permission of the publisher.)*

Fig. 2.1a *A hypothetical curve linking the stimulus intensity to the absolute threshold. Theoretically, below 4 units of stimulus intensity no stimulus is detected, whereas above 4 units the stimulus is detected 100% of the time.*

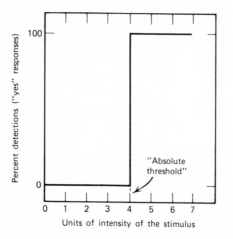

The concept of an absolute threshold assumes that there is a precise stimulus point on the intensity or energy dimension that when administered, becomes just perceptible. Accordingly, a stimulus one single unit weaker will not be detected. If this were the case, then some form of the hypothetical curve such as that shown in Figure 2.1a would result. That is, the subject would not detect the stimulus until a certain energy level was reached (e.g., 4 energy units, in the figure) at which point and beyond the stimulus is detected 100% of the time. In the case of tones, for example, there would either be a sound heard or complete silence would result. However, this rarely if ever happens. Rather, laboratory investigation typically yields *ogival* or *S-shaped* curves like that shown in Figure 2.1b. This indicates that as the energy level is increased there is also an increase in the probability that a stimulus will be detected.

Thus, we must conclude that there is no single immutable or absolute value that represents the minimum stimulus energy necessary for a detection response, that is, no fixed point separating the energy levels that *never* yield a detection response from those that *always* do. As an approximation of the threshold value, psychologists have adopted a statistical concept. By convention the absolute threshold value is assumed to correspond to that stimulus magnitude eliciting a detection response on half the test trials, that is, 50% of the time. This hypothetical point is shown in Figure 2.1*b*.

THEORY OF SIGNAL DETECTION

The observation that the value of the stimulus required for a threshold or detection response shows some variation suggests that factors additional to the observer's discriminative capacity or the magnitude of the stimulus may play some role in the observer's response. For example, in the forced choice method of constant stimuli (i.e., saying either "yes, the stimulus is perceived" or "no, it is not") the observer may say he detects the stimulus when, in fact, he is relatively uncertain. If the stimulus was *not* actually present, his "yes" response would be a *false positive* or a "false alarm"; an opposite error, that of not reporting the stimulus when it is, in fact, present, is also possible (a "miss").

Based on certain theoretical considerations as well as a good deal of research it is held that the proportion of correct detections of a stimulus (especially a weak one) depends on not only the observer's discriminative capacity but on certain nonsensory factors (called response bias), that is, by the criterion set for deciding whether a stimulus was present or not. Thresholds estimated by the classical methods are subject to a number of response bias variables, such as the observer's interpretation of the task instructions, his level of

attention to the stimulus (or the *signal,* as it is typically called in such contexts), his motivation for the task, and other nonsensory factors that might affect the observer's decision as to whether a signal is present or absent. Hence, when the threshold response for a constant stimulus intensity varies for a given observer, we do not know for sure whether his discriminative capacity has correspondingly shifted or whether he has merely changed the decision criteria on which he bases his response.

An approach to this conception of the detection problem, called the *Theory of Signal Detection* or *TSD,* rejects the traditional threshold notion completely (Green & Swets, 1966; Swets, 1973). In its specific details, TSD requires a discussion of statistical concepts and topics that cannot be treated here. However, it is our objective to outline its general scheme and to indicate the significance of TSD for the concept of the threshold and stimulus detection.

A basic assumption of TSD is that every stimulus presentation induces some change in the observer. However, there is ever present a constellation of interfering background or "noise" factors (noise as used here is in no way restricted to the auditory modality), factors whose presence may vary from trial to trial. Noise factors may consist of actual sensory stimuli such as "white noise" (a form of acoustic energy that contains a great number of different frequencies with intensities that take on random values and sounds like a background "hiss"). Noise may also include random effects of fatigue and attention or merely spontaneous or random neural activity. It is further assumed that the effects of background noise (or N) on the observer's sensation can be plotted as a normal probability distribution and that the effects of the signal plus the noise (or SN) on the observer's sensation can also be represented as a normal probability distribution. The normal distribution of N and SN means that on a series of constant energy noise trials (in which case no signal is present) or SN trials, the stimuli administered do not give rise to constant or stable sensory effects. Rather, the sensory effects from the same signal and noise or noise alone stimulation vary from presentation to presentation giving rise to the usual bell-shaped curves. The effects of N and SN can be graphically depicted on the same coordinates as shown in Figure 2.2. The abscissa represents the magnitude of the sensory effects—the sensation continuum.

The observer's task in the typical TSD experiment is to decide on each trial whether the stimulus administered contains the signal or is a trial with noise alone. Indicated on Figure 2.2 is the decision point or sensory criterion adopted by the observer, which determines whether he says "yes" or "no" as to the presence of the signal on a given trial. The criterion, thus, is the sensation level set by the observer for deciding whether a signal was administered or not. According to the criterion point plotted in Figure 2.2 he will say "yes" when the magnitude of the sensory effect, shown on the abscissa, exceeds that point and "no" when the sensory effect is less. In both instances he may be in error. This follows because usually the SN and N distributions have some overlap, making it impossible for an observer to set a sensory criterion or cut-off point that permits a correct response on every presentation of the signal. In fact, the form of the overlap is such that on some SN trials the sensory effects

Fig. 2.2 *Distribution of N and SN effects in TSD theory. The N and SN effects are normally distributed. The height of each curve represents the relative frequency with which a sensory effect of a given magnitude will occur, and the abscissa represents the magnitude of the sensory effect. The vertical lines through the center of each curve indicate the average effects of N and SN. The average effect of SN is slightly greater than the average effect of the N, hence in marking the average of the SN effects the line is displaced to the right of the one for N. The two curves for N and SN overlap so that on some trials the effects of the SN is less than that of the N. The decision point indicated on the abscissa represents the cut-off on the sensory continuum at which the observer decides whether he will report a "yes" or "no" response as to the presence of the signal on a given trial. Any number of criterion points could be adopted. In the hypothetical one employed below, all signals that produce effects that lie to the left of the criterion are responded to by a "no" response; all signals whose effects lie to the right are responded to by "yes". Clearly, the observer cannot always be correct. That is, there is no perfect criterion because some sensory effects can be caused by either the N or SN (shown where the N and SN curves overlap) and errors of "misses" and "false alarms" are possible. The meaning of d′ is described later on in the text. (Source: Galanter, 1966, p. 175. Reprinted by permission of the publisher.)*

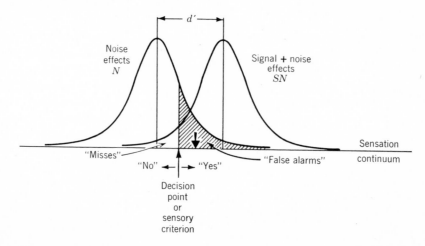

Table 2.2
THE STIMULUS-RESPONSE OUTCOME MATRIX FOR THE
OBSERVER RESPONDING EITHER "YES" OR "NO" ON EACH TRIAL
OF A DETECTION EXPERIMENT

		RESPONSE ALTERNATIVE	
		"Yes, signal is present"	*"No, signal is absent"*
STIMULUS ALTERNATIVES	*SIGNAL + NOISE*	Probability of a positive response when the signal is present HIT	Probability of a negative response when the signal is present MISS
	NOISE	Probability of a positive response when *no* signal is present FALSE ALARM	Probability of a negative response when *no* signal is present CORRECT REJECTION

may be less than those resulting from the presentation of the noise alone.

As noted above, on a given detection trial the observer's task is to decide whether his sensory impression is due to the actual presence of the signal within a noise background or from noise alone, that is, whether the stimulus presented comes from the *SN* or *N* distribution. His decision (shown as the decision point in Figure 2.2) is determined by the criterion level adopted at the moment. In the situation where the observer reports either "yes" or "no" there are four possible outcomes, shown in Table 2.2, each with a probability of a decision. The probability associated with each class of outcomes is due to two independent measures of the observer's performance—his decision criterion or response bias and his detectability of the signal, or his sensitivity, as it is usually called. One of the important bias factors affecting the setting of the criterion is the observer's *expectation* as to the presence of a signal. This may be created during the course of the experiment: If the signal occurs on almost every trial, then the observer will come to expect a signal almost always and the probability of false alarms will be higher than if

no such expectation was created. In contrast, if the signal is rarely present, the result might be many more "no" responses to the *SN* presentations. Table 2.3a presents some reported response probabilities for the case when the signal is presented on 90% of the trials and no signal on 10% (Galanter, 1962, p. 102). Table 2.3b shows the outcome probability for the case when no signal is presented on 90% of the trials and a signal is presented on 10%. It thus appears that variation in the proportion of signal presentations markedly affects the expectations of the observer; consequently he produces systematic changes in the proportions of hits (reporting "yes" when the signal is present) and false alarms. Significantly, the changes in the apparent value of the detection "threshold" occur without change in the stimulus energy.

Another factor that affects the criterion level is the observer's *motivation* toward detecting a specific outcome, that is, his concern with the consequences of his response. For instance, if the observer is motivated toward always detecting the signal, never missing it, he will likely lower the criterion level for reporting its presence and thereby increase his number of "yes" responses.

Table 2.3a
RESPONSE PROBABILITIES FOR A SIGNAL
PRESENTED ON 90% OF THE TRIALS AND
NO SIGNAL ON 10%[a]

		RESPONSE	
		Yes	No
S I G N A L	On	0.97	0.03
	Off	0.62	0.38

Table 2.3b
RESPONSE PROBABILITIES FOR A SIGNAL
PRESENTED ON 10% OF THE TRIALS AND
NO SIGNAL IS PRESENTED ON 90%

		RESPONSE	
		Yes	No
S I G N A L	On	0.28	0.72
	Off	0.04	0.96

[a] Source: Galanter, *New Directions in Psychology*, 1962, p. 102, Holt, Rinehart & Winston.

This amounts to raising the number of false alarms. The adoption of a more conservative criterion might yield fewer false alarms, but there would also be less hits. Thus, there appears to be no simply observed absolute threshold; rather, the observer adjusts his response criterion to both the signal strength and to certain subject variables such as his motivation and expectation concerning the signal's occurrence.

The detectability of the signal and the observer's sensitivity are generally analyzed in terms of the relationship between the proportion of hits and the proportion of false alarms—a relationship that shifts as the criterion the subject employs is

varied. Typically, the proportion of correct detections, hits, is plotted on the ordinate and false alarms on the abscissa. The resultant curves, called *receiver operating characteristic curves* or *ROC curves,* show the relationship between the proportions of hits to false alarms (see Figure 2.3*a*). As shown by Figure 2.3*b*, the form of these curves for any observer depends on two factors: the observer's sensitivity and his response bias. Notice that all points on a given ROC curve represent performance in detecting the same signal relative to the constant background noise. That is, the entire curve is generated without any change in the physical characteristics of the situation: The *N* and *SN* levels are the same for all points. The different points result from a shifting decision criterion exercised by the observer—a

Figure 2.3a *ROC Curves for three signals that are detectable to different degrees. Proportion of hits is plotted against false alarms. The value of d' is a measure of the observer's sensitivity or of the signal's detectability. Graphically, it is the distance between the means of the distributions of SN and N divided by the standard deviation of the common N distribution. (From Signal Detection Theory and Psychophysics, by D. M. Green & J. A. Swets, Wiley, New York, 1966, p. 60. Reprinted by permission of the publisher.)*

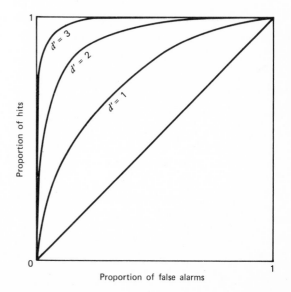

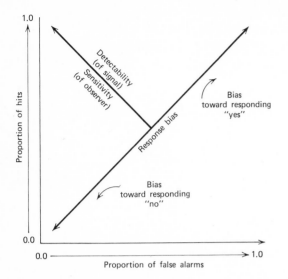

Fig. 2.3b *The features of an ROC curve. Indicated are the two components of a detection task: the observer's sensitivity and his response bias.*

matter of the observer's response bias. ROC curves are also referred to as *isosensitivity* curves (Galanter, 1962) because every point plotted on a given ROC curve results from the same measure of detectability. A measure of the sensitivity of the observer to a given signal strength is estimated by the linear distance of the ROC curve to the 45°

diagonal "chance" line (a line representing chance performance on a detection task). This distance is given by a single statistic known as d', and it is independent of the observer's response bias. The equation for computing d' is:

$$d' = \frac{M_{(SN)} - M_{(N)}}{\sigma_{(N)}}$$

which is the difference between the mean of the underlying probability distribution associated with signal and noise [$M_{(SN)}$] and the mean of the distribution of noise alone [$M_{(N)}$] in units of the standard deviation of the common noise distribution [$\sigma_{(N)}$]. The d' value is an index of the observer's sensitivity that is independent of response bias. A d' representation was shown in Figure 2.2 as the distance between the two vertical lines, representing the means of the N and SN distributions.

Figure 2.3a shows the ROC curves for signals that are detectable to differing degrees. For $d' = 1$, the distributions of N and SN lie relatively close together, and the signal is difficult to detect, whereas for $d' = 3$ the signal is quite easy to detect. These distributions of SN and N are suggested by the representation in Figure 2.4. Thus with increasing signal intensity the distribution of SN is displaced further from the distribution of N, resulting in a larger value of d'. When

Fig. 2.4 *A schematic graphic representation of the distributions of N and SN for the three ROC curves (d' = 1, 2 and 3, respectively) of Figure 2.3a. Here the value of d' is shown to vary with signal intensity relative to noise intensity as indicated by the distance between the averages of the distributions of N and SN. Thus, for d' = 1 the N and SN distributions lie close together, and the signal is difficult to detect relative to the case of d' = 2 or 3. For d' = 3, the means of the distributions for SN and N lie comparatively far apart and the signal is more easily detected. The relative detectability for d' = 2 lies between d' = 1 and d' = 3. The value of d', then, represents a measure of signal strength and the observer's sensitivity to the signal, independent of response bias.*

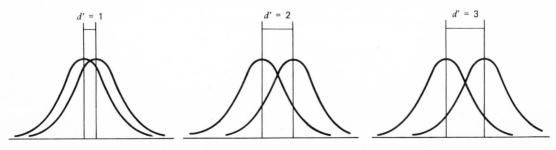

the signal strength is fixed, d' varies with the observer's sensitivity. Hence, d' is a measure dependent only on the signal intensity and the observer's sensitivity (for a lucid discussion of the logic and procedure of TSD see D'Amato, 1970, Chap. 5, and Green & Swets, 1966).

Perhaps the most significant feature of TSD is that it makes possible the isolation and evaluation of the separate effects of the observer's sensory capacity and response bias on his performance. Clearly, there is no single and absolute minimal magnitude value of a stimulus for its detection, no true sensory threshold. However, a threshold notion, as a statistical average, is a very useful concept that has a widespread application, and in terms of energy values, it provides an important approximation of the range and limits of the sensory systems. Moreover, there is an enormous literature on threshold determinations that must be dealt with. The directive made here is that we must interpret threshold statements cautiously: They serve as statistical approximations suggesting an average magnitude and/or a range of magnitude rather than a single energy value.

THE DIFFERENTIAL THRESHOLD

The *differential threshold* (or *difference limen*) is a measure of the smallest difference between two stimuli that can be detected. It is traditionally defined as the difference in the magnitude between two stimuli, usually a standard and a comparison stimulus, that is detected 50% of the time. For instance, if two tones of the same intensity are presented, one immediately following the other, the subject will generally report that they are identical in loudness. However, as we gradually increase the intensity difference between the two tones, a difference in intensities will be reached at which a "difference" judgment on half the trials will be reported. The magnitude

of this difference defines the differential threshold. Like the absolute threshold this judgment will be performed many times and a statistical measure of the difference between two stimuli that "on the average" is just noticeable will be computed. Like the absolute threshold, the differential threshold is a statistical concept of some questionable validity.

A psychophysical measure related to the differential threshold is a measure of the estimate that the magnitude of two stimuli are perceptually equal: It is called the *point of subjective equality* (PSE). PSE's have a wide range of applicability. For example, in the case of illusions two lines may appear equal when, in fact, there is a significant physical difference in their magnitude. The PSE is defined as that magnitude of a comparison stimulus that is equally likely to be judged greater or less than the magnitude of a standard stimulus. In practice the PSE lies halfway between the stimulus just noticeably smaller than the standard and the one just noticeably larger. Many variations in design, experimental methodology, and statistical procedures exist for the determination of the differential threshold and related measures such as the PSE.

Some of the background on this issue is quite significant in the history of the measurement of sensation. In 1834 E. H. Weber, a German physiologist, investigated the ability of subjects to perform discrimination tasks. What he noted was that discrimination is a *relative* rather than an absolute judgment matter. That is, the amount of change, increase or decrease, in a stimulus necessary to detect it as different is proportional to the magnitude of the stimulus. For example, whereas the addition of one candle to 60 lit ones results in a perception of a difference in brightness, one candle added to 120 does not. For the differential threshold to be reached for 120 candles, at least two candles are required. Extending this, then, the differential threshold (or the just noticeable change) for the brightness of 300 candles requires five or more lit candles and for 600 candles, 10 additional ones are required, and so forth. There is a fundamental principle of relative sensitivity involved referred to as *Weber's fraction* (or *ratio*) symbolized as follows:

$$\frac{\Delta I}{I} = k,$$

where I is the magnitude of the stimulus intensity at which the threshold is obtained, ΔI is the differential threshold value or the increment of intensity which, when added to the stimulus intensity I, produces a *just noticeable difference (jnd)*, and k is the resultant constant of proportionality, which differs for different modalities. The equation states that the smallest detectable increment (ΔI) in the intensity continuum of a stimulus is a constant proportion (k) of the intensity of the original stimulus (I). Thus, in the example of the brightnesses of candles, the Weber fractions for 60, 120, 300, and 600 lit candles would be 1/60, 2/120, 5/300, and 10/600, respectively or $k = 1/60$. In general, k is solved by computing the proportion a stimulus must be changed in order to yield a just noticeable difference. The smaller the fraction, the greater is the discriminative capacity of the observer for that task. Some representative Weber fractions for different modalities are given in Table 2.4.

Weber and others who followed him thought that the fraction remained constant across the intensity continuum for a given modality. However, in the course of much research, his view on the constancy of the fraction has been corrected and it does not have the broad validity claimed by Weber and others. In general, the constancy of the ratio has not been found to hold at all levels of intensities for any sensory modality. It holds reasonably well in the middle ranges, but the constancy of the fraction breaks down at weak and strong intensity levels for all modalities (see Boring, 1942). This is not to say that Weber's fraction should be discarded. Under certain conditions in the middle range of intensities the fraction provides a useful measure of discriminability, and we will encounter it in subsequent chapters. Without a doubt it has

Table 2.4
REPRESENTATIVE (MIDDLE-RANGE) VALUES OF THE WEBER FRACTION FOR THE DIFFERENT SENSES[a]

	Weber fraction ($\Delta I/I$)
Vision (brightness, white light)	1/60
Kinesthesis (lifted weights)	1/50
Pain (thermally aroused on skin)	1/30
Audition (tone of middle pitch and moderate loudness)	1/10
Pressure (cutaneous pressure "spot")	1/7
Smell (odor of India rubber)	1/4
Taste (table salt)	1/3

[a] Source: *Fundamentals of Psychology,* by F. A. Geldard, Wiley, New York, 1962, p. 93. Reprinted by permission of the publisher.

played an important role in the measurement of sensation, and it stands as one of the broadest empirical generalizations in the history of psychology. As Geldard (1962) comments, "Its inaccuracy is not the most important thing about it" (p. 92).

FECHNER'S LAW

In 1860 the physicist-physician-philosopher Gustave Fechner published *The Elements of Psychophysics,* a treatise that has had a profound effect on the measurement of sensation and perception. In it he proposed that the differential threshold or the jnd as described by Weber could be used as a standard unit to measure the subjective magnitude of sensation. His inquiry led to a formalization and extension of Weber's ratio into an epochal equation relating the magnitude of sensation to the magnitude of the stimulus. He began with the assumption that for a given sensory modality all jnd's represent subjectively equal units of sensation. According to Weber's

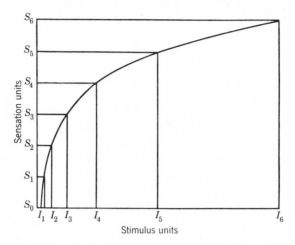

Fig. 2.5 *The relationship between the sensation continuum and the stimulus continuum according to Fechner's Law. As the sensation increases in equal steps (arithmetically), the corresponding stimulus continuum increases in physically unequal but proportional or ratio steps (geometrically). Thus, equal stimulus ratios, $I_2/I_1 = I_3/I_2 = I_4/I_3$, and so on correspond to equal increments on the sensation scale. A logarithmic function represents the relationship between an arithmetic and geometric series; hence, $S = k \log I$. (Source: Guilford, 1954, p. 38.)*

constant fraction, a given jnd corresponds to a constant proportional increase in the stimulus. If the basic intensity is low the increment for the jnd is small; if the initial intensity is high the stimulus increment necessary for the jnd will be large. Under the assumption that all jnd's are psychologically equal, it follows that as the number of jnd's grows arithmetically, stimulus intensity increases geometrically (see Figure 2.5). In other words, relatively larger and larger outputs in stimulus energy are required to obtain corresponding sensory effects. "The sensation plods along step by step while the stimulus leaps ahead by ratios" (Woodworth, 1938, p. 437). This arithmetic to geometric progression reduces mathematically to a logarithmic relation, that is, the magnitude of a sensation is a logarithmic function of the stimulus or

$$S = k \log I.$$

This states that the subjective magnitude or sensation (S) is proportional (k, a constant, which

includes the Weber fraction) to the logarithm of the physical intensity of the stimulus (I).

Just as the Weber ratio holds only marginally to the body of empirical findings, Fechner's law also is only an approximation of the relationship of sensory magnitude to physical magnitude. In fact, not all jnd's are found to be subjectively equal. For example, a tone 20 jnd units above the absolute threshold sounds more than twice as loud as one 10 jnd units above the absolute threshold (Geldard, 1962). However, according to Fechner's statement, "twice the loudness" is the only appropriate judgment.

STEVEN'S POWER LAW

More recent considerations of this issue contend that the relation between stimulus magnitude and sensory magnitude is not logarithmic. Indeed, one paper disputing Fechner's logarithmic equation is pointedly titled: "To honor Fechner and repeal his law" (Stevens, 1961). The mathematical relationship called *Steven's Power Law* (after S. S. Stevens, its originator and until his death in 1973, its principal proponent) shows a reasonably good fit for a wide range of data relating the magnitude of the stimulus dimension to the magnitude of sensation. Some of the sensory and perceptual phenomena that conform to a power law relation are shown in Table 2.5. According to the power law, sensory or subjective magnitude grows in proportion to the physical intensity of the stimulus raised to a power or mathematically stated:

$$S = kI^b,$$

where b is an exponent that is constant for a given sensory dimension and set of experimental conditions, and S, I, and k stand for sensation, intensity, and a constant (a scale factor that takes into account the choice of units used in the intensity dimension), respectively. By using a power law formulation, it is possible to show that

Table 2.5

REPRESENTATIVE EXPONENTS OF THE POWER FUNCTIONS RELATING PSYCHOLOGICAL MAGNITUDE TO STIMULUS MAGNITUDE[a]

Continuum	Measured exponent	Stimulus condition
Loudness	0.67	3000-hertz tone
Brightness	0.33	5° target in dark
Brightness	0.5	Very brief flash
Smell	0.6	Heptane
Taste	1.3	Sucrose
Taste	1.4	Salt
Temperature	1.0	Cold on arm
Temperature	1.5	Warmth on arm
Vibration	0.95	60 hertz on finger
Vibration	0.6	250 hertz on finger
Duration	1.1	White noise stimuli
Finger span	1.3	Thickness of blocks
Pressure on palm	1.1	Static force on skin
Heaviness	1.45	Lifted weights
Force of handgrip	1.7	Hand dynamometer
Vocal effort	1.1	Vocal sound pressure
Electric shock	3.5	Current through fingers
Tactual roughness	1.5	Rubbing emery cloths
Tactual hardness	0.8	Squeezing rubber
Visual length	1.0	Projected line
Visual area	0.7	Projected square
Angular acceleration	1.41	5-second stimulus

[a] These are approximations and average values. That this is the case has been pointed out by Marks (1974), who summarized the exponent determination from 40 studies on loudness. Depending on the method employed the exponents varied from 0.13 to 0.85. Source: Stevens, *Science,* 1970, *170*, p. 1045, December 1970. Copyright © 1970 by the American Association for the Advancement of Science.

the sensory modalities and perceptual tasks differ from each other in the extent to which the rate of sensation changes with changes in intensity. It is the exponent of the equation that reflects this particular feature of the relation between sensation and stimulation. For example, for the judged length of a line, the exponent is very close to 1.00 and the power equation reduces to $S = k$. This means that apparent length grows very nearly in direct proportion to physical length. This is depicted in Figure 2.6 as a straight 45° line. Thus, a 20 cm line looks about twice as long as one 10 cm long. For apparent brightness the exponent is about 0.33, and when a power function is plotted in arithmetic or linear coordinates, the

Fig. 2.6 *Power Functions plotted in Linear Coordinates. The apparent magnitude of shock, length, and brightness follow different growth curves because their power-law exponents are 3.5, 1.1, and 0.33, respectively. Notice that when plotted in linear coordinates the curve is concave upward or downward depending on whether the exponent is greater or less than 1.0. The power function for apparent length is almost straight in linear coordinates because its exponent is close to 1.0. The units of the scales have been chosen arbitrarily to show the relative form of the curves on a single graph. (Reprinted from "Psychophysics of Sensory Function," by S. S. Stevens, in Sensory Communication, by permission of the MIT Press, Cambridge, Mass.)*

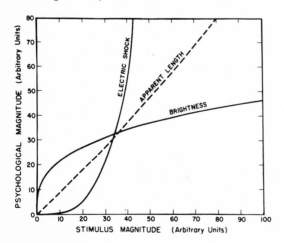

line representing the function is concave downward. This means that in order to double the apparent brightness of a light a considerable amount of stimulus energy, clearly in excess of a doubling of the stimulus magnitude, must be expended. In short, apparent brightness grows much more slowly than does stimulus intensity.

In contrast, the exponent for the apparent intensity of electric shock applied to the fingers is about 3.5, and as shown in Figure 2.6 its power function is represented by a curve that is concave upward. Clearly, a doubling of the electric current flow through one's finger results in considerably more than a mere doubling in the reported sensation (more like a tenfold increase). In general the exponent of the power function determines its curvature. An exponent close to 1.00 results in a straight line curve; a power function with an exponent greater than 1.00 is represented by a curve that is concave upward, whereas if the exponent is less than 1.00 the curvature is concave downward.

In logarithmic form the power law reduces to $\log S = b \log I + \log k$. When plotted in log-log coordinates (logarithmic scales on both axes), this equation describes a straight line whose slope (or measure of steepness) is b. That is, when both the ordinate (S) and abscissa (I) are plotted in logarithmic scales (with an intercept of $\log k$), the curvature disappears and the slope of the resultant straight line becomes a direct measure of the exponent. Accordingly, as shown in Figure 2.7 when the power function curves of Figure 2.6 are replotted in log-log coordinates, they become straight lines whose slopes are the exponents of the power equation. In log-log coordinates the high exponent for the sensation of electric current gives a steep slope, visual brightness gives a flat slope, and the nearly linear function for perceived length results in a slope close to 1.00.

The power function shows that the following relationship between the sensation and stimulation holds: "Equal stimulus ratios produce equal subjective ratios" (Stevens, 1972, p. 7). In other words, for continua conforming to the power law

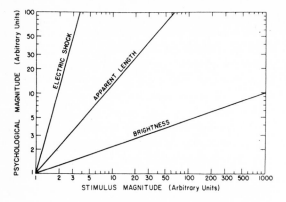

Fig. 2.7 *Power Functions plotted in logrithmic coordinates. When the curves in Figure 2.6 are plotted in log-log coordinates, they become straight lines. The slope of the line corresponds to the exponent of the power function governing the growth of the sensation. (Reprinted from "Psychophysics of Sensory Function," by S. S. Stevens, in Sensory Communication, by permission of the MIT Press, Cambridge, Mass.)*

a constant percentage change in the stimulus produces a constant percentage change in the sensation.

A number of methods are available for determining the power function for a given sensory dimension. Although it is not our task to present this methodology in detail, a general indication is warranted. One of the most often employed methods, called *magnitude estimation,* requires the random or irregular presentation of a series of stimuli that vary only along a single dimension, say, physical intensity. The experimenter (or the subject) assigns a number to a standard stimulus (called the *modulus,* a value of moderate intensity relative to the series)—say, 10 or 100—and the subject is required to produce numbers that express his judgment of the stimuli relative to the standard or modulus. For the example of loudness, if a stimulus in the series seems 10 times as loud as the modulus, the subject assigns a number 10 times as large. If it appears one-fourth as loud, the subject assigns a number one-fourth as large as the modulus, and so forth. In short, the subject

attempts to match the perceived intensity of each stimulus with a number relative to the modulus. Because there is but a short step between the observer's judgment and the final scale, such techniques are often referred to as "direct methods."

Based on a vast body of research, this procedure yields a clear estimate of the relation between subjective experience (sensation) and physical stimulation. Indeed, the method of magnitude estimation was used to obtain most of the exponents listed in Table 2.5. Although it is not unanimous, (e.g., Warren & Warren, 1963), there is general agreement that for many scaling tasks Steven's power law is a better representation of the relation between sensation and stimulation than Fechner's logarithmic equation. In nearly all domains where effective quantification of the sensory dimension is required one finds an application of the power law. We will note this on many occasions in the chapters that follow.

ADAPTATION LEVEL THEORY: THE RELATIVITY OF PSYCHOPHYSICAL JUDGMENT

As we noted, judgments made in psychophysical measurement tasks are significantly influenced by more than the factors that characterize the immediate stimulus. Helson (1947; 1964; Michels & Helson, 1949) proposed an approach to this issue called *Adaptation Level Theory,* which differs markedly from TSD. Adaptation Level Theory contends that when an observer makes judgments of the magnitude of a given stimulus attribute such as size, weight, loudness, color, area, and so on, he establishes a personal or subjective scale upon which the stimuli are judged. Helson has proposed that within a given stimulus series, there exists a magnitude that elicits a "neutral" or indifference response—a "medium" or norm value that he calls the *Adaptation Level* or *AL*. Depending on the attribute investigated, stimulus values above the AL are perceived (or judged) as "large," "heavy," "loud," "bright," and the like, and those below it in stimulus magnitude are perceived as "small," "light," "weak," "soft," "dim," and so forth. The AL represents the "centering" of the observer with respect to the range of stimuli confronting him, and it provides a measure of the frame of reference to which all judgments in a given series are related.

Helson's basic premise is that the AL, the neutral stimulus value, is the result of the interaction or "pooling" of all the internal and external factors confronting the observer in the experimental situation. In Helson's words, the AL is ". . . a weighted mean of all stimuli affecting behavior, past as well as present. . . ." (p. xvi). Helson has identified three classes of stimulus factors that affect the establishment and maintenance of the AL. Two are concerned with factors residing in the external environment, designated by Helson as the *focal stimuli* and the *background stimuli*. The focal stimuli refer to the stimuli to which the subject is directly and concurrently responding—those stimuli that are in the immediate focus of attention. Background stimuli refer to all other stimuli that occur within the confines of the experimental task, primarily the stimuli that provide the context or background within which the focal stimuli occur (e.g., the judgment of prior stimuli; the background on which the focal stimulus is placed). The third class of stimuli refer to internal organismic factors called *residual stimuli*. Usually residual stimuli do not fall under direct experimental control; they are comprised of such effects as the observer's past experience, practice, constitutional factors, and physiological states.

In Helson's detailed mathematical formulation the weights applied to each of the three classes of stimuli are assigned a quantitative expression. However, for our purposes it suffices to take note of a basic premise of AL theory, which is that under many conditions the general background in which psychophysical judgments are made affects the outcome of the judgment; that is, an observer's judgments reflect his adjustment to the total class of stimuli confronting him. By this reasoning judgments are always *relative* to some reference value.

An interesting account of the effects of the background and residual stimuli on the judgment of age and height was reported by Rethlingshafer and Hinckley (1963). Groups of individuals of different average ages and heights served as the subject-judges. It was assumed that the judges' own age and height served as the background and residual stimuli. In the age study the range of ages presented in the series extended from six to 108 years. The judgments were made on a nine-point scale, from "very, very young" to "very, very old." The AL in this context referred to a medium age, "neither young nor old" (a scale value of 5). Predictions were also made of the AL's based on Helson's formulation in which the judge's age was assigned as the value for the background and residual term. The result of the empirical AL's was that the younger the judges, the lower were the AL values. For boys and girls whose average age was 9.7 years the AL was found to be 36 years. For a group of men and women with an average age of 23.4, the AL was 42 years, and for men and women in their seventies the AL was set at 52 years. The theoretical or predicted AL's based on Helson's mathematical formulation was, in increasing age for the three groups, 36.3, 41.2, and 48.9, clearly a reasonably good fit of the predicted to the obtained data.

For the attribute of height, "short" men whose average height was 169.9 cm (66.9 in.) gave an AL or "medium" height that was 171.4 cm (67.5 in.), whereas for "tall" judges, whose average height was 186.2 cm (73.3 in.), the obtained AL was 172.7 cm (68 in.). The predicted AL for these two groups was 170.9 cm (67.3 in.) and 173.4 cm (68.3 in.), respectively—again a good fit. Both these findings support the assertion that characteristics of judges serve as a background factor in determining the values assigned to a series of stimuli and to the establishment of the AL.

Clearly, the quantitative approach of Adaptation Level Theory has identified three significant influences on psychophysical judgment, in particular on the establishment of an observer's frame of reference or standard against which other stimuli are judged. In addition to sensation and perception, Adaptation Level Theory has been applied to many substantively diverse areas of psychology, among them social behavior, cognitive processes, and personality (see especially Parducci, 1968). However, the theory has been criticized on a number of specific methodological (e.g., Fillenbaum, 1963) and general conceptual issues (e.g., Stevens, 1958, 1961). In addition certain modifications in its original formulation have been required in order to conform with a significant body of psychophysical data (e.g., Parducci, 1963).

The objective of this chapter was to outline some of the main issues of *psychophysics*—the relation between the physical dimension and subjective experience. To this end notions of both the *absolute* and *differential threshold* were described. The absolute threshold is traditionally and generally defined as the minimum amount of stimulus energy required for the detection of a stimulus. Although there is a vast literature on the absolute threshold, there are many factors that make a notion of a single immutable stimulus value for stimulus detection untenable. In short, the weight of empirical evidence is against a true threshold value. Pertinent to the threshold notion was an outline of the Theory of Signal Detection (TSD). This stressed that an observer's response bias, owing to many nonsensory factors such as expectation and motivation, determines the criterion exercised by an observer in his report as to whether he detects a stimulus (signal) or not. Furthermore, the TSD makes possible the isolation and evaluation of the separate effects of the observer's sensory capacity and response bias on his performance.

The differential threshold refers to the amount of change in stimulus energy necessary to produce a detectable difference between two stimuli. This led to *Weber's fraction,* which states that the amount of change in a stimulus necessary to detect it as different is proportional to the magnitude of the stimulus. Fechner extended Weber's work and formulated a mathematical equation linking sensation to stimulation. Fechner's equation states that the magnitude of a sensation is proportional to the logarithm of the physical intensity of the stimulus. Although both Weber's fraction and Fechner's equation have been questioned, their impact on measurement in psychology in general has been significant.

An alternative to Fechner's law was presented: *Steven's Power Law* holds that the relation between sensation and stimulation for many kinds of sensory and perceptual phenomena conforms to an exponential expression; that is, sensation grows in proportion to the physical intensity of the stimulus raised to a power. This formulation probably expresses the relationship between sensation and stimulation that has the greatest degree of recent application in many diverse domains of psychology.

Finally, we described the notion that judgments in psychophysical tasks are relative by outlining *Helson's Adaptation Level Theory.* According to this theory, the past and present stimuli evaluated by an observer produce a neutral point, the AL, which serves as the frame of reference against which all judgments are made.

The Orienting System   3

To survive most organisms must move about and maintain a particular physical orientation to their surroundings. To effectively locomote and to orient themselves to their environment most animals, whether they are terrestrial, avian, arboreal, or aquatic, must possess positional information on their body in space.

It is likely that for all animals gravity serves as the basic plane of reference. Organs and receptors sensitive to gravitational force are very old in the evolutionary scale. They are found in every animal phylum, and their general mode of functioning is quite similar (Fraenkel & Gunn, 1961; Gibson, J. J., 1966). The receptors share in common the fact that their excitation is dependent on mechanical deformation. Accordingly, they are called *mechanoreceptors*. In their simplest form, in invertebrates, gravity detectors are known as *statocysts* (*otocysts* in vertebrates), and they are perhaps the earliest specialized sense organs to develop in the entire animal kingdom. Although the physical mechanisms of statocysts observed among animal groups are anatomically diverse, their general sensory equipment operates on the same basic principle. Anatomical structures, generally free moving, called *statoliths* or *otoliths* (*oto* = ear, *lith* = bone) lie within the statocyst cavity (see Figure 3.1*a*). The statoliths are

heavier than the material (generally a fluid) of the statocyst cavity and are free to move. Due to inertial forces (gravity and acceleration), linear bodily movements produce a shifting or displacement of the statolith relative to a sheet of receptor tissue lined with ciliated receptors or hair cells

Fig. 3.1a *Highly simplified schematic drawing of a statocyst cavity, statolith, receptive hair cells and a theoretical set of nerve fibers. (Source: Gibson, J. J., 1966, p. 60; modified by Buss, 1973, p. 162. Reprinted by permission of the publisher.)*

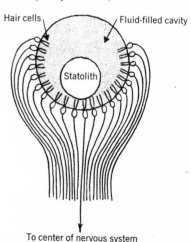

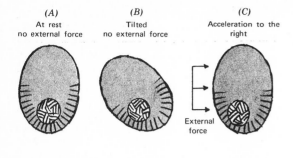

(A)
At rest
no external force

(B)
Tilted
no external force

(C)
Acceleration to the
right

External
force

Fig. 3.1b *The statocyst in three conditions: (A). at rest; (B). tilted; (C). linear acceleration to the right. (From Psychology: Man in Perspective, by A. Buss, Wiley, New York, 1973, p. 163. Reprinted by permission of the publisher.)*

(see Figure 3.1b). The statoliths thus react to gravity or linear movement—up-down, forward-backward, and left-right—by pressure on sensory receptors, which discharge when bent.

An interesting example of the operation of a statocyst is provided by observing some Crustacea. The crayfish regularly molts (sheds) the lining of its statocyst along with the rest of its exoskeleton (external covering). The statoliths, which for the crayfish are grains of sand, are also shed. After the molting process is complete, the crayfish, with its claws, replaces new grains of sand within the new statocyst cavity. As with all statoliths, the grains of sand react to inertial forces and serve to stimulate the sensory cells as the crayfish moves about. If the only replacement statoliths provided are iron filings, the crayfish will place them in its statocyst cavity. If a magnet is now moved about the head of the crayfish, the replacement statoliths will be correspondingly attracted, and the crayfish will alter its bodily orientation accordingly (the classic demonstration is by Kreidl in 1893; see Howard & Templeton, 1966, p. 108).

THE MAMMALIAN ORIENTING SYSTEM

The evolution of the organ for detecting orientational information probably proceeded from primitive organs consisting of cells covered with sensory cilia (hair-like structures) located in pits in the skin of aquatic animals. These were receptive to mechanical stimulation; that is, they were sensitive to movements and vibrations of the fluids filling the depression. In evolution these depressions became specialized and account for the bony cavities of the inner ears of mammals (sometimes called the *labyrinth*). The advanced development of the statocyst mechanism is seen in the mammalian structures, the *saccule, utricle,* and *semicircular canals,* collectively labeled the vestibular organs (see Figure 3.2a and b).

The function of the saccule is obscure; perhaps it has a minor auditory role or it is a vestigial organ (Wendt, 1951; Howard & Templeton, 1966). On the other hand, the utricle acts as a statocyst. It is a membranous sac filled with a fluid called *endolymph.* The utricular receptor is called the *macula,* and it is composed of cilia imbedded in the inner surface of the utricle. The cilia extend as nerve fibers to the vestibular nuclei in the brain. The statoliths in the utricle sac are calcium carbonate crystals that range up to 14 microns in diameter for mammals. In operation the cilia are bent by the statoliths in accordance with the extent and direction of linear displacement and bodily position with respect to gravity. Presumably when the body is speeding up or slowing down in a straight-line motion or when the head is tilted, that is, with linear acceleration (*changes* in the rate of motion), the inertia of the statolith particles brings about a bending of the hair cells with a consequent discharge by attached nerve fibers.

The functioning of the utricle overlaps with the operation of a second dynamic vestibular organ whose primary function is to register the direction and extent of *rotary acceleration* about any head axis. (Theoretically the utricle can

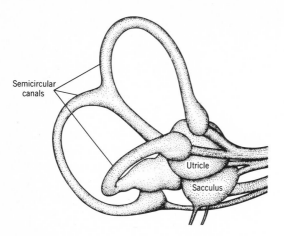

Fig. 3.2a *A drawing of the human vestibular organs. (Conrad C. Mueller, Sensory Psychology, © 1965. Reprinted by permission of Prentice-Hall, Inc., Englewood Cliffs, N.J.)*

register rotary motion as well as linear motion, but functionally this would produce a very complex pattern for a single receptor organ. The addition of a second receptor system for rotary motion enables the separation of functions and yields a greater sensitivity to movement.) The detection

Fig. 3.2b *Position of vestibular apparatus in head. (Source: Krech & Crutchfield, 1958, p. 187. Reprinted by permission of the authors.)*

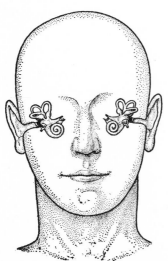

of rotary acceleration is available to few invertebrates, but most vertebrates from fish upward have developed specialized structures for its detection called *semicircular canals.* The semicircular canals, which vary from 15 to 22 mm in length and average 0.8 mm in width, are fluid (endolymph)-filled enclosures that lie at approximately right angles to each other (see Figure 3.3) and share a common cavity in the utricle. Each canal, functionally a complete and independent fluid circuit, relates to a major plane of the body. Thus together the canals form a three-coordinate system to which gross bodily motion of a rotary nature can be referred. Within each canal is a set of sensory hair cells. These receptors are stimulated when pressure is exerted on the fluid of the canal, such as during rotary acceleration resulting from movement of the head. Each canal widens at its base into a somewhat spherical, fluid-filled chamber called an *ampulla,* which contains the vestibular receptors (see Figure 3.4). Each of the ampullae contains a tongue-shaped protuberance, a sensory structure called the *cupula.* It is composed of crests of hair cells and tufts from the vestibular nerve and is encased in a gelatinous mass (see Figure 3.5a). The

Fig. 3.3 *Highly schematic drawing of semicircular canals. The semicircular canals in the head are at approximately right angles to each other. (Conrad C. Mueller, Sensory Psychology, © 1965. Reprinted by permission of Prentice-Hall, Inc., Englewood Cliffs, N.J.)*

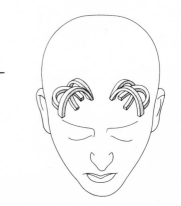

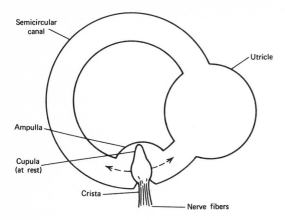

Fig. 3.4 *Schematic of a semicircular canal with ampulla, cupula, and crista. The dotted arrows indicate the potential deflection of the cupula by displacement of the endolymph produced by appropriate rotation of the head.*

Fig. 3.5a *Cross section of the cupula, showing the transverse ridge of hair tufts and cells fixed at the base (crista). The small insert shows the position of the ampulla of the semicircular canal. (From Foundations of Psychology, by E. G. Boring, H. S. Langfeld, & H. P. Weld, Wiley, New York, 1948, p. 376. Reprinted by permission of the publisher.)*

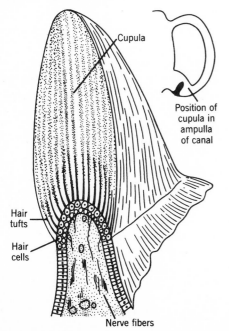

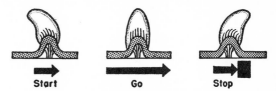

Fig. 3.5b *Representation of activity at the crista during various head movements. When the head starts moving or turning, the endolymph liquid of the ampulla at first lags behind, bending the cupula and the hair tufts in the direction opposite to the head movement. As the movement of the head continues, the ampullar liquid and the cupula move at the same rate as the movement of the head, and the hair tufts become erect (which is the case when there is no head movement). As long as the head is moving in a constant direction and at a constant speed, the hair tufts will remain erect. However, when the head movement stops, inertial force of the ampullar liquid carries the cupula forward and the hair tufts are bent in the forward direction. Thus, starts and stops and changes in direction move the liquid in the semicircular canals, bend the cupula, deform the hair tufts, and stimulate the hair cells, whereas constant motion, as shown in the center figure, produces no deformation and no neural impulses. (Source: Krech & Crutchfield, 1958, p. 187. Reprinted by permission of the authors.)*

cupula is fixed at its base, the *crista*, but swings freely into the ampullar cavity and is capable of being bent by pressure of the endolymph. This movement at the crista stimulates the hair cells, which transmit a series of impulses to the brain. Indeed, this is what occurs when the head is turned or rotated on a given axis (see Figure 3.5b). The endolymph fluid of the canals circulates and becomes displaced appropriate to the head rotation, creating hydraulic pressure. This resultant pressure causes a bending of the cupula, its deflection being proportional to the force of the head turn. The rotary movement thus causes differential deformation of the hair-cell receptors and is analyzable into its spatial components. When the rotation ceases or its rate stabilizes, the deflection is canceled and the cupula returns to its

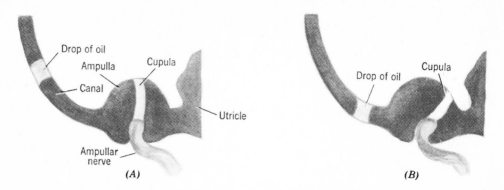

Fig. 3.6 *The effect of angular acceleration on the position of the cupula. The displacement of the endolymph was revealed by an injected droplet of colored oil. A. The cupula in its normal position at rest before rotation of the preparation. B. Change in position of the cupula as a consequence of rotary acceleration. (After Dohlman, 1935, page 1374, Reprinted by permission of the Proceedings of the Royal Society of Medicine.)*

normal position. In contrast, linear acceleration and gravitational force have little effect on the cupula.

The movements of the cupula have been measured directly in fish by dyeing the cupula so it could be photographed (Dohlman, 1935). Injection of a small drop of oil into the fluid of the canal enabled observation of the change in the position of the cupula in response to rotation. As Figure 3.6 shows, angular displacement of the endolymph produces pressure on the cupula and results in its bending.

The Vestibular Stimulation

The basic orienting system evolved as an adaptation to the conditions that normally confront animals, such as active movements and brief passive movements. It is not surprising, then, that the system is not well suited to cope with novel spatial conditions—ones that rarely or never occur in nature. For example, the vestibular system does not register sustained passive movements at a constant rate. If the velocity is kept stable or uniform, as in high-speed vehicular transport (e.g., trains, planes, or elevators), motion as such is not detectable. This follows from the fact that with constant motion the fluids, statoliths, and receptors will soon all move at the same speed, inertial forces will be overcome, and there will be no relative movement between the components of the vestibular mechanism, hence no stimulation.

The kinds of motion that the vestibular receptors are responsive to are acceleration or deceleration—*rate of change* of motion. In other words, the vestibular organs are suited to detect starts and stops and changes of motion, not constant velocities.

We should note that whereas adequate stimuli for the vestibular organs are head movements, it is possible to stimulate the receptors experimentally by electrical, mechanical, caloric (thermal), and even chemical stimuli. For example, with the caloric method stimulation is produced by irrigation of the external auditory canal with water, either warmer or colder than the canal wall (generally cold water is used). This produces a heat exchange that is readily transmitted to the vestibular organs, particularly to the fluid of a semicircular canal. The heating or cooling of the endolymph, producing expansion or contraction, causes an upward or downward movement of the fluid, which then deflects the cupula (Wendt, 1951).

VESTIBULAR PHENOMENA

Vestibular Nystagmus

Stimulation of the vestibular nerve reaches to the lower centers of the brain (medulla and cerebellum) from which connections are made with motor fibers to the neck, trunk, limb, and ocular muscles. The concern in the present discussion is with the relation of bodily position to patterns of ocular reflexes. When an individual is rotated about his body axis, stimulation of the vestibular canals and utricle initiate rhythmic and reflexive movements of the eyes. The eyes move slowly in a direction opposite to the movement of the rotation and rapidly back. This series of movements is termed *nystagmus*. When observed directly after rotation, these ocular movements are referred to as *post-rotational nystagmus*. The nystagmic reflex occurs when the subject is in the dark and is therefore not dependent on vision. However, nystagmic reflexes become complex if vision intervenes. When the eyes are open, another visually induced form of nystagmus occurs called *optokinetic* nystagmus, which becomes dominant over vestibular nystagmus. With the eyes opened during rotation, the nystagmus is more geared to the speed at which the retinal image moves. Vision during rotation may also inhibit post-rotational nystagmus (Wendt, 1951). It is thought that the vestibular response initiates the nystagmus, but optokinetic nystagmus takes command when the eyes are opened to compensate for movements of the retinal image so as to maintain a stable image on the retina. The dominance of vision over vestibular nystagmus is seen in the fact that the latter is almost completely inhibited if a rotating subject fixates on a target attached to his head (Marler & Hamilton, 1966).

In lower animals nystagmus may be lacking. However, in some instances similar responses to angular acceleration have been observed. For example, the turtle shows a smooth head-turning response which, upon analysis, occurs reflexively and serves to maintain its eyes toward a fixed point in space (Crampton & Schwam, 1962). A similar phenomenon has been shown with arthropods. When placed within a rotating, vertically striped cylinder, an insect, for example, turns its body in the same direction as the rotation of the cylinder. This response, called the *optokinetic reaction,* is apparently an attempt to stabilize the stripes in the visual field (e.g., see Davis & Ayers, 1972).

Oculogyral Illusion

There are visual effects, often correlated with nystagmic reflexes, that are sensitive indicators of vestibular stimulation. During or just after a period of rapid rotation about the body's longitudinal axis, objects in the visual field appear to move, either in phase with or against the direction of the rotation of the body. If a subject is rotated in the dark and fixates on an illuminated light source that rotates with him and that is stationary in space relative to the subject, the perceived movement of the light will be in the direction of the rotation at the start of acceleration (in accordance with the movement of the cupula). However, the apparent visual movement of the light will cease when the velocity of rotation becomes stabilized (owing to the cupula's returning to a normal resting position during constant velocity) and deceleration will reverse the apparent direction of the movement of the light. That is, negative acceleration will produce a deflection of the cupula, in a direction opposite to that of acceleration, falsely specifying the direction of rotation of the light. The result is an illusory perception of movement produced by stimulation of the semicircular canals, and it is called the *oculogyral illusion* (Graybiel & Hupp, 1946; Graybiel, Clark, MacCorquodale & Hupp, 1946).

An illusion similar to the oculogyral effect occurs in which observers report that they are moving when in actuality they are stationary and the visual field is in motion. Perhaps the most common experience of this occurs when an observer, looking from the window of a stationary train and viewing only a nearby moving train, perceives that his train is in motion. What occurs is that there is no vestibular stimulation of movement, but there is ambiguous visual stimulation. The visual scene is such that either train can be perceived as moving. Since the tendency is to perceive a consistent environment, the viewer attributes the movement to his train and perceives the visual field as stationary. In addition, under certain conditions, gravitational changes may be simulated by moving visual fields (Dichgans et al., 1972). These are further indications in man of the dominance of vision over vestibular information.

Notice should be taken of the fact that the conditions that produce these illusions are quite unnatural. Commenting on vestibular illusions obtained in the laboratory, J. J. Gibson (1966) states: "For millions of years animals moved by rhythmic pushes, not as Newtonian bodies and not in railroad cars or airplanes. It is therefore reasonable that an individual should be susceptible to vestibular illusions when passively transported in a vehicle" (p. 69).

And further, "The organ (cupula) was evolved for the needs of active locomotion, not for swiveling chairs. The illusion is hardly the fault of the organ, in view of its structure; the psychologist has simply *overstrained the capacity of the organ to register information.* Man has invented a great number of situations in which the natural information-gathering function of his perceptual systems is exceeded" (pp. 70–71).

Vestibular Adaptation and Habituation

The vestibular system is subject to adaptation or habituation. That is, if acceleration of rotation is sustained, the feeling of motion will gradually decrease and eventually may subside. Technically the phenomenon in which vestibular effects decrease for long periods of time with prolonged exposure is termed *vestibular habituation,* while *adaptation* effects are considered to be rapidly in-

duced and dissipated. However, it has been pointed out that the distinction between the two processes is not clear, and they will be treated as the same process (Marler & Hamilton, 1966).

Nystagmus may habituate with extended exposure to the abnormal vestibular stimulation that characteristically occurs to individuals who experience durations of continual motion, for example, sailors, airmen, acrobats, and dancers. Other consequences of rotation, for example, illusions of movement, vertigo, nausea, and dizziness, also habituate. For example, figure skaters were reported' to be able to walk straight after being rotated in a chair. The tendency to veer off had completely habituated out (McCabe: in Marler & Hamilton, 1966).

There are a number of procedures that reduce certain vestibular phenomena even when the body remains in motion. Ballet dancers, for example, are known to reduce nystagmus while spinning by "spotting," that is, by fixating on some distant point generally in the audience. A dancer keeps his head pointing to the audience as long as possible and then flicks his head around faster than his body until it again faces the same way. Though the vestibular organs of the dancer are continually stimulated by his spinning, the visual sense, providing a somewhat stable environment through spotting, overrides this. Furthermore, the more or less stable visual input obtained by spotting during rotation ensures that post-rotational nystagmus will not occur.

Deficiencies of the Vestibular Mechanism

A cat or rabbit suspended upside down by its paws and then released, whether in a light or dark environment, will right itself during the fall and land on its feet (see Figure 3.7). This is known as the *air-righting reflex* (Warkentin & Carmichael, 1939). This feat of bodily orientation in mid-air, physically extremely complex, is controlled by the functioning of the vestibular organs. An animal lacking proper vestibular functioning

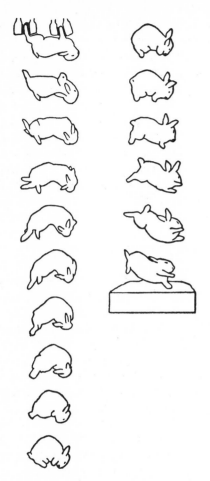

Fig. 3.7 *Tracings of successive frames of a motion picture (64 frames per second) of a 20-day-old rabbit dropped while upside-down. (Source: Wendt, 1951; from Warkentin and Carmichael, Journal of Genetic Psychology, 1939, 55, 77.)*

organs may be totally degenerate (due to the proximity of the vestibular organs to the auditory ones), equilibrium and postural adjustment are effective. However, when the use of vision is reduced or visual cues are ambiguous, general bodily orientation is sharply reduced. Boring (1942, p. 542) writes that some deaf people do not go under water when swimming because what is "up" and "down" get confused and there is danger of drowning.

Individuals both deaf and blind face a more serious problem in maintaining equilibrium. Of a group of 10 deaf-blind subjects studied with regard to their vestibular functioning, nine were unable to maintain balance more than a second or two when standing on one foot (Worshel & Dallenbach, 1948). Furthermore, the same nine deaf-blind subjects showed no post-rotational responses after 30 seconds of rotation in a chair. There was no nystagmus, nausea, dizziness, or illusion of movement. It is likely that the vestibular function was completely lacking in these subjects. It follows that individuals who suffer total loss of vestibular function are not susceptible to motion sickness.

Persons with certain vestibular defects of the utricle are not prone to an illusion that normal subjects experience called the *inversion illusion* (Simons: in Kellogg, 1971). It has been described that while testing the effectiveness of magnetic shoes for walking along the ceiling of an aircraft at zero gravity, a researcher had the strange visual experience of looking forward in the craft and perceiving the pilots sitting upside down. That is, the immediate spatial orientation of "down" conformed to where the feet were. In a systematic study of this phenomenon (see Figure 3.8) some of a group of normal subjects but none of a group who suffered otolithic defects experienced a reversal of their own orientation with regard to the locus of up and down (Graybiel & Kellogg: in Kellogg, R. S., 1971). This is probably due to the fact that in a zero gravity condition the normal subjects were denied the usual vestibular stimulation that enables them

does not show this adaptive reaction to falling and lands in a heap-like fashion.

In man the loss of vestibular function is accompanied by a general disorientation that eventually subsides. Initially the individual cannot stand upright steadily with his eyes closed and may suffer from vertigo. However, with use of vision he appears eventually to compensate for the loss. In congenital deaf-mutes, whose vestibular

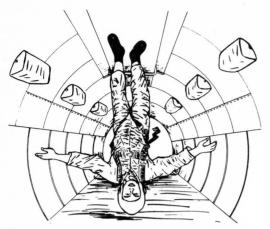

Fig. 3.8 *Subject orientation during investigation of the inversion illusion. (Source: Kellogg, 1971, 88, 220. Reprinted by permission of the author and the New York Academy of Sciences.)*

to perceive their orientation. Hence, they relied on themselves as the reference for the upright position. The group with defective otoliths were accustomed to a lack of vestibular stimulation and always perceived orientation with respect to the visual surroundings.

Evidence indicates that there is an interaction between the vestibular and visual modalities in man (e.g., Witkin, 1959). Indeed, as we have previously pointed out, the visual input for man dominates the input from the vestibular mechanism. As we ascend the phylogenetic scale, the vestibular apparatus diminishes in importance as a means of controlling bodily orientation. It follows that damage to the vestibular system of higher mammals is a less serious matter than in simpler animals where a substitute mechanism is not available. On the other hand, there are substitute positional mechanisms in lower animals that are not available to man. For example, modified mechanoreceptors are found in many fish that are receptors ("electroreceptors") specialized for the detection of electric fields and that may be useful for orientation (Bennett, 1971; Rommel & McCleave, 1972). In addition, fish possess a spe-

cialized mechanism that is extremely susceptible to low frequency vibrations or pressure changes in the surrounding water. It appears as a line running along the side of the body from head to tail and is called the *lateral line*. A small fluid-filled tube that runs under the skin beneath the line contains bundles of sensory cells (*neuromasts*) that respond to faint vibratory stimuli. It has been suggested that in the course of evolution the labyrinth (the auditory and vestibular organs) was derived from the lateral line organ (see Wersäll & Flock, 1965; Bergeijk, 1967).

Motion Sickness

Perhaps the most immediate and distressing feature of abnormal vestibular stimulation is motion sickness. In man (though motion sickness is not confined to man), it manifests itself in dizziness, nausea, vertigo, "cold sweating" and often it is accompanied by vomiting. Motion sickness can be produced by repeated vertical motion of a relatively moderate frequency—for example, that pattern of motion occurring to the seated aircraft passenger in rough air or in transit on a heaving ship in rough water. In one instance, a seven-foot wave of 22 cycles per minute, experienced as if on a ship, produced sickness within 20 min in 53% of a group of naval officers (Wendt, 1951). A series of short, self-imposed, rapidly repeating movements, as in walking and running, are not effective.

During experimental rotation of the body the potential for motion sickness is reduced if the position of the head is fixed relative to the body. It is higher if independent head movement is allowed. In the latter case very complex forces act on the vestibular organs due to the interaction of the movements of the rotation and those of the head. It was previously noted that, because motion sickness is primarily a result of unusual vestibular stimulation, individuals lacking vestibular function are not likely to suffer it.

An important factor in the initiation of motion sickness is whether or not the subject is actively or passively moved. Motion sickness is less common when the subject is in control of the movement. Thus the driver of a car is less likely to become sick than is his passenger. Perhaps this occurs because the active member, as the inducer of the movement, can anticipate the movement and produce compensatory motor adjustments toward maintaining proper orientation. Other events from common experience also appear to affect motion sickness: visual disorientation, visual illusions of movement, unpleasant odors, uncomfortable warmth, drugs (e.g., alcohol, narcotics), and certain emotional factors such as anxiety may facilitate motion sickness. Fortunately from an experiential point of view stimuli that initially produce motion sickness are eventually habituated to. Drugs are also available that inhibit the distressing symptoms of motion sickness.

In this chapter we have dealt with the mechanism by which organisms maintain a particular physical orientation to their surroundings. The sensory structures for this mechanism in mammalian forms of life are the utricle and semicircular canals, collectively labeled the vestibular organs. The utricle reacts to gravity or linear acceleration, whereas the semicircular canals register the direction and extent of rotary acceleration.

It was noted that the effective stimulation for the vestibular organs is accelerations or decelerations—changes in the rate of motion; constant or uniform motion is not detectable.

A number of vestibular phenomena were described: vestibular nystagmus, the oculogyral and inversion illusion, vestibular habituation, deficiencies of the vestibular mechanism, and finally, motion sickness.

The ability to receive mechanical stimulation does not cease with the vestibular system. Indeed, it is from the vestibular structures that the auditory system evolved, carrying with it the general principle of hair-cell stimulation by some mechanical agent.

The purpose of this chapter is to identify the characteristics of auditory stimuli and to describe the sequence of physiological events and processes of the auditory system that ultimately result in the perception of sounds.

THE PHYSICAL STIMULUS

The "sounds" we hear are actually patterns of successive pressure disturbances occurring in some molecular medium, which may be gaseous, liquid, or solid. If a guitar string is plucked, it vibrates back and forth compressing the air. Successive vibrations produce a pattern of periodic condensations or compressions and rarefactions of the surrounding air (see Figure 4.1). The pressure variations generated by vibrating bodies travel in wave form within the medium. The simplest kind of sound wave is one that causes successive pressure changes over time in the form of a single repeating sine wave. A graphic plot of the periodic compressions and rarefactions of a simple sound wave is shown in Figure 4.2. Though sound waves move progressively from place to place within the medium, the medium itself does not necessarily move. A visual analogy to sound wave propagation occurs when the surface of a pond is observed after throwing a rock into it. The entry of the stone causes disturbances that are seen as radiating circles of ripples that move progressively from place to place in the water without carrying the water with them.

The velocity of sound is calculated by measuring the time required for a compression to move a known distance. The velocity of sound propagation varies with the physical characteristics of the medium. For example, at 15° C, the rate of sound transmission in air is about 1100 ft/sec (340 m/sec), about four times this in water, and another four times as fast in steel or glass (Karplus, 1969; Hagelberg, 1973; see Table 4.1). In general, the velocity of sound is inversely proportional to the density of the conduction medium. The velocity of sound transmission changes with temperature variation: In air, it increases about 2 feet (61 cm) per second for every centigrade rise in temperature.

The principal physical properties of sound

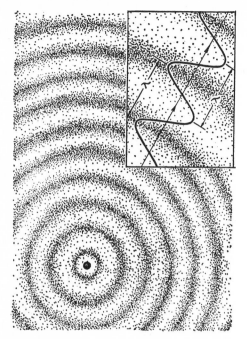

Fig. 4.1 *The molecules of air around a sound source are distributed as in the figure. Some molecules are grouped closely and some loosely, representing compression and rarefaction of pressure, respectively. A graph of this variation in pressure, shown in the insert, appears as a sine wave. The Greek letter, λ, represents wavelength. (Source: Griffin, D. R., 1959, p. 39. Reprinted by permission of the author.)*

waves may be characterized by their frequency, amplitude or intensity, and complexity.

Frequency

It is conventional in acoustics to characterize sound waves by the number of cycles or pressure changes completed in a second, that is, how rapidly the pressure changes. This measure is referred to as *frequency.* The experiential or psychological attribute corresponding to frequency is called *pitch.* The number of cycles per second is usually denoted by the term, *Hertz* (Hz), named for the nineteenth century German physicist Heinrich Hertz. The linear distance

between two successive compressions is called the *wavelength.* Wavelength and frequency are inversely related in that wavelength equals sound propagation speed divided by frequency (see Figure 4.3). Thus a 1100 Hz sound wave traveling at 1100 ft/sec (340 m/sec) has a wavelength of 1 foot (30.48 cm). A higher frequency means more pressure changes occur in a given unit of time and occur closer to each other in space, thus producing a shorter wavelength. Normally the maintenance of a sound of constant frequency is unexpected. Rather, sounds emitted from the environment, in particular animal vocalizations and speech, manifest patterned changes in frequency. Changes in the frequency of a continually vibrating body are referred to as *frequency modulations.* The frequencies of some familiar sound sources are indicated in Figure 4.4.

Amplitude

As Figure 4.2 indicates, sound waves also vary in their *amplitude,* which refers to the extent of displacement of the vibrating particles in either direction from the position of rest. The psychological attribute of *loudness* depends on the amplitude of the sound. Amplitude, which corresponds to the intensity of the vibration, is a function of the force applied to the sound-emitting source; in practice, the fundamental measure of amplitude is pressure variation. (Technically, the

Table 4.1
SPEED OF SOUND TRANSMISSION FOR SOME REPRESENTATIVE MEDIUMS

Medium	Speed (m/sec)
Air	340
Helium	960
Water	1500
Brass	3500
Marble	3800
Iron	5000
Fused silica	5960

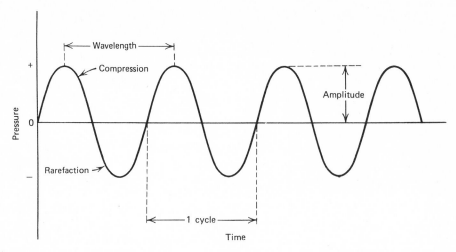

Fig. 4.2 *A graphic sinusoidal representation of successive compressions and rarefactions produced by a simple acoustic wave plotted as a function of time. The frequency of the sound wave is the number of cycles or pressure changes completed in a second. The amplitude of the sound, shown as the height of the wave, indicates the degree of compression (or rarefaction) of the sound wave.*

intensity or energy of a sound is proportional to the square of the amplitude of the pressure changes.) Pressure is force per unit area and sound pressure is measured in dynes per square centimeter (dynes/cm^2); sometimes sound pressure is stated in the equivalent term, *microbar*. A more recently employed unit of pressure variation is Newtons per square meter (N/m^2); one N/m^2 equals 10 dynes/cm^2. The ear is sensitive to an enormously wide range of pressures. The range in sensitivity from the strongest to the weakest sound that man can hear is of the order of 100 billion to one (Corso, 1967). Because of this immense range it has been found convenient to use a logarithmic scale of pressures called the *decibel* (*db*) scale. In essence the scale compresses or abbreviates the tremendous range of values that is possible so that the entire auditory amplitude scale is contained within a range of values from 0 to 160, approximately. The decibel is defined as one-tenth of a *bel,* which, in turn, is defined as the common logarithm of the ratio between two intensities or energies. The number of decibels is thus defined as 10 times the

logarithm of the ratio of two energies. However, decibels can also be used to express the ratio of two pressures that are related to energy flow by the square law. That is, in a sound wave, energy is proportional to the square of the pressure. The decibel formulas for sound energy and for pressure are:

$$N_{db} = 10 \log_{10} \frac{P_1^2}{P_2^2}$$

or

$$20 \log_{10} \frac{P_1}{P_2},$$

where N_{db} is the number of decibels, P_1 is the sound pressure to be measured and P_2 is a standard reference pressure, 0.0002 dynes/cm^2 (2 × 10^{-4} dynes/cm^2 or 2 × 10^{-5} N/m^2), chosen because it is close to the average threshold of human hearing (for a 1000 Hz tone). (Notice that the logarithm of any number squared is equal to two times the logarithm of the number; accordingly in the second formula, we have transposed the 2 from the exponents of the energies to the coefficient of

10.) Stimulus amplitude, utilizing the reference pressure of 0.0002 dynes/cm^2, is conventionally termed *sound pressure level (SPL)*. Use of the decibel scale, of course, eliminates any absolute zero reference point; the threshold level is taken as the starting level. As an example, a sound with a pressure of 0.02 dynes/cm^2, 100 times the reference pressure, corresponds to 40 *db* since

$$N_{db} = 20 \log_{10} \frac{0.02 \text{ dynes/cm}^2}{0.0002 \text{ dynes/cm}^2}$$
$$= 20 \log_{10} 100 = 40 \ db.$$

Fig. 4.3 *Wavelength as a function of frequency (measured in air at 15° C).*

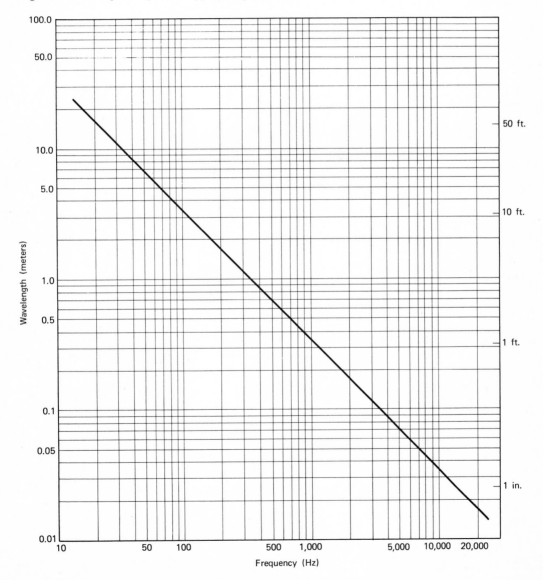

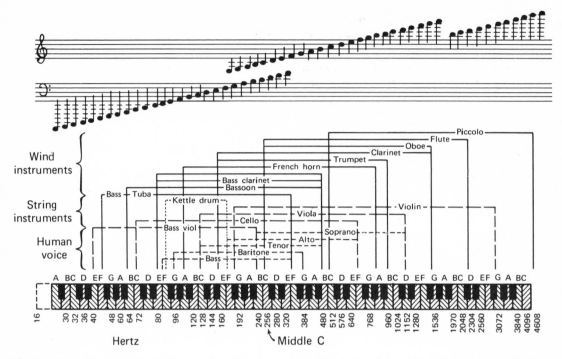

Fig. 4.4 *Tonal frequencies of various orchestral instruments and the human voice. (After the Principles of Radio, by K. Henney, Wiley, New York, 1938. Reprinted by permission of the publisher. Reproduced from Human Senses, by F. A. Geldard, Wiley, New York, 1972, p. 156.) (Notice that the scale notes corresponding to 1970 Hz and beyond should be one octave higher than indicated.)*

Accordingly, a sound with a pressure of 0.002 dynes/cm^2 equals 20 *db*, and a sound whose pressure level is 0.2 dynes/cm^2 equals 60 *db*. Thus a sound ten times the reference pressure corresponds to 20 *db*, a sound 100 times the reference pressure corresponds to 40 *db,* and a sound 1000 times the reference pressure corresponds to 60 *db.* In other words, for each ten-fold increase in sound pressure, we must add 20 *db*. Table 4.2 shows the relationship between sound pressure ratios (SPL) and decibel values. Some common sound sources and their decibel values are given in Figure 4.5.

It should be stressed that the critical component in the calculation of the decibel is the reference pressure against which other sound pressures are compared. We have described decibels with respect to a reference pressure that ap-

proximates the least pressure necessary for the *average* human observer to hear a 1000 Hz tone [i.e., 0.0002 dynes/cm^2 (SPL)]. Another reference employed is the value of the threshold pressure for hearing at the frequency of the tone. That is, the sound pressure for a tone of a given frequency is specified relative to the threshold pressure for that frequency. Notice that because the threshold sound pressure varies as a function of frequency, a different reference pressure is necessary for each frequency. When the threshold for each frequency is used as a reference, the sound pressure ratio in decibels is referred to as the *sensation level* or *SL.* A third reference pressure, employed primarily in research on physiological acoustics, is 1 dyne/cm^2 or 1 microbar (zero decibels on the SPL scale corresponds to 73.8 below 1 dyne/cm^2). The point of

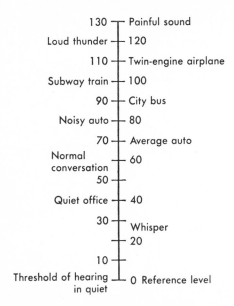

130 — Painful sound
Loud thunder — 120
110 — Twin-engine airplane
Subway train — 100
90 — City bus
Noisy auto — 80
70 — Average auto
Normal conversation — 60
50
Quiet office — 40
30
Whisper
20
10
Threshold of hearing in quiet — 0 Reference level

Fig. 4.5 *Sound pressure levels in decibels (SPL) of various common sounds (From Hearing: Its Psychology and Physiology, by S. S. Stevens & H. Davis, Wiley, 1938, p. 31. Reprinted by permission of the publisher.)*

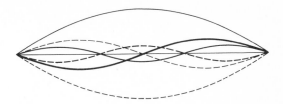

Fig. 4.6 *The figure shows the complex way in which a plucked string vibrates. In addition to the full length vibration, which produces the string's fundamental tone, there are simultaneous vibrations of shorter lengths (harmonics) that are precise divisions of the string's length—in this example, one-half and one-third. (Modified from Stevens & Warshofsky, 1965, p. 14. Reprinted by permission of Time-Life Books, Inc.)*

all this, of course, is that the reference pressure should be given in order for the decibel to have precise meaning.

Complexity

The sounds that occur in nature rarely if ever possess the simple sinusoidal form of Figure 4.2. Indeed, a sound described by a perfect sine curve is usually a laboratory achievement requiring special equipment such as tuning forks or an audio oscillator. Most natural sound-producing sources emit tones that possess a complex waveform. The psychological dimension corresponding to the sound's complexity is termed *timbre*. Complex sounds result because vibrating bodies do not do so at a single frequency. In general, a body vibrates simultaneously at frequencies that are multiples of the *fundamental* one or *first harmonic*, that is, the lowest tone of a series of tones. If a violin string is plucked, it vibrates as a whole,

alternately compressing and rarefying the air molecules. However, in addition to the full length of vibration (the fundamental tone) there are simultaneous vibrations of shorter lengths (*overtones* or *harmonics*) that are precise divisions of the string's length (see Figure 4.6). It is on the basis of tonal complexity that we are able to differentiate between musical instruments that emit tones at the same frequency and amplitude. Some examples of complex waveforms are shown in Figure 4.7.

One of the tools of complex sound wave

Table 4.2
RELATION BETWEEN SOUND PRESSURE RATIOS (SPL) AND DECIBEL VALUES

Pressure Ratios (P_1/P_2)	Decibels (SPL)
0.0001	−80
0.001	−60
0.01	−40
0.1	−20
1.0	0
10.0	20
100.0	40
1000.0	60
10,000.0	80

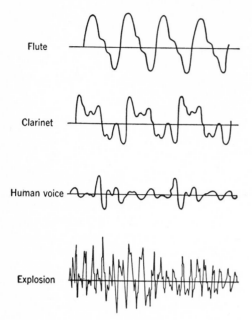

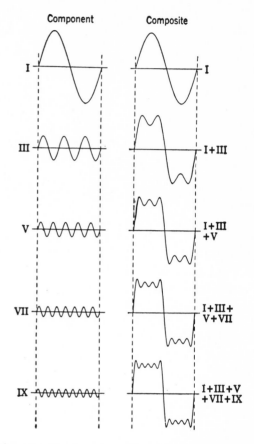

Fig. 4.7 *Typical sound waves. The first three are periodic waves, repeated regularly. The last is highly irregular. (Source: Foundations of Psychology, by E. G. Boring, H. S. Langfeld, & H. P. Weld, New York, 1948, p. 315. Reprinted by permission of the publisher.)*

analysis is based on a mathematical theorem devised in the early nineteenth century by the French physicist-mathematician, Jean Baptiste Fourier. Briefly, Fourier's theorem states that it is possible to express any periodic wave form as the sum of a series of simple sine waves, each with its own frequency and amplitude. The breakdown of a complex waveform into its components is called *Fourier analysis*. As an example of how a complex wave is so constructed, examine Figure 4.8. A complete cycle of the complex wave is shown at the lower right (roughly a square wave produced by some sirens). A Fourier analysis of this tone reveals that five components, illustrated by the left column of Figure 4.8, comprise it. In the right column are shown the composite waveforms as each component is added in successive steps. Mathematically, Fourier analysis

Fig. 4.8 *Simple waves add up to a complex wave. The first five harmonic components of a single cycle of a "square wave" are shown in the left column. The column at right shows the progressive change from a simple sine wave as each component is added. The relative frequency of each component corresponds to the numbers I, III, V, VII and IX, to the left of each line. If enough additional odd harmonics were added, the "square wave," a rectangular form that is already apparent in the form at the lower right corner of the figure, would be even more closely approximated. (From Foundations of Psychology, by E. G. Boring, H. S. Langfeld, & H. P. Weld, Wiley, New York, 1948, p. 316. Reprinted by permission of the publisher.)*

begins with a fundamental frequency that is the same as the frequency of the complex wave. To the fundamental frequency are added sine waves of higher frequencies that are multiples of the fundamental frequency.

The ear appears to be able to perform a crude Fourier analysis on a complex wave in that the ear can detect in a complex tone many of its frequency components. This fact, known as *Ohm's acoustical law,* states (with certain qualifications) that when exposed to two tones simultaneously we hear each tone separately. In practical terms, Ohm's law refers to a true aspect of hearing. For example, individuals who can identify the notes of a piano when they are sounded one at a time may identify the two notes when they are simultaneously sounded.

The sine waves that represent a musical note, then, bear a simple relationship to each other. Each is an overtone or harmonic of the fundamental note, and the frequency of each overtone

is a multiple of the fundamental frequency. Plucking the A string (A above middle C) of a violin produces not only the fundamental A note of 440 Hz but also the first overtone one octave (the interval between two tones, one of which is exactly twice the frequency or half the wavelength of the other) higher of 880 Hz, a second overtone of 1320 Hz, and so on. An example of the relative contribution made by each of the harmonics is given in Figure 4.9. The upper waveform represents the note of a plucked piano string of C (128 Hz, one octave below middle C). The components of the tone, shown in the lower part of the figure, are seen to extend over a considerable frequency range. The greatest contribution, of course, is made by the fundamental frequency (128 Hz), and the higher overtones or harmonics show smaller magnitudes. Observe, however, that in this example the fifth overtone (768 Hz) contributes slightly more than half the amplitude of the fundamental frequency. What is revealed in

Fig. 4.9 *The waveform produced by a piano playing c = 128 Hz. The relative contribution made by each of the components is shown in the lower graph. [Source: Speech and Hearing, (revised ed.) by Harvey Fletcher, © 1952. Reprinted by permission of D. Van Nostrand Company, Inc.]*

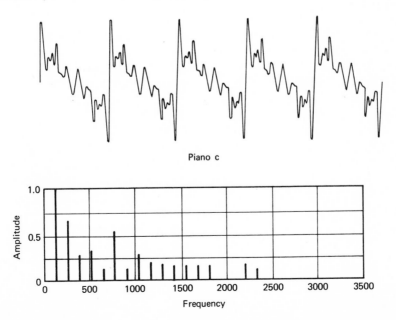

this example is a pattern of harmonics specific to this note. All notes of musical instruments are complex in different ways. Other instruments emphasize different overtones in a different way. Both the number of overtones and their amplitudes are to be determined by the physical properties of the vibrating body and the forces acting upon it.

Phase

A complete sound pressure wave or cycle extends from a position of rest to compression to rest to rarefaction and to rest again (refer to Figure 4.2). Generally, a complete cycle is specified as extending for 360°. The beginning is taken as 0°, the first compression peak as 90°, rest as 180°, rarefaction as 270°, and rest again as 360°. Two sounds of the same frequency, simultaneously sounded, will move alike at every instant and their waveforms will be "in phase." However, if two sounds are produced of the same frequency but displaced slightly in time, their waveforms

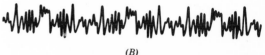

(A)

(B)

Fig. 4.11 *The effect of phase difference on complex sounds: The waveforms for two complex sounds are shown by A and B. Each complex wave is the result of the same thirty-two component sine waves of different frequencies. However, the complex wave forms differ because the peaks of the component sine waves for each complex wave have different relative phases. Thus, the relative phases of the component sine waves were adjusted so that their arrivals were at different times relative to one another, and the complex sound waves are heard as very different. The upper wave, at A, sounds harsher, lower in pitch, and somewhat louder than the wave at B. (Source: Bergeijk, Pierce and David, 1960, p. 86. Reprinted by permission of Doubleday & Co., Inc.)*

will differ in the time at which the waves rest or reach compression. These sounds will be "out of phase" and the phase difference is expressed in degrees. Some examples of phase differences are given in Figure 4.10. If one sine wave is in compression one-quarter of a cycle sooner than another, the waves are 90° out of phase (Figure 4.10*b*). If one wave occurs one-half of a cycle sooner than the other, they are 180° out of phase (Figure 4.10*c*). In this case, if both waves have the same frequency and amplitude, they would exert opposite effects on the air pressure, canceling each other's effects, and no sound would be heard. With respect to Figure 4.10, wave *C* is said to have the "reverse" phase of wave *A*.

Although in certain instances we may be aware of the vibratory nature of sound (e.g., a very low frequency note of a pipe organ), we do not generally perceive the time of arrival of compressions of high frequency waves. However,

Fig. 4.10 *Phase differences · The phase difference between two waves is produced by differences in the time at which the waves reach compression. In the above example, the phase differences are calculated relative to Wave A. For example, Wave B reaches its peak compression 90° after Wave A; Wave C reaches compression 180° after Wave A, and so on. (Source: Bergeijk, Pierce, & David, 1960, p. 85. Reprinted by permission of Doubleday & Co., Inc.)*

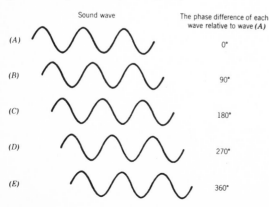

there is a perceptible effect of phase with complex sounds. In part, the waveform of a complex sound depends on the relative times of arrival of the wave crests of the component frequencies comprising it (see the example of Figure 4.11). Although the frequencies and intensities of the components remain constant, altering the relative phases of the components—having their compressions occur at different times relative to one another—alters the waveform and the quality of sound.

ANATOMY AND MECHANISMS OF THE EAR

We now turn to an analysis of the mechanisms of the ear that enable the complex pressure variations described above to produce the perception of sound. Specifically, our concern is with the receptor organs and mechanisms that transduce sound energy into nerve impulses and how these organs function. Though there are nu-

merous structures in nature for picking up acoustic energy, we will focus primarily on the human ear (Figure 4.12a). As shown in Figure 4.12b, this auditory system can be grossly divided into three major structural components: the outer ear, the middle ear, and the inner ear.

The Outer Ear

The outer ear of mammals consists of an earflap called the *pinna*, or *auricle*, the *external auditory canal* (or the *external auditory meatus*), and the *eardrum* (or *tympanic membrane*). The pinna, a wrinkled or convoluted vestigial flap that lies on the side of the head, functions to protect the sensitive and delicate inner structures, to prevent foreign bodies from entering the ear passage, and to collect and funnel air vibrations into the external auditory canal. It has been reported that pinnae may aid slightly in the localization of sounds (e.g., Batteau, 1968; Freedman & Fisher, 1968). Although man normally does not have functional control over the muscle system that controls the pinnae, many mammals possess

Fig. 4.12a *A semischematic drawing showing the gross anatomy of the ear. Vibrations entering the external auditory canal affect the eardrum. Vibrations of the drum are transmitted through the middle ear by the chain of bones [malleus (hammer), incus (anvil), stapes (stirrup)]. The foot of the stapes carries the vibration to the fluid of the cochlea. (Source: Davis, Hearing and Deafness: A Guide for Laymen, 1947, Murray Hill.)*

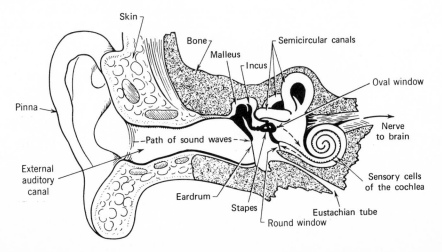

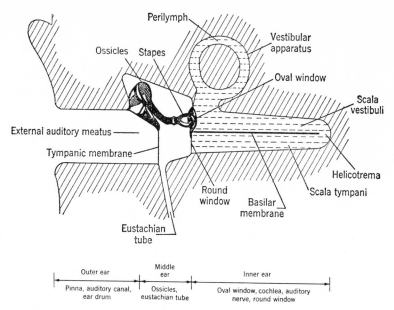

Fig. 4.12b *Schematic drawing of the ear. Notice that the cochlea is uncoiled in this drawing (as Figure 4.12c illustrates). When the footplate of the stapes moves inward, the fluid inside the cochlea flows in the direction of the helicotrema and makes the round window membrane bulge outward. (Source: Békésy & Rosenblith, 1951, p. 1076. Reprinted by permission of the publisher.)*

highly mobile ones; it is common to observe many lower mammals orient their pinnae toward the direction of a sound source. Pinnae are not found in all mammals. Sea-dwelling mammals such as the dolphin and whale do not possess pinnae, perhaps because they are so close to the density of the liquid transmitting medium, thus transparent to sound; moreover, the protuberance created by earflaps would undermine the streamlining of their outer body surface and hinder mobility. This may also be the reason lower vertebrates such as frogs, reptiles, and birds lack pinnae. In fact, some birds have a covering of feathers over their ear passage that may even hinder their hearing, but it is required to reduce wind noise during flight (Marler & Hamilton, 1966).

The external auditory canal is a cylindrical cavity about 2.5 to 3 cm long and 7 mm in diameter, open on the outside and bounded on the inside. It functions primarily to conduct vibra-

tions to the ear drum, but it also acts as a protective device against foreign bodies and it serves the purpose of controlling the temperature and humidity in the vicinity of the eardrum. The auditory canal acts like a horn, especially for sound frequencies around 3000 Hz, amplifying the sound pressure by induced vibrations. At this resonant frequency the sensitivity of the ear can be increased by as much as 8 to 10 *db* (Békésy & Rosenblith, 1951; Gulick, 1971). Of interest is the fact that in man this frequency corresponds closely to the frequency to which the ear is most sensitive.

The eardrum, a thin membrane pulled slightly inward at its center, is stretched across the inner end of the auditory canal and seals off the cavity of the middle ear. The eardrum vibrates in response to the pressure waves of sound. It is at the eardrum that pressure variations are transformed into mechanical motion. The displacements of the eardrum by pressure waves required to produce hearing are minute. It has been cited that for the detection of some sound frequencies near 3000 Hz the vibrations of the ear drum are as small as one billionth of a centimeter, which is about one-tenth the diameter of a hydrogen atom (Békésy, 1957a).

The Middle Ear

The general function of the middle ear is to transmit the vibratory motions of the eardrum to the inner ear. The eardrum closes off the air-filled cavity of the middle ear. Attached to the eardrum and vibrating with it is the *hammer* or *malleus,* the first of a chain of three small bones called *ossicles* (known by both their English and Latin names) that link the inner ear to the middle ear. The hammer connects to the *anvil* or *incus,* which in turn connects to the *stirrup* or *stapes,* whose footplate finally connects to the oval window of the inner ear. The ossicles are firmly connected by ligaments and transmit the vibrations acting on the eardrum by a lever system—with the motion of the stirrup footplate acting as a piston—to the *oval window.* It has been noted that the ossicular linkage in the middle ear of mammalian

life is of special importance to the reception of high frequency sounds (Masterton, Heffner, & Ravizza, 1968).

The eardrum (with an average area of about 70 mm^2) is considerably larger than the area of the foot of the stirrup (3 mm^2). Thus, comparatively large motions at the eardrum are transformed to smaller motions at the oval window. This difference produces an increase in pressure on the oval window about 25 to 30 times as great as that acting on the eardrum. In brief, small air pressure variations, distributed over the relatively larger eardrum, are concentrated on the smaller oval window with an increase in pressure. Notice that this increase in pressure' is a requirement owing to the change in sound wave medium from the aerial vibrations of the middle ear cavity to the fluid-filled inner ear chambers. In other words, the eardrum vibrates in response to small changes in pressure in the air, an easily compressible medium, whereas the oval window must move against the fluid of the inner ear, which requires much more pressure to be set in motion, since fluid is considerably more resistent to movement than is air.

In addition to making the incoming sound waves more effective, the middle ear protects the

Figure 4.12c   *Schematic of the cochlea uncoiled to show the canals. (Source: Stevens & Warshofsky, Sound and Hearing, p. 44. Reprinted by permission of Time-Life Books, Inc.)*

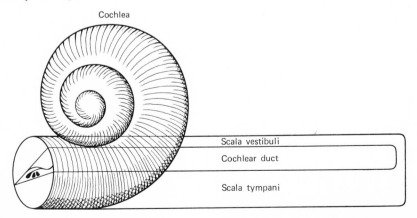

Cochlea

Scala vestibuli

Cochlear duct

Scala tympani

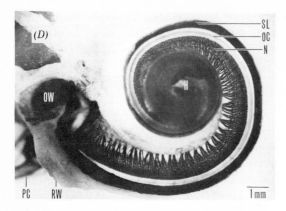

Figure 4.12d *Photograph of the human cochlea structure (25-year-old white female). H–helicotrema; OC–organ of Corti; N–auditory nerve fibers; OW–oval window; RW–round window. (Source: Johnsson & Hawkins, 1972, 81, 181. Reprinted by permission Annals of Otology, Rhinology and Laryngology.)*

inner ear from very intense sounds (hence very intense pressure changes). The middle ear chamber, though sealed off from outside atmospheric pressure changes, connects with the back of the mouth cavity through the *Eustachian tube.* This connection permits pressure from the outside to be equalized with air pressure in the middle ear. When the mouth is open, air pressure on both sides of the ear drum is equalized. Extreme pressure differences on both sides of the ear drum may produce abnormal and painful membrane displacements. When one is confronted with extremely loud sound or abrupt air pressure changes as from altitude dislocations, the sudden pressure change may burst the ear drum unless the mouth is kept open.

The Inner Ear

Next in the relay of pressure variations is movement in the inner ear, specifically the movement of the *stapes* exerted on the fluid of the inner ear. The inner ear is a small, tubular structure about 25 to 35 mm in length, resembling a snail shell, and for this reason it is called the *cochlea* (Latin

for snail). The cochlea is coiled on itself about three turns. Figure 4.12c shows a schematic of the cochlea, uncoiled to show the parts (see also Figure 4.12d). The cochlea contains three chambers or canals. Along most of its length it is divided by the *cochlear duct* or partition (also referred to as the *scala media*) into two chambers. The upper canal, the *scala vestibuli* (or vestibular canal), starts at the oval window and connects with the lower canal, the *scala tympani* (or tympanic canal), at the tip or apex of the cochlea by way of an opening called the *helicotrema*, a small opening of 0.25 mm^2 in area. A membrane-covered opening called the *round window*, which expands to accommodate fluid displaced by the stirrup against the oval window, is found at the basal part of the scala tympani. The two chambers are filled with a liquid called *perilymph*. The cochlear duct is filled with fluid *endolymph*, and it does not directly communicate with the other two canals. The cochlear

Figure 4.13 *Schematic drawing of the inner ear with the cochlea uncoiled. Notice that the basilar membrane increases in width as it extends toward the helicotrema. (Source: Békésy, 1960c; also, Békésy, 1967, 137. Reprinted by permission of the publisher.)*

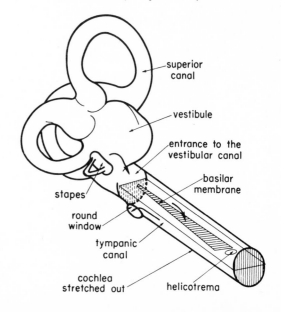

duct is bounded by two membranes. It is divided from the scala vestibuli by *Reissner's membrane* (vestibular membrane), and it is divided from the scala tympani by the *basilar membrane,* a tough but flexible membrane anchored to a bony shelf on one side of the wall of the cochlea and by a ligament on the other. It is the basilar membrane that is considered to differentially displace in response to the frequency of the sound; the displacement of the basilar membrane near 3000 Hz is about one-hundredth the diameter of a hydrogen molecule (Stevens & Davis, 1938, p. 56). Whereas the cochlea narrows toward the apex, the basilar

membrane becomes progressively wider (see Figure 4.13). At the base it measures about 0.08 mm wide, near the apical or helicotrema end it broadens to 0.52 mm. In addition, the basilar membrane at the base of the cochlea is about 100 times stiffer than it is at the apex.

It is within the cochlear duct that the specialized sensory structures, nerves, and supporting tissues for transducing vibrations to nerve impulses are found. Collectively these form a receptor structure called the *organ of Corti,* which rests on the basilar membrane and extends from the basal to the apical tip of the basilar

Fig. 4.14 *Diagrammatic cross section of the canals of the cochlea. The cochlear duct, bounded by Reissner's membrane, contains the organ of Corti with its hair cells that are the receptors for hearing. (Source: Davis et al., 1953. Reprinted by permission of the senior author and publisher.)*

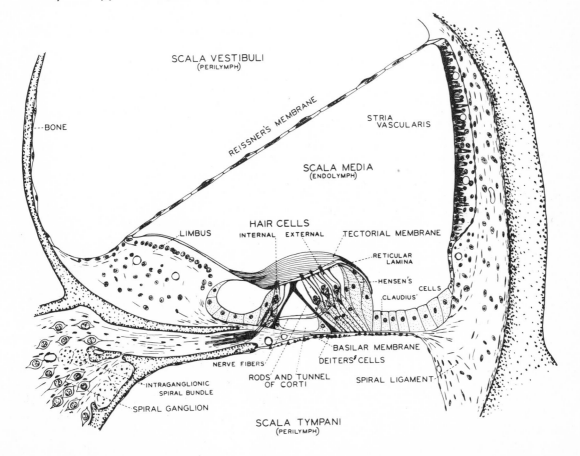

membrane. The organ of Corti is shown in Figure 4.14. It contains columns of specialized hair cells arranged in two sets, divided by an arch (*arch of Corti*), that are called the *inner hair cells* and the *outer hair cells* and number 3500 and 20,000, respectively. These sensory hair cells are the ultimate transducers of mechanical vibrations into nerve impulses. At the basal end, the hair cells are about 0.05 mm in length, whereas at the apical end they extend between 0.085 to 0.1 mm in length (Geldard, 1972). The filaments or cilia of the hair cells attach to an overhanging *tectorial membrane*. The tectorial membrane is attached at only one end and does not extend entirely across the cochlear duct. Motion of the basilar membrane that occurs in response to vibrations produced in the cochlea, initiated by movement of the *stapes* against the oval window, bend the cilia and the hair cells against the tectorial membrane in a shearing action (see Figure 4.15). This produces stimulation of the nerve endings and initiates the neural conduction process whereby mechanical

Fig. 4.15 *Schematic of shearing action between the tectorial membrane and the basilar membrane. Shearing action occurs when two flexible strips are joined at one end and then bent; the strips move in opposite directions relative to each other. It is the operation of this principle that produces the shearing action within the cochlear duct. That is, the motion of the basilar membrane produces a bending of the cilia and hair cells against the tectorial membrane in a shearing action. (Modified from Stevens & Warshofsky, Sound and Hearing, 1965, p. 47. Reprinted by permission of Time-Life Books, Inc.)*

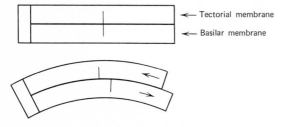

energy in a vibratory form is transformed into the nerve impulse.

Nerve fibers from the hair cells of the organ of Corti originate all along the basilar membrane from the base to the apex and make up the auditory nerve. The separate fibers are bundled together in such a way that fibers from neighboring regions on the basilar membrane remain together as they ascend to the brain. This spatial organization of neural elements—corresponding to the separation of different frequencies—produces a point-for-point projection of the basilar membrane in the cortex.

Bone Conduction

An alternative route of sound transmission is available, called *bone conduction*. This involves a direct contact between the head and a vibrating body bypassing the eardrum, ossicles, and other middle ear structures. In bone conduction, the vibration of the skull produces compression in the bones and stimulates the cochlea directly. It is quite easy to experience the effects of bone conduction: Close the auditory canal with ear plugs or even the finger tips and hum or speak. The vibrations of the air in the oral cavity are transmitted to the cheeks and from there to the lower jaw. The sounds heard are bone-conducted sounds that have reached the cochlea without access to the outer portions of the auditory system. This explains why the playback of a tape-recorded voice sounds strange and less familiar to the speaker than to his friends. Actually, it is not the voice that he usually hears when he speaks. Normally he hears not only the air-conducted sounds that others hear but also the sounds transmitted by bone conduction; however, only air-conducted sound has been recorded.

Animals living close to the ground like the snake, who is without eardrums, and some amphibia, have little need for the reception of airborne sounds; however, low frequency vibrations from the ground are received by these animals by a form of bone conduction.

FUNCTIONING OF THE INNER EAR

The chain of vibration transmission that produces the phenomenon of hearing normally proceeds from the eardrum to the ossicles to the oval window and then to the cochlea. However, it is the movement of the cochlear duct that activates and differentially affects the sense cells and associated nerve fibers. Thus, to understand the production of auditory messages we must primarily focus on how the basilar membrane and the organ of Corti respond to incoming sound waves.

Pitch Mechanisms in the Inner Ear

There are two main theories to account for the way in which the sensory structures of the ear function to enable frequency reception. Although there are a number of variations, they are conventionally referred to as the *place* theory and the *frequency* theory.

The *place theory* assumes that the organ of Corti is organized in a *tonotopic* fashion. Specifically, sensory cells near the base of the basilar membrane are more affected by tones of high frequency, and sense cells located near the apex or helicotrema are more likely to be stimulated by low frequency tones. Place theories thus maintain that different regions of the basilar membrane are stimulated by different frequencies—in short, different frequencies excite different auditory nerve fibers.

Evidence for a Place Theory

The Nobel laureate (1961, for medicine and physiology) Georg von Békésy has traced and documented the operation of the inner ear and has reported a number of research findings that support a place theory of hearing. His fundamental research findings concern the hydrodynamics (i.e., transmission in a fluid medium) of the inner ear. The basilar membrane is a flexible membrane not under tension. When vibrated by fluid motion, it shows *traveling wave* motion. As Figure 4.16a shows, a traveling wave is a wave form whose point of maximal displacement moves within an envelope. According to Békésy, the general operation of the auditory process is that a traveling sound wave of fluid-conducted vibration, produced at the oval window by the action of the stirrup, moves up the cochlea stimulating the cochlear canal and displacing its components, the basilar membrane and hair cells. In particular, high frequency vibrations create traveling waves whose points of maximal displacement are near the *stapes* (see Figure 4.16b), whereas low frequency vibrations produce traveling waves with peaks near the helicotrema.

A number of ingenious experiments by Békésy support the notion of the transport of vibrations by traveling waves. The sensory effects of much of the physical activity that occurs in the cochlear duct has been graphically illustrated by a

Fig. 4.16a *Various momentary positions within a cycle and the envelope formed of a traveling wave along the basilar membrane for a tone of 200 Hz. (Source: Békésy, 1953, 25, 770–785.)*

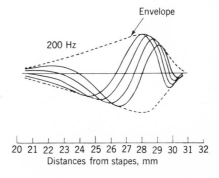

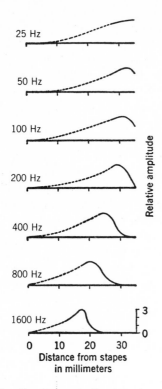

Fig. 4.16b *Envelopes of vibrations for various frequencies over the basilar membrane in cadaver of man. The maximum dispacement amplitude moves toward the stapes as frequency is increased. (Source: Békésy, 1949, vol. 21, pp. 245–249.)*

series of mechanical models designed by Békésy (1955) that accurately reproduced many of the elastic properties and couplings among components of the ear. Only some of these can be considered here. Figure 4.17 depicts one of the models of a portion of the uncoiled cochlea. Under the assumption that the basilar membrane is derived embryonically from skin, the model was designed to be used with the arm.

The model was essentially a fluid-filled brass tube enclosed in plastic with a narrow longitudinal slit covered with a plastic membrane. The width of the slit was held constant but the membrane's elasticity (in keeping with a model of the basilar membrane) was changed as shown in the figure by altering its thickness from the basal end (stapes–hand) to the apical end (helicotrema–elbow). In the center of the membrane a ridge was formed on which the skin of the arm rested. A bellows or piston that could be expanded and compressed (40 to 160 Hz) by a vibrating rod to set the fluid in the tube in motion was inserted in the right side of the tube (see Figure 4.17b). The forces in the fluid produced waves that traveled from the position of the hand to that of the elbow.

In operation the model works as follows. If an observer's arm is placed in contact with the ridge, he feels that as the frequency of the bellows

Fig. 4.17a *Two cross sections of a dimensional model of the cochlea, (B) made near the driving end and (A) made near the other end. (Source: Békésy, 1955, 27, p. 832. Reprinted by permission of the American Institute of Physics.)*

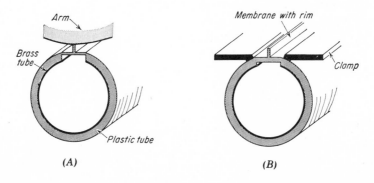

(A)   (B)

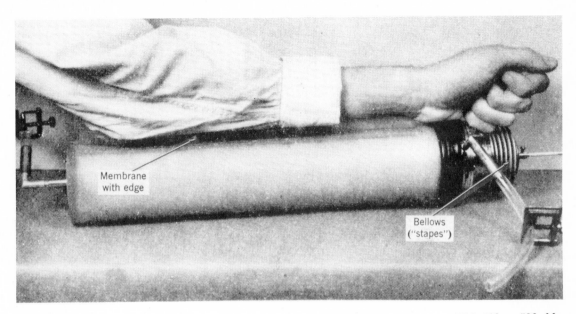

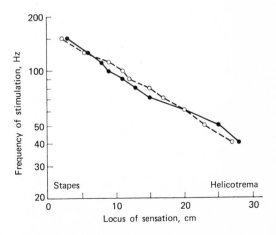

Fig. 4.17b *Mechanical model applied to the skin of the arm. (Source: Békésy, Science, 1956, 123, p. 783, May 1956. Reprinted by permission of the American Association for the Advancement of Science.)*

action is changed the locus of maximum stimulation moves from one end of the model to the other. Although the distribution of vibrations along the membrane is relatively broad, only a small section of the membrane seems to vibrate (about 2 to 4 cm). Figure 4.18 shows the relation between stimulation frequency and the location points of maximal perception for two successive sets of measurements on the left arm with the hand close to the "stapes" and the elbow near the "helicotrema."

To the extent that the model reflects cochlea activity, the action of the basilar membrane is rather flat or broad. How is it possible then for subjects to discriminate between frequencies that are only 3 Hz apart? Indeed, within a frequency range of 1000 to 4000 Hz we can detect frequency changes of less than 1%. Localization of the vibrations on the basilar membrane for various frequencies does not, at first glance, appear to be sharp or specific enough to account for this degree

Fig. 4.18 *The two curves represent two successive sets of measurements on the left arm with the hand close to the "stapes" region and the elbow near the "helicotrema." Intensity level was set at 25 db above threshold (SL). (Source: Békésy, Science, 1955, 123, 779–783. Reprinted by permission of the American Association for the Advancement of Science.)*

of acuity. It would appear that our ability to discriminate between frequencies is based on more than merely the separation of sound waves on the basilar membrane. A mechanism suggested to account for this was demonstrated by another mechanical model devised by Békésy (1957*b*). It consisted of a set of small vibrators placed in a box shown in Figure 4.19*a*. Each vibrator could be adjusted in intensity and was driven at the frequencies shown. With the forearm placed on the model and all the vibrators switched on at once at the same intensity, the impression is of a single vibratory event which corresponds to that of the 80 Hz vibrator activated alone. That is, the sensation produced is perceived as coming only from the middle vibrator. The frequencies of the other vibrators are inhibited but they contribute to the intensity of the central sensation (see Figure 4.19*b*). What is held to occur is that the nervous impulses corresponding to the peripheral vibrators are inhibited as far as specifying frequency or "pitch" information; however, their inputs are somehow channeled into and contribute to the "loudness" of the central vibrator in a sort of neural interaction that Békésy (1958) termed "funneling." Funneling is a phenomenon in which

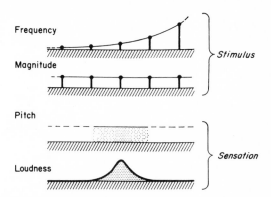

Fig. 4.19*b* *A representation of the sensory effects of stimulation of the skin surface with the apparatus shown in 4.19a. The physical aspects of the stimulation are schematized in the top part of the figure whereas the bottom part represents the psychological experience. (Source: Békésy, 1957b, Vol. 29, pp. 1059–1069.)*

a central summatory action and a lateral inhibitory action occur simultaneously, which serves to sharpen the pitch discrimination of sound. It is as if the vibrators on the side shift their apparent locus to the middle and in this way increase the "loudness" of the center vibrator. To the extent that this phenomenon occurs within the ear—on the basilar membrane, in particular—then the broad response of the basilar membrane is converted into a narrow one.

In addition to his construction of analogue models, Békésy attempted to observe the activity of the cochlea directly. Békésy observed wave motion of the basilar membrane in fresh and preserved specimens of human and animal cochleae. His techniques of preparing and observing the specimens are themselves studies worthy of examining for their precision and inventiveness, but they can only be summarized here. In some investigations he placed particles of fine metals or carbon in the cochlea and observed their movements during stimulation under magnification or with stroboscopic illumination. He also cut windows into the human cochleae at various locations and noted the vibration pattern of the basilar membrane for selected frequencies. The results of

Fig. 4.19*a* *Arrangement of a series of vibrators operating at different frequencies to show the neural interaction of "funneling" in which summation and inhibition occur simultaneously. (Source: Békésy, 1957b, Vol. 29, pp. 1059–1069.)*

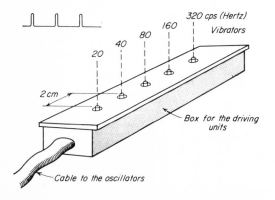

some of these investigations were presented in Figure 4.16*b*. The patterns of movement revealed by direct observation were in close correspondence with those obtained with the mechanical models: In short, the locus of maximal displacement of the basilar membrane varies progressively with changes in the frequency of stimulation at the oval window.

A place theory explanation of loudness assumes that the more intense a sound, the larger the proportion of basilar membrane called into action (e.g., Glaser & Haven, 1972). More specifically, the loudness of a tone depends on the number of hair cells and nerves stimulated, regardless of the location of the displacement along the basilar membrane. As we noted earlier, the organ of Corti includes two sets of hair cells (see Figure 4.14). The inner set has a single column of hair cells, whereas the outer set has three columns. It is held that the outer set (for a number of plausible neural and mechanical reasons) has a different response threshold for innervation than does the inner set. The inner hair cells require more intense stimulation to the ear to set them off, whereas the outer hair cells are located so that they respond to minimum intensity levels. Because of the difference in the innervation of the inner and outer hair cells it has been speculated that they function as pitch and loudness detectors respectively (see Dallos, Billone, Durrant, Wang, & Raynor, 1972).

In summary, then, loudness may depend not only on the number of nerve impulses produced by basilar membrane displacement but on the nerve fibers' connection with the outer or inner hair cells.

The Frequency Theory

The major opponent of the Békésy place theory is called the *frequency* or *periodicity* theory (Wever & Bray, 1930). It holds that the basilar membrane vibrates as a whole reproducing the vibrations of the sound. Frequency thus is transmitted directly by the vibrations of the cochlea ele-

ments much like the telephone or microphone diaphragm transduces sounds. The pitch heard, according to this theory, is determined by the frequency of impulses traveling up the auditory nerve, which in turn is correlated with the frequency of the sound wave. The brain, then, serves as the analyzing instrument for pitch perception. Some evidence in support of a frequency theory comes from studies on pitch discrimination in fish, an animal lacking peripheral frequency analyzers such as a cochlea or basilar membrane. Results indicate that fish do possess this discriminative capacity (Fay, 1970; see also the brief review on this matter by Bergeijk, 1962, p. 35–36).

Volley Principle

A major criticism of the frequency theory is that a single nerve fiber cannot directly respond more than 1000 times per second—hence, transmit frequencies above 1000 Hz—so it certainly cannot transmit all the frequencies within the audible range. Modifications by Wever & Bray (1937) of the frequency theory have been made under the assumption that every nerve fiber does not fire at the same moment, but rather the total neural activity is distributed over a series of auditory nerve fibers (see Figure 4.20). It is held that a cooperation exists between fibers so that squads or volleys of fibers fire at different times; the overall effect is that the neural pattern of firing is in direct correspondence to the frequency of the stimulus. Thus, groups of fibers that have a staggered discharge rate together yield impulses synchronized with the frequency of the stimulus. This explanation is called the *volley principle* (see Wever, 1949). Some sort of volley phenomenon has been reported from the responses of single element neurons (e.g., for frequencies up to 1050 Hz; Galambos & Davis, 1943).

Loudness is explained by increased firings in each volley as shown in Figure 4.21: More fibers may enter in the volleys and fibers may fire more frequently. The total effect of increasing intensity

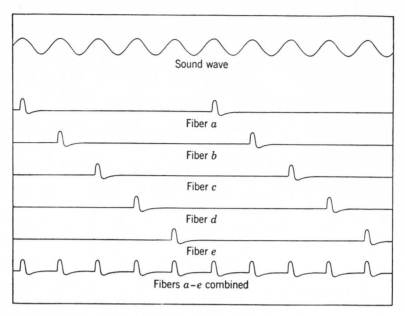

Fig. 4.20   *The volley principle. Each fiber responds to certain of the sound waves, and their total responses (fibers a to e, combined) represent the full frequency of the wave. (From Theory of Hearing, by E. G. Wever, Wiley, New York, 1949, p. 167. Reprinted by permission of the publisher.)*

is to produce more impulses per volley without changing frequency.

It should be noted that the final word on a theory of pitch perception has yet to be written. Although modern hearing theory generally stresses a place notion, many accounts of hearing favor a compromise theory drawing from aspects of each theory. E. G. Wever (1949), a major proponent of the frequency theory, has written: ". . . the low-tone region is that in which frequency holds sway, the high-tone region that for place representation, and the middle-tone region one where both frequency and place work side by side" (p. 190). Békésy (1963) has likewise commented that only the frequency mechanism is active below 50 Hz, the place mechanism alone signals pitch above 3000 Hz, and between 50 and 3000 Hz, both appear to play a role.

Of interest is research that supports this compromise. For example, Simmons et al. (1965) implanted electrodes in different parts of the audi-tory nerve of a subject's deaf ear and found that different pitch effects were produced from differently located electrodes; that is, in support of a place mechanism, pitch effects were produced that correlated with the place of stimulation. However, support of a frequency mechanism also occurred in that variations of stimulus frequency from about 20 to 300 Hz, independent of electrode location, produced changes in the pitch of the resulting sound.

AUDITORY PATHOLOGY

Auditory pathology may take a number of diverse forms—from various hearing impairments that produce systematic distortions to a complete failure of the auditory mechanism to respond to acoustic energy. In this section we can consider only some of the major forms of pathology of the auditory system.

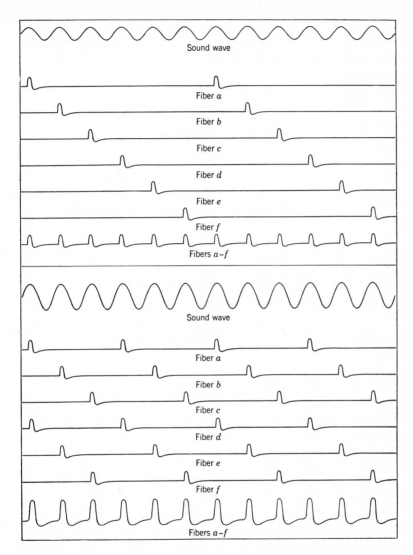

Fig. 4.21 *The effect of stimulus intensity on the volley principle. The upper part of the figure shows the discharge of nerve fibers at a relatively low intensity; each fiber fires at every sixth wave. The lower part of the figure shows the pattern of nerve firing for a more intense tone; here each fiber fires at every third wave. At the lower intensity the total discharge of these few fibers gives rise to only one impulse per wave, which is barely sufficient to represent the stimulus frequency. At the greater intensity there are two impulses per wave, yet the composite frequency is un-changed. (From Theory of Hearing, by E. G. Wever, Wiley, New York, 1949, p. 173. Reprinted by permission of the publisher.)*

Tinnitus

The most obvious manifestation of tinnitus is a ringing in the ears, usually of a relatively high pitch. It may have a variety of causes and may also occur in the absence of pathology. Tinnitus is often encountered clinically as a prominent symptom of a number of ear disorders, accompanying ear infections or high fever.

Displacusis

Displacusis—literally "double hearing"—is a common, although usually transient, abnormality of hearing. In its usual form, a single tone is perceived as different in pitch by the two ears. Like tinnitus, displacusis may often be a prominent symptom of a number of ear disorders.

Presbyacusis

There is a progressive loss of sensitivity to high frequency sound with increasing age (see Figure 4.22). Although the upper limit for frequency reception may be beyond 23,000 Hz in children, it decreases with age. In one citation, individuals in their forties were observed to drop in a regular fashion 80 Hz from their upper limit of hearing every six months (Békésy, 1957a). In support of a place theory of hearing is the observation that nerve degeneration characteristic of presbyacusis is mainly at the basal end of the cochlea—presumably the region responsible for the reception of high frequency sounds (e.g., Johnsson & Hawkins, 1972). Whether presbyacusis occurs as a result of deterioration in neural structures directly related to the biology of the aging process, or only indirectly due to aging—that is, from the collective influence of infection, occasional abnormal noise exposures and other damaging events that occur in the course of one's life—is unclear. However, the latter is quite possible since some individuals reach an advanced age without any deterioration of their hearing.

Deafness

There are two main types of deafness: *conduction* or *transmission* deafness, and *nerve* deafness. Conduction deafness results from deficiencies in the conduction mechanism of the auditory system particularly involving the structure and function of the external auditory canal, the eardrum, or the ossicles. Nerve deafness occurs from deficiencies or damage to the auditory nerves or to the basilar membrane or other closely linked neural connections in the cochlea.

An important instrument for studying deaf-

Fig. 4.22 *Age and auditory acuity. Five age groups were tested under similar conditions, and the results are presented with respect to the youngest group (20 to 29 years). The curves show for each group the relative sound pressure required for threshold perception, as a function of frequency. (From Theory of Hearing, by E. G. Wever, Wiley, New York, 1949, p. 364. Reprinted by permission of the publisher.)*

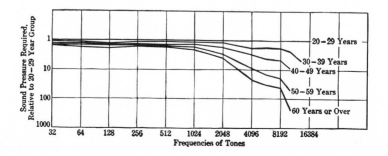

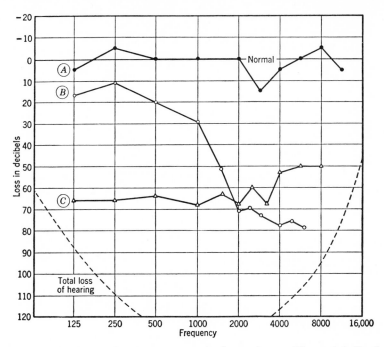

Fig. 4.23 *Typical Audiograms. Normal is the line at zero level near the top. The straight line for zero hearing loss represents the average results obtained from a great many individuals. Curve A lies within the normal limits of these average data. Complete loss of hearing is shown by the dashed line near the bottom. (A) Typical normal ear. (B) Sloping loss, maximal in high frequencies. (C) Flat loss with all frequencies cut down nearly the same. (Modified from Foundations of Psychology, by E. G. Boring, H. S. Langfeld, & H. P. Weld, Wiley, New York, 1948, p. 340. Reprinted by permission of the publisher.)*

ness is the *audiometer*. It usually consists of a tone generator that provides pure tones at a number of different frequencies and allows for setting the intensity at levels at which the tone is just audible. At each test frequency the intensity necessary for the tone to be barely audible is measured and is compared with previously established standards. The resulting graph from the manipulations is called an *audiogram* and shows any departure from normal sensitivity, that is, hearing loss, in decibels, for the different test frequencies. Typical audiograms are given in Figure 4.23. The curve for a person with normal hearing (shown by curve A) remains close to the zero in hearing loss in all frequencies. However, the other curves are typical ones for persons with hearing deficiencies. Curve B in the figure is an

example of the hearing loss for a person with nerve deafness. It is characteristic of this form of auditory pathology for hearing loss to be very pronounced in the high frequencies and much less for the lower frequencies. Curve C is an example indicative of a person with conduction deafness. The curve shows that the person has approximately the same severe hearing loss at all frequencies.

The causes of deafness vary. They may involve chronic infection of the middle ear, prolonged exposure to intensive industrial noise, and perhaps the overall effect of aging. One result of abnormal exposure to sounds is called *stimulation deafness*. Exposure to excessive and prolonged acoustic stimulation can produce severe effects on hearing (see Burns, 1973; Anthrop,

1973; Lipscomb, 1974). Hirsh (1952) has written that over time hearing loss increases as the intensity increases. The effects of intense sounds may be specific to the frequency of the sound (e.g., intense high frequency tones may produce damage near the basal end of the cochlea, as a place theory would predict). However, it has been noted that impairment effects of intense stimulation to one tone, particularly a low frequency tone, may uniformly occur to the perception of all frequencies, regardless of the specific frequency of the insulting tone (Gulick, 1971).

COMPARATIVE AUDITORY STRUCTURES

The functioning of the ear and its psychological consequence, hearing, is more fully understood when considered in a general biological context. In order to do this it is necessary to consider hearing from a comparative view. This can be very useful since the widely different degree of structural elaboration in the auditory mechanisms of vertebrates enables many properties of hearing to be analyzed with respect to anatomy.

The vestibular and auditory structures of a turtle, a bird, and a mammal are sketched in Figure 4.24. Shown are the semicircular canals, the otocysts and the otoliths, and the auditory nerve endings along the basilar membrane. From an evolutionary perspective, the semicircular canals appear invariant with phylogenetic ascension whereas there is an increase in the length of the basilar membrane. As Figure 4.24 shows, the increase in length of the cochlea in birds and mammals (*B* and *C*) appears as an elaboration of the lowest otolithic structure seen in the turtle (*A*).

The size of the cochlea and especially the length of the basilar membrane within it can be related to some aspects of auditory reception (See Table 4.3). Elongation of the basilar membrane presumably occurred in the evolution of avian and mammalian life. Generally the basilar membrane is shortest in amphibia and reptiles, somewhat longer in birds, and it is longest in mammals (Manley, 1971). A conjecture as to the significance of these phylogenetic differences is given by Masterton and Diamond (1973): "Because sounds of different frequencies result in stimulation at different places along the basilar membrane, this lengthening of the receptor organ almost certainly means that there existed a strong and persistent pressure on the ancestors of mam-

Fig. 4.24 *The vestibular and auditory organs of a turtle (A), a bird (B), and a mammal (C). The vestibular organ is fully developed in fish, and there has been no further evolutionary development in higher animals. However, in higher animals the length of the basilar membrane shows a decided increase from the turtle to the mammal. The dotted ellipses represent otoliths; the parallel dashes represent the auditory nerve endings along the basilar membrane. (Source: Békésy, 1960b; and Békésy & Rosenblith, 1951, p. 1102. Reprinted by permission of the publisher.)*

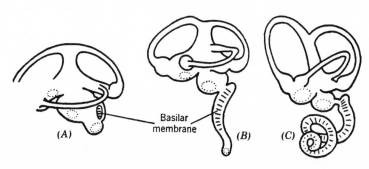

Table 4.3

LENGTH OF THE COCHLEA AND LOWER FREQUENCY LIMIT FOR VARIOUS ANIMALS[a]

Animal	Length of Cochlea from Stapes (mm)	Lower Frequency Limit
Chicken	5	100
Mouse	7	400
Rat	10	200
Guinea pig	18	200
Man	35	20
Cow	38	50
Elephant	60	30

[a] After Békésy, 1960*b*.

mals for wider range and finer discrimination of frequency" (p. 411).

Structures other than those of the inner ear are important to the extents of hearing. Masterton, Heffner, and Ravizza (1968) have pointed out that high frequency hearing (above 32,000 Hz) is a characteristic unique to mammals and due to the evolution, in mammals only, of the middle-ear ossicles.

Of interest to the present discussion is the relationship of hearing to gross bodily dimensions. Békésy (1960*a*) has surmised that the physical size of the animal bears some relationship to the minimum frequency that is detectable. Specifically, he has suggested that the lower frequency limit is shifted downward with increases in animal size. This is related to the general enlargement of the ear. When sound is transmitted along the ear's main surfaces, the sound absorption is less for low frequency tones than for high ones. Accordingly, when auditory passages are relatively large, there is an advantage to the reception of low frequency tones. According to Békésy and Rosenblith (1951), the favoring of

low frequency tones offers an ecological advantage to large animals: "The wisdom of nature is evident in all this, because it is certainly important for large animals to hear over great distances. If the sound is propagated along the ground, the absorption will in general affect low-frequency sounds less than high-frequency sounds. Hence the usefulness of favoring the low frequencies" (p. 1104).

In this chapter we described the physical characteristics of the auditory stimulus and its representation in waveform. The principal physical properties of sound waves are characterized by their variation in frequency, amplitude or intensity, complexity, and phase.

The main anatomical structures and mechanisms of the three main divisions of the ear (the outer, middle, and inner ear) were identified and the sequence of physiological events and processes of the auditory system that result in the perception of sound were discussed. In the context of describing the functioning of the inner ear we considered two main theories of pitch perception: Békésy's place theory and the frequency theory (and volley principle); in addition we presented some of the significant findings that bear on these. Although modern hearing theory favors some form of place notion, we noted that a compromise is possible in that the reception of low frequency tones may be explained by a volley frequency notion and high frequency reception by a place theory.

Some common conditions of auditory pathology were outlined: tinnitus, diplacusis, presbyacusis, and certain forms of hearing deficiencies and deafness.

Finally, a brief section was given on comparative auditory structures. We noted that increased length of the basilar membrane evolved with phylogenetic ascension.

In this chapter our focus will be on the perception of certain psychophysical features of auditory phenomena. In particular, much of our discussion will concern the relationship of the subjective dimensions of hearing to the measurable physical events that produce them. We have briefly noted that the psychological dimensions of hearing are loudness and pitch; these are functionally related to the physical dimensions of intensity and frequency, respectively. We now turn to some of the quantitative relationships between these dimensions.

PERCEPTION OF INTENSITY

The sensitivity of the vertebrate auditory system to the intensity of a sound is extraordinary. The human threshold—the lowest intensity level that produces a sensation of hearing—at frequencies around 3000 Hz begins to approach the reception of the sounds made by random movement of air molecules (Békésy & Rosenblith, 1951). Yet at higher frequencies, say 13,000 Hz, a cat requires an intensity level only one-thousandth as much as man to detect the

presence of a sound (Milne & Milne, 1967). As we noted earlier, with man near 3000 Hz hearing can occur with movements of the ear drum of one-tenth the diameter of the hydrogen atom (10^{-9} cm), and the amplitude of the displacement of the basilar membrane may be as small as 10^{-10} cm (Stevens & Davis, 1938, p. 56). Measures of the ear drum displacement at threshold levels of stimulation are shown in Figure 5.1. Geldard (1972, p. 184), in his review of sensitivity measurement, suggests that in the case of the cat's auditory threshold the amplitude of the vibrations of its ear drum for a 5000 Hz tone is close to 10^{-11} cm.

Figure 5.2 shows the results of two measures used to determine the thresholds of intensity as a function of frequency for man. The basic difference between them is the way the tones are delivered to the ears. Measures may be made of the minimum audible pressure (MAP) on the ear drum itself, or of the intensity in the free sound field in which the observer is located, called the minimum audible field (MAF). In the latter method, stimulation may be either monaural or binaural—the binaural threshold may be from 3 to 6 *db* lower than that for the monaural threshold (Stevens & Davis, 1938, p. 52; Reynolds & Stevens, 1960). It is clear from the

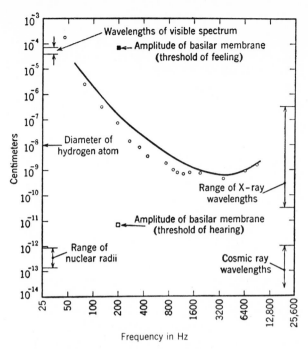

Fig. 5.1 *Amplitude of vibration of the eardrum at threshold. Where the ear is most sensitive the amplitude of vibration of the eardrum is less than one-tenth of the diameter of a hydrogen atom. (Source: Békésy & Rosenblith, 1951, p. 1081, based on data of Wilska.)*

Fig. 5.2 *Auditory threshold as a function of frequency. M.A.P. stands for "minimum audible pressure," M.A.F. for "minimum audible field." Notice that the ordinate is plotted in decibels from 1 dynes/cm². The arrow at −73.8 db shows the standard reference pressure. Curve 1 represents the threshold of hearing when measurement is made of sound pressure at the ear drum. Curve 2 represents the threshold intensities of a sound field when the observer faces the source and listens with both ears. Curve 3 represents threshold values when the sound reaches the observer from all sides. (After Sivian and White, 1933, Vol. 4, pp. 288–321, modified by Geldard, 1972, p. 183.)*

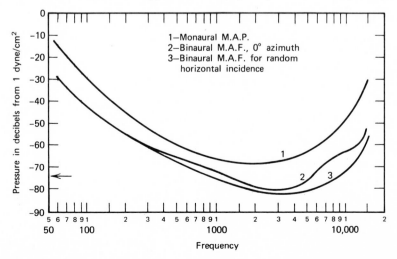

59

figure that the human ear is differentially sensitive to pure tones of different frequencies; thus each frequency has its own threshold value. Although there are differences in the results from the two methods of threshold determination, there is good agreement between curves that maximal sensitivity is for those frequencies in the region of 3000 Hz. [A similar function for rats would show a threshold minimum at 40,000 Hz (Gourevitch & Hack, 1966), for some species of bats at 20,000 to 60,000 Hz (Dalland, 1965), and for the monkey at 1000 Hz (Stebbins, Green, & Miller, 1966).] With intensity held constant, a sound of 3000 Hz sounds louder than other frequencies. This corresponds to the natural resonance of the external ear canal noted earlier. From an ecological perspective the benefit to man of this particular frequency-related sensitivity lies perhaps in the alarming and piercing quality of a cry that occurs in the 3000 Hz range. For the most part aspects of language remain principally in frequencies less than 1000 Hz, which is below that part of the audible band to which man is most sensitive. Perhaps as Milne and Milne (1967) speculate, we leave a ". . . channel open— as though reserved for emergencies—for any high-pitched scream" (p. 43).

Intensity Discrimination

An important aspect of intensity reception concerns the degree to which the stimulus intensity of a sound must be changed, either increased or decreased, in order to perceive a discriminable difference (referred to as the differential threshold, often noted as ΔI, see Chapter 2). Not unexpectedly, the ΔI is dependent on a number of factors, chiefly among them the frequency of the sound on which the measurement is made. Empirical determinations of the differential sensitivity indicate that when the base intensity is below 30 db, the frequency range in which the differential sensitivity is greatest is also approximately that frequency region (2500 to 3000 Hz) in which maximal sensitivity occurs, and it

becomes progressively worse as frequency is raised or lowered. In short, the frequency region that requires minimal intensity for threshold detection is also the frequency range with the greatest differential sensitivity.

Loudness

Loudness refers to a psychological dimension of audition—an aspect of experience—and as we have previously noted, loudness is generally determined by the physical intensity of the sound. However, the relationship between loudness and intensity is an imperfect and complex one in that the perception of loudness does not correspond solely to physical intensity.

A method used to investigate this relationship is Steven's magnitude estimation (described in Chapter 2). A subject is given a standard stimulus tone and a set of tones that vary in intensity, but all tones are presented at the same frequency (1000 Hz). The standard is assigned a modulus value, say 10 or 100, and the subject's task is to assign numbers to the variable tones that reflect its sensory magnitude in proportion to the standard. The result is the construction of a subjective scale of loudness that is a power function of physical intensity. Specifically, Stevens (1956) has shown that the psychological dimension of loudness (L) is related to the physical intensity of the sound (I) (times a constant, k), by a power law of the form:

$$L = kI^{0.3}.$$

This means that loudness increases approximately as the cube root of sound intensity. [It must be noted that other exponents have been reported for the scaling of loudness, for example, 0.54 for monaural (one-ear) loudness and 0.67 for binaural loudness, see Reynolds & Stevens, 1960.] Thus increases in intensity produce lower proportional increases in loudness. In other words, loudness grows more slowly than physical intensity.

It has been useful to adopt a standard unit of

loudness. Stevens and Davis (1938) used the term *sone*, one sone defined as the loudness of a 1000 Hz tone at a 40 *db* intensity level. Both the term and its referents have been universally adopted as the standard of loudness. A function relating intensity level to the sone scale is given in Figure 5.3.

Loudness and Frequency

Specifying only the decibel level of a sound will not fully describe its loudness. Loudness is not solely a matter of physical intensity but it is also dependent on the frequency of the sound. The dependence of loudness on frequency is apparent when two tones whose frequencies differ are matched for loudness and their respective intensities are compared. Using psychophysical methods, it is possible to specify the different frequencies and intensities of sounds that are perceived as equally loud. For example, subjects listen to two tones that differ in frequency and intensity. One has a fixed frequency and intensity and it is called the standard tone. A second, comparison tone is presented at a different frequency

Fig. 5.3 *Relationship between intensity level (db) and loudness (sones) Notice that in this function a 10 db increase in the intensity scale increases loudness by a factor of 2. (Source: Lindsay & Norman, 1972, p. 257. Reprinted by permission of the authors and publisher.)*

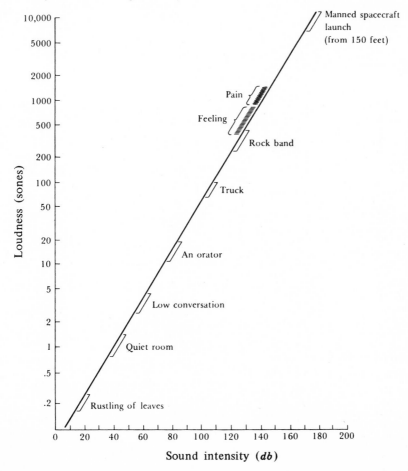

and intensity and the subject's task is to listen alternately to the standard and comparison tones and adjust the intensity of the comparison until it matches the loudness of the standard tone. When this is done for a number of comparison tones, a curve may be plotted that describes the intensity at which tones of various frequencies appear equally as loud as the standard tone. Each curve of Figure 5.4 shows the result of such a procedure for a different standard. The family of curves relate perceived loudness to intensities and frequencies and shows to what extent loudness is affected by frequency. The curves are labeled in *phons,* a measure of the loudness level of a tone specified as the number of decibels of a standard 1000 Hz tone of equal loudness. That is, the number of phons of a tone is numerically equal to

the number of decibels of a 1000 Hz tone that sounds equally as loud as the tone. For example, consider the curve labeled 30 on Figure 5.4. Any sound whose frequency and intensity lies on this curve appears equally as loud as any other sound on the curve although their frequencies and intensities will differ. It follows that a 300 Hz tone at a 40 *db* intensity level appears equal in loudness to a 1000 Hz tone at a 30 *db* (or 30 phons) intensity level and a 6000 Hz tone at a 35 *db* intensity level. Thus, the 300 and the 6000 Hz tones at 40 and 35 *db,* respectively, have a loudness level of 30 phons and any sound whose frequency and intensity falls on this curve (i.e., 30 phons) has a loudness level of 30 phons. Appropriately the curves of Figure 5.4 are called *equal-loudness contours* (or isophonic curves).

Fig. 5.4 *Equal Loudness Contours. The values by each curve refer to the loudness levels in phons. The bottom curve shows the absolute sensitivity of the ear as a function of frequency. Presumably tones below this curve are not audible. (Source: Berrien, 1946, 43, p. 143.)*

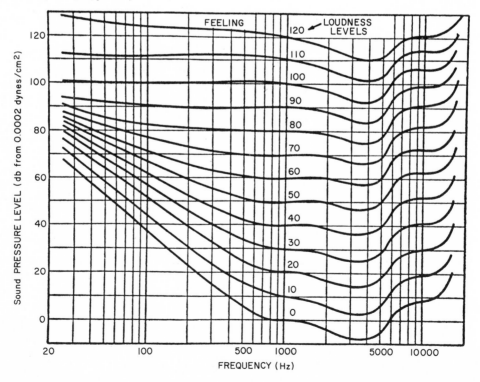

Figure 5.4 points out a number of important facts about the perception of loudness. The effect of frequency on loudness is greatest at low levels of intensity; at high intensity levels frequency does not play a significant role in the perception of loudness and the equal-loudness contours are relatively flat. In other words, if tones are sufficiently intense, they tend to sound equally loud, irrespective of frequency. At relatively low intensity levels frequencies lower than about 1000 Hz and higher than 4000 Hz sound softer than intermediate frequencies for the same intensity level. The bow-shaped curves indicate how low and high frequencies must be boosted in intensity in order to maintain a constant loudness level. This relationship appears not only with laboratory produced sounds but occurs in ordinary listening experiences. For example, many high-fidelity amplifiers possess a compensatory adjustment circuit for listening at low intensity levels called a "loudness compensator" (or simply "loudness"), which overemphasizes the very high and low frequencies. It is necessary because in turning the "volume" (a misnomer) of the amplifier down the relative loudness of various frequencies is changed in the manner shown by Figure 5.4.

PERCEPTION OF FREQUENCY

Although the perception of a sound involves the interaction of intensity and frequency, there are a number of aspects of frequency reception that bear analysis. In the case of "normal" human hearing, the limits of hearing for frequency extend between 20 and 20,000 Hz. Below 20 Hz only a vibration feeling or a fluttering-like sound is perceived, whereas above 20,000 Hz perhaps only a "tickling" is experienced. We have seen from Figures 5.2 and 5.4 that the threshold of hearing varies with both intensity and frequency and that at the extremes of frequency reception the sounds must be quite intense in order to be audible.

Of course, the range of frequency reception is quite different for different species. It was previously noted that the range of frequency reception varies with a number of biological and ecological demands; high frequency reception (above 32,000 Hz) is unique to mammals (Masterton, Heffner, & Ravizza, 1968).

Frequency Discrimination

The discrimination question raised for intensity can also be asked for frequency; namely, how much of a change in frequency, (Δf) must occur in order to be detected by the observer? Precise measurements of this aspect of sound discrimination are very difficult to obtain. In one instance, investigators smoothly modulated a tone back and forth between two frequency points and noted the frequency separation at which the listener could just detect a pitch variation (Shower & Biddulph, 1931). The findings indicate that the human observer can detect a change in frequency of about 3 Hz for frequencies up to about 2000 Hz (at a 40 db level). Above this frequency Δf rises sharply; for example, at about 10,000 Hz a 40 Hz change is required for a change to be perceived. For frequencies above about 2000 Hz, frequency discrimination is a constant fraction of the frequency. In general, the lower the stimulus frequency, the more sensitive the ear is to frequency differences. In one study, frequencies from 60 to 4000 Hz were employed and discriminability to frequency differences improved continuously as frequency was decreased (Harris, J. D., 1952).

Important among the variables that affect the determination of the minimal discriminable change in frequency is the intensity level of the sounds at which the measurements are taken. The Δf for frequency increases with decreases in stimulus intensity (especially for high frequencies). In other words, as a sound appears softer it becomes more difficult to detect it as different from other sounds close in frequency.

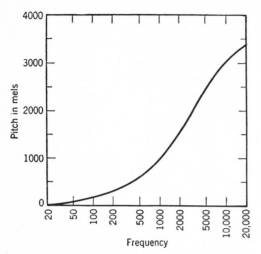

Fig. 5.5 *The frequency-pitch function. The curve shows how the perceived pitch of a tone in mels changes as a function of the frequency of the stimulus. This pitch-function was determined at a loudness-level of 40 db. (Source: Boring, Langfeld, & Weld, 1948, p. 323; after Stevens & Volkmann, 1940, 53, 329–353.)*

Pitch

Pitch is a subjective tonal dimension of hearing that refers to how high or low a sound appears, and it is principally but not exclusively determined by the frequency of the tone reaching the ears. Typically, high pitch sounds are heard from high frequency tones, low pitch sounds result from low frequency tones, but the cor-

respondence is not precise (e.g. see Wightman & Green, 1974). The dimension of pitch has been scaled using an arbitrary unit called the *mel*. By definition the subjective pitch of a 1000 Hz tone at 40 *db* is assigned a value of 1000 mels. The relationship between pitch and frequency was determined by the employment of a psychophysical procedure called the method of *fractionation*. For example, an observer was presented alternately with two tones at a constant intensity level but only one tone at a fixed frequency. The other tone was varied in frequency by the observer until its pitch was perceived to be one-half of the pitch of the fixed tone. In this case 1000 mels was assigned to the pitch of a 1000 Hz tone and the number 500 mels to the frequency of the tone that sounded half as high in pitch. Similarly, a sound that appeared twice as high in pitch as the 1000 Hz tone was assigned a value of 2000 mels. Extending this procedure for other frequencies and extrapolating the results produced the numerical pitch scale of Figure 5.5. The curve of Figure 5.5 expresses the relationship between pitch and frequency at a constant 40 *db* level. Figure 5.6 shows how a piano keyboard would appear if each key was adjusted in size to represent the number of mels it includes.

Pitch and Intensity

Although intensity has not been shown to influence the pitch of complex tones (for reasons not

Fig. 5.6 *The Mel Keyboard. The piano keyboard is distorted so that equal distance represents equal amounts of pitch rather than equal units on the musical scale. This shows why melodies are so much clearer when played in the treble than when played in the bass. (From Foundations of Psychology, by E. G. Boring, H. S. Langfeld, & H. P. Weld, Wiley, New York, 1948, p. 323. Reprinted by permission of the publisher.)*

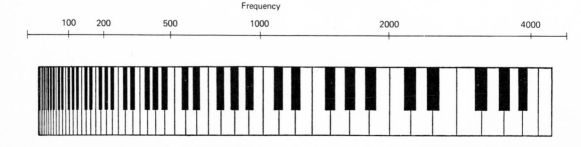

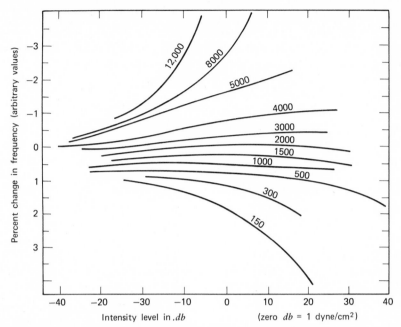

Fig. 5.7 *Equal pitch contours. Contours showing the dependence of pitch on intensity. The percentage change in frequency necessary to keep the pitch of a given tone constant as its intensity is changed can be taken as a measure of the effect of intensity on pitch. It is important to note that the ordinate was chosen so that the curves tend toward a common origin and that a contour with a positive slope shows that pitch increases with intensity and a contour with a negative slope shows that pitch decreases with intensity. (Source: Stevens, 1935, Vol. 6, p. 151.)*

well understood), it does have a measurable effect on the pitch of relatively pure tones. In an often cited study, Stevens (1935), using a single trained observer, determined the effect of intensity on the pitch of tones for 11 frequencies ranging from 150 to 12,000 Hz. Two tones of slightly different frequencies were presented in succession to the observer who adjusted the intensity of one of the two tones until both were perceived as equal in pitch. In short, the observer compensated for frequency differences by means of a difference in intensity. The results can be seen by the family of curves shown in Figure 5.7—called *equal pitch contours*—each of which relates to the different frequencies and intensities that must be maintained in order to keep a pure tone at a constant pitch level. It should be pointed out that the ordinate of the figure was arbitrarily chosen so that the slope of the curve indicates a decrease or

increase in pitch. For high frequencies, an increase in the intensity of a tone requires a decrease in its frequency in order for it to sound at a constant pitch; similarly, an increase in the intensity of a relatively low tone requires an increase in its frequency for it to remain at a constant pitch. Stated differently, when intensity is increased the pitch of high tones increases and the pitch decreases for low tones. For frequencies in the middle range, pitch does not vary with intensity.

More recently, Gulick (1971, pp. 138–141) reported findings on the effect of intensity on pitch by using a technique in which the observer adjusted the frequency of a comparison tone so that it matched the pitch of a standard tone. In all, ten observers made pitch matches to each of nine standard tones (at a 30 *db* intensity level) when the intensity levels ·of the comparisons, at corresponding frequencies, were 30, 50, and 70 *db*. Figure 5.8 shows the results. The ordinate gives the intensity of the comparison tone, and the abscissa shows the change in frequency of the comparison to produce a pitch match with the standard. As the figure shows, for tones of 2500 Hz or above, it was necessary to reduce the frequency of the comparison to maintain equal pitch with the standard, and the degree of the reduction varied with the intensity level. For example, when the standard and comparison for the 4000 Hz tone were at the same intensity level, namely 30 *db,* there was a perfect pitch match, that is, no adjustment of the comparison tone was required. However, when the 4000 Hz comparison tone was at 50 and 70 *db,* pitch matches were produced by lowering the frequency by approximately 12 Hz and 80 Hz respectively. The figure also shows that for tones below 2500 Hz, it was necessary to raise the frequency of the comparison tone to maintain equality of pitch, although the absolute magnitude of the required changes were of a much smaller order than was the case for frequencies exceeding 2500 Hz. Finally, the figure indicates that the minimal effect of intensity on pitch perception occurred for the 2500 Hz tone. In general, the results are in agreement with the earlier study by Stevens (1935) except that the effect of intensity on pitch perception is not as great.

Hearing and Temporal Effects

Since hearing is largely a matter of stimulus reception over time, we would expect certain temporal factors to influence the perception of sound. Indeed, recognizable tonal quality requires some minimal duration of the acoustic stimulus. For example, if a tone of an audible frequency and intensity is presented for only a few milliseconds, it will lose its tonal character and be heard as a "click." According to Gulick (1971, p. 142) the length of time a given frequency must last in order to produce the experience of a stable and recognizable pitch for tones above 1000 Hz is 10 msec. In the case of loudness, for tonal durations shorter than 200 msec, intensity must be increased to maintain a constant level of loudness (see Figure 5.9). Thus although the sound heard depends primarily on the frequency and intensity of the sound, both its pitch and loudness are secondarily affected by the duration of the ex-

Fig. 5.8 *Equal-pitch contours for each of nine standard tones of 200, 500, 700, 1000, 2000, 2500, 3000, 4000, and 7000 Hz, all at 30 db. The intensity of the comparison tone was 30, 50, and 70 db, and the changes of the comparison tone at each intensity in order to match the pitch of the standard is shown in Hz. The db level is specified with reference to the absolute threshold for each frequency. (Source: Gulick, 1971, p. 140. Reprinted by permission of Oxford University Press.)*

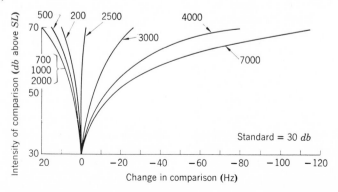

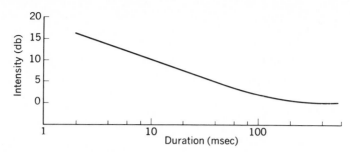

Fig. 5.9 *Equal loudness contour for middle frequency tones showing the changes in intensity required to maintain a constant loudness as a function of tonal duration. Intensity is expressed in decibels relative to a standard tone of long duration. As durations become briefer than 200 msec, intensity must be increased to maintain constant loudness. (Source: Gulick, 1971, p. 148. Reprinted by permission of Oxford University Press.)*

posure. Within limits, the loudness and pitch increase as a brief burst of sound is lengthened.

EFFECTS OF MULTIPLE TONAL STIMULATION

Beats

When simultaneously listening to two tones that are of similar intensity but slightly different in frequency, one may perceive the occurrence of beats—perhaps best described as the perception of a single throbbing tone with a single pitch midway between the two tones but periodically varying in loudness: In short, an alternate waxing and waning in loudness. The frequency with which the loudness fluctuates for the beating phenomenon is precisely the difference between the frequencies of the two sounds that are combined. The reason that beats occur is that there is a continuous change in the relative phase of two simultaneously applied tones so that the tones alternately reinforce and cancel each other. For example, when two tones that differ by 3 Hz are simultaneously produced, the sound waves generated by each will be in compression at the same time three times each second and be out of phase at the same time three times each second;

that is, the tones will reinforce and cancel each other three times a second. The ear hears this phase alternation as periodic variations in loudness, that is, as beats. Indeed, one tone is said to be "beating" against the other.

As the difference between tones increases, beats become faster and they soon lose their individuality. With sufficient increases in the frequency difference (at about 30 Hz) the resultant sound begins to assume a "roughness." The upper limit for the perception of beats is dependent on the absolute frequencies and intensities of the tones, but under proper circumstances tones separated by as much as 250 Hz may produce beats (Geldard, 1972).

Combination Tones

When the frequency difference between the two tones is sufficiently great to eliminate beating phenomena, other tones in addition to the primary pair may be heard. The frequencies of these tones are the sums and differences of the frequencies of the primary tones and their simple multiples. These are termed *combination tones* and they are of two types: *difference tones* and *summation tones,* both of which may occur from the simultaneous stimulation of the ear by two pure tones. The sound of a difference tone has the pitch that corresponds to the frequency difference of the two primary tones, whereas summation tones occur from the frequency summing of the two primary tones. Unlike beats, the basis for the occurrence of combination tones is not in the physical stimulus; rather, they are a result of the ear's distorting action. Many combination tones may result from two primary frequencies and their resultant harmonics. For example, an examination of the combination tones present in the cochlear response of a cat stimulated by a 700 and 1200 Hz tone at 90 *db* yielded 66 different tones, that is, various combinations of the two tones and their upper harmonics (Newman, Stevens, & Davis, 1937, cited in Stevens & Davis, 1938, pp. 198–199).

Masking

When two tones are applied to the ear that are close in frequency but one is of greater intensity, the more intense tone will reduce or eliminate the perception of the softer one. It is familiar to experience one sound drowning or masking out another. This phenomenon is termed *masking* and is defined as the rise in the threshold of one tone in the presence of a second (masking) tone.

The classic study of masking is by Wegel and Lane (1924; see also Zwicker & Scharf, 1965) and many of the findings are summarized in Figure 5.10. The figure shows the masking effects of a 1200 Hz tone (sounded at three intensity levels) on tones of various frequencies ranging from 400 to 4000 Hz. Each curve represents the degree of masking, measured as the rise in the intensity level necessary for test tones (whose frequencies are distributed along the abscissa) to be heard in the presence of the 1200 Hz masking tone. The numbers assigned to each curve, 40, 60, and 80 *db*, represent the three levels of intensity that were applied to the 1200 Hz masking tone. The curves themselves represent the masking results—the amount that the thresholds were raised due to the presence of the masking tone. As the figure shows, a masking tone raises the threshold of hearing by an amount

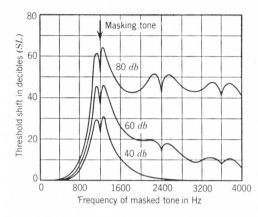

Fig. 5.10 *Auditory masking. The curves show how much the threshold is raised at each frequency as a result of the masking by a 1200 Hz tone at 40 db, 60 db, and 80 db. (Source: Boring, Langfeld, & Weld, 1948, p. 327; after Wegel, R. L., & Lane, C. E., Physiological Review, 1924, 23, 271. Reprinted by permission of the publisher.)*

that varies with intensity and frequency. More specifically, tones close in frequency to the masking tone are more strongly masked than those far removed in frequency. By examining the collective results for the three intensity levels of the masking tone, it is clear that a greater amount of masking results when the masking tone is more intense.

Apparent from the figure is the asymmetry of the 80 and 60 *db* curves with respect to the frequency range of the masking effects. This suggests that the effect of masking is greater on tones whose frequencies exceed the masking tone than for those below it. However, this is manifest only with relatively high intensity masking tones and is held to be due to the masking effect of overtones produced by the masking tone (e.g., Geldard, 1972). These overtones are evident on the curves as scallops or minor peaks of masking at multiples of the masking tone, for example, at 2400 and 3600 Hz (the second and third harmonics) respectively. When the results with lower intensity masking tones are examined, the disproportionate influence of certain frequencies on masking is no longer observed. For example, the curve for the 40 *db* masking tone shows little skewness. Notice also that the sharp dips in the minor masking peaks, representing the occurrence of beats, result at those frequency points that lie close to the fundamental or the harmonics of the masking tone and serve to lower the detection threshold.

Sound-induced Hearing Loss (Auditory Fatigue and Adaptation)

The effects of masking on threshold levels of hearing are not necessarily voided when the masking tone is eliminated. Ordinarily normal threshold sensitivity to a premasking threshold level is restored very soon after the termination of the masking tone. However, when very intense masking stimulation has been applied for long durations, the effects may extend for a number of hours. To the extent that the threshold remains elevated above a premasking threshold *after* termination of the masking stimulus, we have a measure of sound-induced hearing loss (also called *auditory fatigue* or *adaptation*). Like the effects of masking, this form of hearing loss is manifested by an upward shift in the threshold for a given tone or a reduction in its loudness. However, masking is a temporary loss in sensitivity to a tone *during* exposure to another tone, whereas fatigue is a loss in sensitivity to a tone *following* exposure to another tone. Not unexpectedly, the length and severity of the hearing loss or fatigue depend on the duration and intensity of the inducing tone.

This is observed when the ear is subjected to intense acoustic stimulation. In principle, the hearing loss or change in threshold sensitivity at a number of frequencies, measured immediately following exposure to the intense sound, is compared with preexposure measures of threshold sensitivity. The shift in threshold at different frequencies is taken as the measure of temporary hearing loss. Figure 5.11 shows the amount of hearing loss induced by prior exposure to *white*

noise (a form of noise containing a mixture of all audible frequencies of similar intensities). The horizontal zero line represents the preexposure sensitivity of the ear. The curves specify temporary hearing loss for various rest periods after exposure to the noise. The figure shows clearly that temporary hearing loss due to exposure to the intense noise is more pronounced for high frequencies and as the rest period increases, hearing sensitivity approaches normalcy.

Consonance and Dissonance

For most observers, when two tones are sounded together the resultant combination sounds either pleasant or unpleasant. Those combinations that sound pleasant—that tend to fuse or blend well together—are characterized as *consonant*. Those combinations that sound discordant or harsh are termed *dissonant*. Although it is likely true that nonauditory attributes such as custom, culture, and related learning factors have a role in the consonance-dissonance attribute of combined tones, other auditory processes are also involved.

An important acoustic consideration as to whether two sounds are heard as consonant or dissonant is their frequency difference. One explanation is that dissonance occurs when the upper harmonics of the two fundamentals are so close in frequency as to produce a roughness in the sound (the basis for this was described in the section on beats), whereas consonance occurs when the harmonics of the two fundamentals differ sufficiently in frequency to be heard as distinct sounds or they coincide and reinforce each other. (See Geldard, 1972, pp. 213-215 or Plomp, 1971, pp. 204-210, for a brief discussion of this phenomenon and its history.)

SUBJECTIVE TONAL ATTRIBUTES

The literature on psychoacoustics contains reference to qualities of pure tones that cannot be accounted for by only pitch and loudness. One of

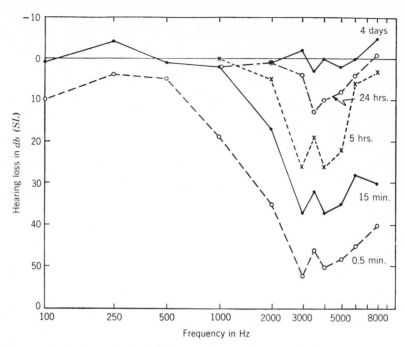

Fig. 5.11 *Audiogram showing changes in auditory sensitivity as a result of exposure to intense noise (115 db) for 20 min. The curves specify the temporary shift in sensitivity (hearing loss) for various rest periods following exposure to the intense noise. (Source: Postman & Egan, 1949, p. 72.)*

these characteristics is termed *volume,* which refers to the size, expansiveness, or voluminousness of a tone. It is based on the assumption that certain sounds, independently matched in pitch and loudness, appear to occupy more space than others. (Notice that the term "volume" as used here is different from the misnamed "volume" control found on radios and amplifiers.) When observers are required to order tones along a large-small dimension, considerable agreement occurs in that tones of high frequency sound smaller or less voluminous than tones of low frequency. Stevens (1934) investigated volume as an independent tonal attribute by having subjects adjust the intensity of each of a series of tones of different frequencies until a match in volume with a standard tone (500 Hz, 60 *db*) was produced. The results are shown by the equal volume contour of Figure 5.12, which represents the com-

binations of frequency and intensity needed to maintain the invariance of volume. Generally, to maintain a fixed volume, higher frequency tones were raised in intensity. For example, tones of 450 Hz at 58 *db,* 500 Hz at 60 *db,* and 550 Hz at about 62 *db* all have the same volume. Thus, as pitch increases the loudness must also be increased to maintain volume equality—volume increases with intensity but decreases with frequency. This general observation has been largely substantiated by Terrace and Stevens (1962) using Steven's magnitude estimation method (described in Chapter 2).

Another tonal quality has also been reported called *density.* Density refers to the compactness or tightness of a sound, and greater density occurs with tones of high frequency. Density appears to be reciprocally related to volume with the exception that both increase with increases in intensity, that is, with sufficient increases in intensity a low frequency tone can be matched in density with a high frequency tone (see also Guirao & Stevens, 1964). This relationship can also be observed from the appropriate contour of Figure 5.12.

The remaining isophonic contours in Figure 5.12 indicate the minor dependence of loudness on frequency, and pitch on intensity, within the range of values employed. Notice that unlike volume and density, the curves for pitch and loudness do not vary greatly with changes in intensity and frequency, respectively.

We have outlined a number of significant facts about psychoacoustics. However, we must note that most of this vast body of research, although extremely useful and informative, has been performed in laboratory settings using precisely controlled tones—usually relatively long

duration pure tones—quite unlike those that ordinarily occur in nature. Perhaps the greatest departure of these laboratory tones from natural ones lies in their purity and duration. Clearly, long duration pure tones are an infrequent natural occurrence. As put by Masterton and Diamond (1973): "... most natural sounds and almost all natural sounds that warn an animal of a potentially dangerous intruder are very brief sounds ... made up not of enduring pure tones or even their simple combinations, but instead, of sounds such as snaps, pops, crackles, thumps, and thuds" (p. 419).

By way of summary, we described some of the relationships of the subjective, psychological dimensions of sounds to the physical dimensions of tones. The psychological dimensions of hearing are loudness and pitch and these are principally determined by the physical dimensions of intensity, and frequency, respectively.

The measurement of intensity, intensity discrimination, loudness, and the effect of frequency on loudness were described. Some of the main findings for man are that, with intensity held constant, a sound of 3000 Hz sounds louder than other frequencies; differential sensitivity is also greatest in that frequency region.

Frequency, frequency discrimination, pitch, and the effect of intensity on pitch were discussed. Pitch refers to how high or low a sound appears, and it is primarily determined by the frequency of the tone reaching the ear.

Finally, a number of phenomena and variables integral to understanding the perception of sound were discussed: the effects of the duration of a tone, the perception of beats, combination tones, masking or the rise in the threshold of a tone in the presence of second tone, sound-induced hearing loss (auditory fatigue and adaptation), consonance and dissonance, and the subjective tonal attributes, volume and density.

Fig. 5.12 *Isophonic contours for volume, density, pitch, and intensity. Each contour represents a set of tones judged equal in the quality specified by the contour, that is, the set of tones whose intensities and frequencies lie along a given contour are judged subjectively equal for that experience. Thus, a tone of 450 Hz at about 58 db is judged equal in volume to a tone of about 550 Hz at 62 db. (Source: after Stevens, 1934.)*

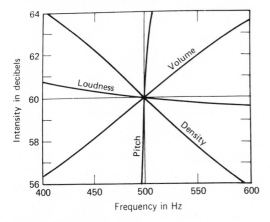

Complex Auditory Phenomena II: Sound as Information

In this chapter we will be concerned with the reception of acoustic energy as an informative, meaningful activity, that is, with sound as potential stimulus information. Sounds in nature may provide sufficient spatial information to enable the perception of features of distant vibratory events, such as location and identification. The pick-up of meaningful sounds may also allow a form of vocal-auditory behavior—communication.

We must emphasize that meaningful natural sounds manifest a vast number of elaborate and complex variations. These variations are far more complex than those observed with the precise experimental manipulations of certain isolated dimensions of laboratory-produced sound stimulation (e.g., frequency and intensity) that we discussed in the preceding chapter. The range of complexities of meaningful sounds in nature has been well put by J. J. Gibson (1966):

> Instead of simple duration, they vary in abruptness of beginning and ending, in repetitiveness, in rate, in regularity of rate, or rhythm, and in other subtleties of sequence. Instead of simple pitch, they vary in timbre or tone quality, in combinations of tone quality, in vowel quality, in approximation to noise, in noise quality, and in changes of all these in time. Instead of simple loudness, they vary in the direction of change of loudness, the rate of change of loudness, and the rate of change of change of loudness. In meaningful sounds, these variables can be combined to yield higher-order variables of staggering complexity. But these mathematical complexities seem nevertheless to be the simplicities of auditory information, and it is just these variables that are distinguished naturally by an auditory system. Moreover, it is just these variables that are specific to the source of the sound—the variables that identify the wind in the trees or the rushing of water, the cry of the young or the call of the mother. (P. 87)

BRAIN ASYMMETRY AND HEARING

In the main we have described the functioning of the auditory mechanism as if it consisted of a single unit—the ear. However, normally one ear is but one-half of the listening apparatus. Moreover, the possession of two ears does not merely reflect a duplication of structure; we cannot assume that the ears function independently of each other. Indeed, the auditory nerves that originate from each ear do not necessarily make independent connections with the auditory receiving part of the brain (auditory cortex). The general scheme of connections is sketched in Figure 6.1. After leaving the ear, the fibers of the auditory nerve make a series of connections at various relay stations along the pathway to the brain. Some of the fibers leaving the internal ear to the brain, aside from connecting with other structures, remain on the same side and interact with fibers from the opposite ear. However, the majority of nerve fibers from one ear (about 60%) cross over to the opposite side. Indeed, this largely *contralateral* (as opposed to *ipsilateral*) connection of neural elements from one side of the body to the opposite side or hemisphere of the brain is characteristic of most of the neural systems of the body. The auditory cortex is primarily dominated by the fibers that cross—conduction is faster and stronger for the crossed pathways—so that each ear is better represented on the opposite cerebral hemisphere of the brain (Rosenzweig, 1961). It has been experimentally demonstrated in the laboratory with cats that the cortical representations of an auditory stimulus presented to only one ear is stronger in the hemisphere opposite to the ear being stimulated than in the hemisphere ipsilateral to that ear (Rosenzweig, 1951, 1954). The effect of this for hearing is that the neural message originating from the right ear is predominantly registered on the left side of the brain and that a message from the left ear is principally registered on the right side of the brain. In operation this means, of course, that a sound produced on one side of the body results in greater cortical activity on the opposite side.

Another lateral difference in the auditory pathways is that the left and right hemispheres of the brain predominate in the perception of different broad characteristics of sound—a functional distinction referred to as *brain asymmetry*. The results of a number of studies have indicated that the auditory cortex of the left hemisphere of the brain predominates in the perception of speech and language-related stimulation whereas the right side of the auditory cortex is more functional in the perception and processing of certain nonverbal sounds. This has been demonstrated with an auditory technique called *dichotic listening* (differential stimulation delivered to the ears is termed *dichotic*). Basically, an observer wearing an independently driven earphone over each ear simultaneously hears two separate messages— a different message to each ear. In one of the initial studies different digits, presented in pairs spaced one-half second apart, were heard by the two ears. When the subjects reported what they heard, more of the digits that had entered the right ear (and as we indicated above, primarily registered on the left hemisphere) were correctly reported than were digits delivered to the left ear (Kimura, 1961). These general findings have been extensively replicated and extended (e.g., Springer, 1971; Shankweiler, 1971). Interestingly, even when speech-like sounds such as those produced by the reverse playback of recorded speech are presented to the left and right ears, the sounds arriving at the right ear are more accurately identified than those arriving at the left (Kimura & Folb, 1968). Kimura (1964, 1967) also reported the related finding that for musical stimuli (solo instrumental passages) a reversal in ear dominance occurred, that is, musical stimuli delivered to the left ear are recalled better than similar stimuli to the right ear. This has also been shown with pure tones as stimuli (Spreen, Spellacy, & Reid, 1970) as well as environmental noise (Curry, 1967). It appears that for verbal stimuli the right ear is dominant, that is, has a better path to the speech-processing area of the left cerebral hemisphere, whereas for nonverbal stimuli the left ear (and right cerebral hemisphere) is more important. However, it cannot be concluded that it is something inherent in the nature of verbal stimuli per se that accounts for left hemisphere dominance. There is evidence that it is the kind or level of analytic processing characteristic of verbal or language-related stimuli that is crucial.

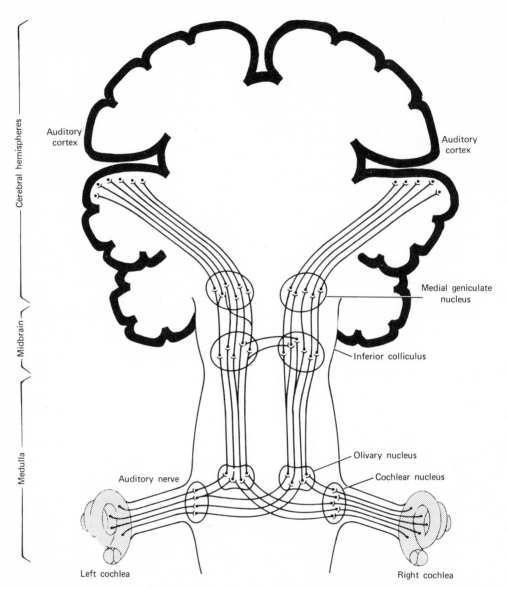

Fig. 6.1 *Semischematic diagram of the conduction pathway of auditory stimulation from the cochlea of each ear to the cerebral cortex. At the olivary nucleus (a relay station) some of the nerve fibers from the cochlear nuclei of both ears converge on the same nerve and thus transmit messages from both ears. At still higher levels there is increasing convergence and interaction between messages from the two ears. Notice, however, that more nerve pathways originating in one cochlear nucleus cross to the opposite side of the brain than remain on the same side.*

Bever and Chiarello (1974) have reported that musically experienced listeners recognize simple melodies better in the right ear than in the left, whereas the reverse is the case for naïve listeners. They hypothesize that the experienced listener performs a level of analysis on the music similar to that typically required for speech perception. In short, the left hemisphere is dominant for analytic processing in general, not only for verbal stimulation (see also Wood, Goff, & Day, 1971).

These behavioral findings bearing on stimuli content and ear-hemisphere dominance have also been given a firm physiological base. Recording auditory responses of the human cortex, Cohn (1971) reported that click noises showed a relatively greater response amplitude over the right cerebral hemisphere and that verbal stimuli produced either an equal or higher response amplitude over the left hemisphere. Using a similar neurophysiological response, it has been shown that the asymmetry of the auditory brain is related to the meaningfulness of the stimuli to the subject (Matsumiya, Tagliasco, Lombroso, & Goodglass, 1972). When made relevant or significant to the subject, certain noises appeared to produce a greater effect in the left hemisphere than did some words.

Still additional evidence of the left-right ear and brain difference is given by the studies of people who have had large portions of the brain or a single lobe removed in order to relieve some of the effects of epilepsy. If the left temporal lobe is removed, the patients show very marked difficulties with verbal-related tasks such as comprehending and remembering verbal stimuli. In contrast, lesions of the right temporal cortex lead to difficulties in the perception of nonlinguistic stimuli (Shankweiler, 1966; Kimura, 1967; Milner, B., 1962). Similarly, patients who have had the connections between the two halves of their brain severed were not able to respond appropriately to verbal stimuli that were presented only to the receptors leading to the right hemisphere (e.g., Gazzaniga, 1967; Gazzaniga & Hill-

yard, 1971). We will briefly return to functions of brain asymmetry in the next section.

Dichotic Listening and Attention

An interesting sidelight of dichotic listening, with respect to the meaning conveyed by the messages, concerns the situation where two independent spoken messages are dichotically transmitted to the listener. Ordinarily, the listener "shadows" or follows one message while ignoring the other. However, under certain conditions of dichotic listening, sound from the ignored ear is heard. Moray (1959) showed that a person fully attending to the message from only one ear will also hear his own name in the message sent to the unattending ear though he might remain quite unreceptive to any other aspect of the message coming to that ear. Moreover, if the content of the ignored ear's message is made relevant to the shadowed message, it may also be perceived (Treisman, 1964).

AUDITORY SPACE PERCEPTION

Functionally the auditory system serves to localize sounds in space. In order to do this precisely both the *direction* and the relative *distance* of sound-emitting stimuli must be perceived and these are given by *monaural* (one-ear) and by *binaural* cues.

Monaural Cues

For the most part, monaural cues may be useful for evaluating an object's relative *distance*. Certainly an important characteristic in judging the distance of a sound source is given by the *intensity* or loudness of the sound wave reaching the ear. The louder the sound, the closer the object appears to be. If two sounds are heard, ordinarily the louder one is perceived as closer. If the intensity of a single sound gradually changes, the perception correspondingly changes. The sound is perceived to approach if it gradually grows louder, and it is perceived to recede if it grows softer. The changing intensity of a siren's wail as a cue to the changing distance of an emergency vehicle in transit relative to a stationary observer is a familiar example.

DOPPLER SHIFT Another cue to the changing distance of a moving object is given by the shift in the frequency (and pitch) emitted by a sound source moving in relation to a stationary observer. It is called the *Doppler Shift,* named after its discoverer, a nineteenth century Austrian physicist, Christian Doppler. The basis of the shift is that as a sound-emitting object moves, each of its successive sound waves is emitted slightly farther ahead in its path. However, the waves, though moving in all directions at a constant speed, do not share a common center (as would be the case with a stationary sound source). Rather, the sound waves tend to bunch up in front of the moving sound source, resulting in a compression of the sound waves—that is, a lessening of the distance between waves, hence an increase in frequency. The perceptual result is that as the frequency of the sound waves that pass a given point increases, the pitch heard at that point increases. After the object passes, a reversal in pitch occurs; that is, the distance between waves is stretched, frequency decreases, and to the observer, the pitch lowers.

A related phenomenon of great practical concern is the "sonic boom." In this case the velocity of the moving sound source is faster than the speed of sound; that is, the sound emitting object races ahead of its own pressure changes. The resultant sound waves in the wake of the moving object join together to generate a single wavefront, which when passing by a listener, is heard as a sharp double clap.

Binaural Cues

Although relative distance information is available, the ability to perceive the *direction* of a sound is seriously affected when using only one ear. To a monaural observer the physical information from a sound-emitting object could specify the sound lying at any number of undifferentiated locations (e.g., Butler, 1971). It appears that localization depends on the relative stimulation of the two ears—on binaural cues.

TIME DIFFERENCES The information contained in dichotic binaural stimulation does enable sound localization. One such cue is the slight time differences produced when a sound, especially one with a sharp onset such as a click, reaches one ear before it reaches the other. As shown in Figure 6.2, any sound from source (*B*) in the head's median plane (the plane passing through the middle of the head from front to back) will produce equal effects on the two ears (called *diotic* stimulation). In contrast, a sound arriving from a lateral location, as from source (*A*), will travel farther to reach the right ear then the left. It follows that the sound waves from (*A*) will have a later time of arrival at the right ear than the left. In general, a sound located closer to one ear than the other sends off waves that reach the nearer ear sooner than the farther one. The difference may be slight, but under certain circumstances it is sufficient to locate the sound source (see Wallach, Newman, & Rosenzweig, 1949). It has been stated that sounds whose time of arrival differ by as little as 0.0001 seconds (without accompanying intensity differences) are sufficient to serve as cues for localizing sound in space; this must be accomplished neurally because such an interval is too small to allow the sounds to be heard as separate stimuli (Rosenzweig, 1961).

Rosenzweig (1951, 1954, 1961) has demonstrated with anesthetized cats that such small differences produce differential responses in

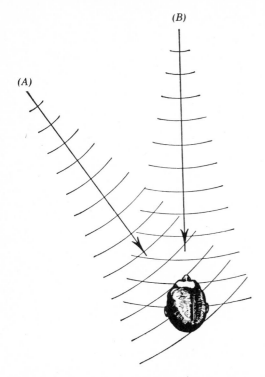

Fig. 6.2 *Cues for Sound Localization. Sound waves coming from source B in the median plane affect both ears equally. A sound from source A reaches the left ear before the right ear, and it is more intense because the right ear is slightly "shadowed" by the head. (From Foundations of Psychology, by E. G. Boring, H. S. Langfeld, & H. P. Weld, Wiley, New York, 1948, p. 338. Reprinted by permission of the publisher.)*

the auditory cortex. Tiny electrodes placed at various points along the auditory neural pathway, including the auditory cortex, recorded signals produced by independent earphones, one on each ear. Although responses occurred at both sides of the auditory cortex, when only the right ear was stimulated the responses at the left side were stronger. When both ears were stimulated but with a small time interval between stimuli (clicks), the resultant cortical responses resembled the responses to the single stimulus. For example,

when a click to one ear preceded one to the other ear by, say, 0.0002 seconds, the amplitude of the cortical response from the initially stimulated ear was slightly larger than that from the other ear. Of course, as previously described, this is based on the fact that each ear is represented more strongly in the opposite side of the brain than in the same side; thus a sound delivered to one ear prior to the other excites more neural activity in the side of the brain opposite to the ear first stimulated and partially inhibits the response to the later one. The neural response pattern therefore reflects the temporal differences in the pattern of stimulation.

INTENSITY A second binaural cue results from the intensity difference between the sounds reaching each ear. A sound, nonequidistant from the ears, not only strikes the nearer ear first but it also delivers a slightly more intense sound to that ear. This is because the head becomes an acoustic obstacle, that is, the head casts a sound "shadow" and the ear opposite to the sound source lies in this shadow (see Figure 6.2). Hence, sound waves that must pass around the head are disrupted and reach the farther ear with a weaker intensity than the nearer one. Because the long wavelengths of low frequency sounds tend to bend around the ear, the influence of sound shadows on binaural intensity differences are greater as frequency increases (i.e., wavelength decreases). For example, due to the head's acoustical shadow under certain conditions, a 10,000 Hz tone will undergo a 20 *db* drop in intensity at the farther ear, a 6 *db* drop in intensity for a 1000 Hz tone, and only about a 2 *db* drop for a 250 Hz tone (Gulick, 1971, p. 189).

Relevant to localization based on binaural intensity differences is the fact that when a tone is presented to both ears simultaneously but made more intense to one ear, the listener hears the tone as coming only from the direction of the more intensely stimulated ear. That is, the tone appears to stimulate only the ear receiving the more intense signal. However, the weaker signal, although not audible, contributes to the overall loudness of the more intense tone in that if the weaker tone is eliminated the more intense tone appears to decrease in loudness.

HEAD MOVEMENTS To binaural listeners the location of sound sources in the horizontal plane is possible, but vertical location (i.e., the location of a sound above versus below the observer) poses a problem. Furthermore, if a sound source is located in the median plane, its direction cannot be correctly determined by a stationary observer. Similarly, an observer may experience confusion in discriminating between sounds originating on the surface of a "cone of confusion," as illustrated in Figure 6.3, although he could tell from which side the sounds come. Confusion in these cases results because no matter where the sounds originate on the median plane or the conical surface, they are always the same distance farther from one ear than from the other, thereby producing the same degree of binaural time and intensity differences. These problems of location can be solved by allowing free movement of the head: When an organism moves its head, temporal and intensity changes in sound reception are produced. It follows, then, that if the head moves to the left of the midline, a sound directly behind is heard sooner and louder by the left ear than by the right ear. Moreover, by moving the head up and down sound-emitting stimuli in the vertical plane can be located.

Much of the foregoing relates to animals with symmetrical ears. However, the ears of the owl, unlike those of all other vertebrates, are not symmetrical. Because of this the owl can easily locate horizontal and vertical sound sources (Matthews & Knight, 1963, p. 176). The openings of their ears (birds do not have pinnae) are modified so that the two sides are asymmetrical. The degree of asymmetry varies with species, but in extreme cases the distortion may be so great that the shape of the skull itself is asymmetrical in the

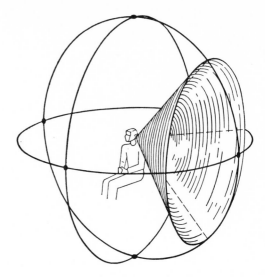

Fig. 6.3 *Cone of confusion. The conical surface on the side of the median plane is called a cone of confusion because the observer cannot discriminate among the sounds lying on its surface although he can tell from which side the sound comes. Confusion results because all points on the cone are the same distance farther from one ear than from the other. Thus, sounds originating at any location on the cone will provide the same difference in stimulation at the two ears. The circles indicate possible positions of the sound source in the three principal planes of the head. (From Foundations of Psychology, by E. G. Boring, H. S. Langfeld, & H. P. Weld, Wiley, New York, 1948, p. 337. Reprinted by permission of the publisher.)*

region of the auditory canal. Thus, to the owl a sound heard in the median plane reaches one ear first, whereas in most other vertebrates both ears would receive the sound at the same instant. No doubt we can assign the asymmetrical placement of the owl's ears as a special adaptation: Characteristically the owl stalks its prey (generally small rodents and insects) on the wing at night, flying about 4 meters per sec, and must locate it primarily on the basis of faint and brief transient sounds (see Konishi, 1973).

STEREOPHONIC LISTENING Almost all individuals are familiar with the striking auditory effects produced by stereophonic recordings that employ a playback system of two loudspeakers. The basis for the stereophonic experience is binaural hearing in which the differences in the recorded stimulation sent to each ear simulate the differences that are normally experienced due to the location of the ears on the head. In this sense stereophonic listening is due to a mild form of dichotic stimulation. Generally this is done by recording the same acoustic event with two microphones placed at different locations. A very realistic sound experience can be achieved by placing a recording microphone close to the auditory canal of each ear (an artificial skull may also be used). The sounds thus recorded preserve all the binaural differences that are ordinarily heard. On playback, wearing stereophonic head phones, the recording sounds strikingly like what was heard during the original recording. Stereophonic effects can be manipulated by a number of factors, such as by changing the microphone placement at the recording site and by varying the location of and the intensity difference between the playback loudspeakers in the listening environment. Reproduction systems using four speakers (so called "quadraphonic" sound systems) are now offered for home use that tend to produce a more displaced and enlarged sound space than that offered by the two loudspeakers of stereophonic sound systems.

Echolocation

The natural habitat of a number of nonterrestrial mammals, including bats, whales, porpoises and perhaps some small terrestrial rodents, requires activity in places where the use of vision is severely reduced or eliminated. For example, bats are active at night and in conditions where the amount of light is negligible; whales and porpoises may dwell at depths to which light does not easily penetrate. Functionally speaking, in order to locomote effectively in visually impeded environments, these animals have evolved the ability to evaluate the reflection or echoes of their own

sounds from objects in their surroundings. The result is that they gain information about the range and direction (and perhaps the velocity, size, and shape) of objects at a distance. In short, they are made aware of the location of objects that they cannot see by means of self-emitted sound waves reflected by them. The use of self-produced echoes to gain location information is termed *echolocation*.

Most of the research on echolocation has been done with bats, whose principal sensory modality appears to be audition. We will briefly focus on the bat's echolocating mechanism. The bat avoids obstacles when flying in the dark, and it can locate and capture prey with near perfect accuracy while it and its prey fly at relatively high speeds. Bats perform these feats by producing and receiving the echoes of extremely brief *ultrasonic* cries or pulses (i.e., sounds above the frequency limit of human hearing) whose frequencies are in excess of 100 kHz (k stands for thousand; see Figure 6.4). The number of pulses emitted varies with the bat's activity. During searching flight, only 10 pulses per second are emitted, whereas during interception maneuvers as many as 200 of these pulses may be produced in a second (Novick, 1971).

The production and reception of ultrasonic sounds are necessary for bats to identify and track prey and avoid obstacles. This is due to several physical considerations of sound transmission: High frequency sounds are propagated and reflected less diffusely than low frequency sounds. In addition, since the returning stimulus carries information of its reflected objects, the wavelength must be smaller than the object of reflection—for the bat, insects and the like are relevant objects—and high frequency sounds (and short wavelengths) are most important. This points out the biological value of the bat's extended upper limit of hearing.

Indeed, there are structural peculiarities of the bat's auditory and vocal anatomy that facilitate the reception of high frequencies. For example, the region of the cochlea concerned with

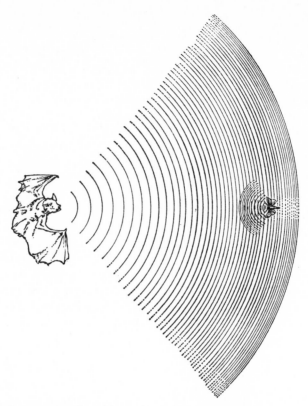

Fig. 6.4 *A flying bat and a representation of its emitted ultrasonic pulse. The curved lines represent individual sound waves in a single pulse. The frequency and wave length of a bat's sound may vary during each pulse. The figure, which according to its author is drawn to scale, illustrates the small amount of sound reflected by one insect. In searching flight bats may emit about 10 pulses per second. The pulse rate is increased to between 25 to 50 per second during a phase in which the bat appears to identify a target. During an approach or interception phase, the rate may be increased to 200 or more pulses per second (Novick, 1971). (Source: Griffin, 1959, p. 86 reprinted by permission of the author.)*

high frequency reception, nearest the middle ear, is unusually large in bats. Similarly, the bat's vocal structures are well engineered for producing ultrasonic pulses (Griffin, 1958; 1959).

The design of ultrasonic pulses for bats varies with family. For example, *horseshoe* bats, an insectivorous group, emit sounds of nearly a single frequency of about 83 kHz—followed by a sweep down to 65 or 70 kHz (Simmons, 1971). The individual sounds may last from 50 to 65 msec. The small brown bats, common to the United States, begin their pulses at 90 kHz and end up at 45 kHz. Their pulse duration lasts only about 2 msec, which means that there is a very

rapid frequency change. As Griffin (1959) points out, in 2 msec, this species of bat passes through a frequency band that consists of twice the whole range of human audibility. This type of sound emission is called *frequency modulated* or **FM**. FM pulse emission can serve as a very sophisticated range-measuring mechanism. The utilization of a pulse whose frequency changes means that echoes returning from targets located at different distances are heard at different frequencies. In the case of a single echo, if it reached one ear prior to the other, it would be heard at a different frequency in each ear. Other pulse designs are also employed (e.g., see Simmons, 1971; Novick,

1971); however, the general mechanism of bat echolocation utilizes an emission of a series of short ultrasonic orientation pulses and a comparison of their echoes with respect to the original pulses. This may involve the evaluation of temporal, intensity, and frequency differences between the emitted pulse bursts and the reception of their echoes. In many respects this mechanism is similar to the man-made instruments for sound navigation in water (i.e., *SO*und *N*avigation *A*nd *R*anging, hence the term, *SONAR*).

In actual operation echolocation is a complex behavioral process. The following excerpt by Novick (1971) on echolocation in goal-directed flight bears this out:

> *The approach phase starts when the bat, having detected an object, begins to devote its attention to it. Generally, the pulses are then shortened linearly with distance, the pulse repetition rate is increased, and the frequency and frequency pattern may be altered. During this phase, the bat seems to identify the direction and distance of the target and to adjust its flight path for interception or avoidance. The terminal phase, often lasting about 100 msec, is characterized by very short pulses, rapidly repeated, and ends as the bat intercepts or passes its target. Probably the cessation of immediate echo input brings the terminal phase to an end. During the terminal phase, the bat is engaged in its final interception maneuvers and appears, for the moment, to sacrifice attention to other objects. (P. 198)*

Obstacle Perception by the Blind

Blind individuals are often able to avoid running into obstacles. Several theories have attempted to account for this ability. A prominent one holds that the touch and temperature senses have developed sufficiently in certain of the blind to enable them to feel air currents as they are affected by the proximity of obstacles. The locus of this ability was attributed to the face hence the

term "facial vision". Auditory cues in the form of echoes from objects has provided another explanation for the perception of obstacles by the blind. A series of experiments in the 1940s was undertaken to choose between these two explanations.

Using blindfolded normally sighted and blind subjects, Supra, Cotzin, and Dallenbach (1944) tested the effectiveness of auditory cues for obstacle perception—the obstacle in this case was a wall of fiber board, about 1.2 by 1.5 meters located along a hallway. A subject was instructed to walk down the hallway and to indicate when he thought he was approaching the wall and to walk up as close as possible to it without striking it. When sound cues were reduced—such as by having subjects walk in their stocking feet over thick carpeting or by stopping their ears—obstacle avoidance was poor or eliminated. In most instances this result occurred although potential sources of touch stimulation were available, that is, the head, arms, and hands were open to stimulation. This indicated that touch is not sufficient for the perception of obstacles. Moreover, when subjects wore earphones that allowed only a 1000 Hz masking tone but were also provided with potential touch stimulation, no obstacle avoidance was observed. Indeed, that sound alone is critical for obstacle avoidance is given in the following experiment in which all sensory channels of stimulation except the acoustic one were eliminated. Subjects were placed in a soundproof room and were instructed to judge the experimenter's approach to the obstacle by means of the experimenter's footsteps. The sounds of the experimenter's footsteps were picked up by a microphone carried by the experimenter at ear height and transmitted to the subject through an amplifying system and earphones. Under these conditions all subjects tested were able to perceive the experimenter's approach to the obstacle and their ability to do so was only slightly inferior to their performances when they themselves walked toward the obstacle. Clearly, these experiments point to the conclusion that blind subjects perceive obstacles on the basis of sound information. Subsequent research with subjects both deaf and blind reaffirmed the conclusion that auditory stimulation is both a necessary and a sufficient condition for the perception of obstacles by the blind (Worshel & Dallenbach, 1947).

Several questions arise: How accurate are sound cues for spatial perception? What additional spatial abilities are possible using sounds? Some research on this has been attempted by W. N. Kellogg (1962) who compared the performance of the blind with that of blindfolded normally-sighted control subjects in a number of spatial tasks. Of particular interest is that subjects were informed that they could make any sound they wanted for the purpose of producing echoes. Although the subjects sometimes employed tongue-clicking, finger-snapping, hissing, or whistling, coupled with headbobbing, the preferred source of self-produced auditory signals was the human voice used in a repetitive fashion—that is, vocalizing the same word over and over.

In one task subjects were instructed to indicate whether a one-foot (30.5 cm) diameter wood disc that was moved silently by the experimenter to one of seven fixed positions [which varied from one to four feet (30.5–122 cm) from the subject] was nearer or farther away than a disc held at a constant two-foot (61 cm) distance. In another task, discs ranging from 14.7 cm to 30.5 cm in diameter, were compared in size to a standard stimulus of 23.9 cm in diameter. In general, blind subjects were able to derive distance and size information from the stimuli whereas the performance of the blindfolded normal subjects was at about a chance level. Texture differences were also discriminable by blind subjects. Six discs, all with different surface characteristics, were presented in all possible pairs to subjects at a 30.5 cm distance. The materials covering the surfaces were sheet metal, glass, plain and painted wood, denim, and velvet. The result was that the echoes from many of the surfaces were sufficiently discriminable for blind subjects to perceive them as different. In contrast, the judgments of the normally-sighted

controls were almost never above chance. For the blind subjects the echoes from hard surfaces, though indistinguishable from one another, were readily distinguishable from soft surfaces. For example, the glass surface was discriminated from the velvet surface 99% of the time whereas metal was discriminated from glass only 47% of the time (50% is pure chance). Curiously, denim was distinguished from velvet approximately 87% of the time. The conclusion is that the perception of echoes reflected from objects provides sufficient information for object detection and avoidance in the human blind.

As to the stimulus factors used by subjects for the acoustic perception of obstacles, Cotzin and Dallenbach (1950) have shown that changes in the pitch rather than the loudness of echoes are the basic cues. In their experiment, the test obstacle was a screen 1.2 meters wide by about 1.5 meters high. A loudspeaker, mounted on an electrically driven apparatus that moved toward the obstacle screen, produced either a pure tone or a loud hissing noise called "thermal noise" (because it arises from the amplification of the random electrical currents resulting from molecular motion). The motor of the apparatus was remotely controlled by the subject as he listened to the changes in the noise through earphones in a soundproof room. The subject stopped the advancing apparatus when he perceived a change in the pitch of the tone. Successful obstacle perception occurred only with the thermal noise (whose frequencies ranged between 100 and 12,000 Hz) and with pure tones whose frequencies were 10,000 Hz. With tones below 10,000 Hz obstacle perception was not obtained.

In subsequent research, Rice (1967) also attempted to specify some of the physical characteristics of usable acoustic signals, but in this case the focus was on sounds self-produced by humans in their sonar-type system of echolocation. The self-generated signals used to provide information on the presence or absence of an object—tongue-clicks or hiss signals—were spectrographically analyzed (a *spectrogram* is a graphic reproduction of the frequency spectrum and duration of an acoustic signal, described in more detail in the next section). The findings were that the frequency limits of spectrograms of the signals covered the range between 170 Hz and 16 kHz. Although not conclusive, it is probable that moderately high frequency sounds are most useful because the higher the frequency, the shorter the wavelength and the better the reflection. Furthermore, as we have previously noted, wavelength size also specifies another limitation: An object must have a size at least as large as a single wavelength in order to reflect an effective echo.

THE PERCEPTION OF SPEECH

Another behavioral function of the auditory system is its role in the form of human communication called speech. Obviously, the perception of speech begins with stimulation of the ear. However, speech perception involves an enormous number of complex psychological variables so that we can only briefly outline the processes involved. Consider how remarkable this ability is. It requires the ability to make very fine discriminations between sounds: For example, a spoken word consists of a short pattern of sounds lasting less than a second. Moreover, the perception of speech persists when the sounds comprising words undergo a number of marked changes. That is, words retain their identity and are accurately perceived under a number of distorting conditions: for example, varying accents and voice qualities, masking background noises and sound omissions, and distortions produced by electrical means such as by telephones or other mass communications systems. Indeed, even when most physical characteristics of speech sounds have been changed to some degree, a measure of identity affording intelligibility may still persist. That meaningful speech occurs under these conditions points out a striking perceptual achievement.

The range of actual speech sounds is limited by the anatomy of the vocal apparatus rather than by the potential of the ear to hear. Human speech is produced by the mechanics of the vocal cords and the variably resonant vocal tract, which includes cavities of the mouth, throat, and nose. The air in the cavities is set into vibration by movement of the vocal cords producing sound waves. Different frequencies may be produced by the combined action of the vocal tract and the relative positioning of the tongue, lips, cheeks, and jaw. The potential for varying frequency is determined by a number of factors. The resonant frequency of the oral cavity is governed by the physical length of the tract and the mass of the vocal cords. For the average man this frequency is close to 500 Hz, for women, 727 Hz and 850 Hz for children (Bergeijk, Pierce, & David, 1960). As Figure 6.5 shows, the highest useful frequencies for speech production lie close to 6500 Hz. Thus, speech sounds occupy about a third of the total range of frequencies audible to humans. With respect to the intensive extents of audibility, the range of produced intensities is likewise narrow. Between the softest sounds (whispers) and the loudest sounds (shouts) that may naturally occur from the human voice is a range of about 70 *db* (Boring, Langfeld, & Weld, 1948). The energy levels at both these extremes are far from the limits of human audibility. Moreover, though some speech sounds may extend to comparatively high frequencies, the major part of speech energy occurs at frequencies below 1000 Hz, regardless of the speaker's gender (refer to Figure 6.6).

Speech Sounds

To comprehend the fine discriminations perceived between words we must focus on the individual sounds upon which a language is built. A familiar division of speech sounds into distinctive features is that between vowels and consonants. Vowels are sounds produced by the vocal cords, the resonance of the throat cavities, and the open mouth. Consonants are produced by constriction of the passage through the throat and mouth. Con-

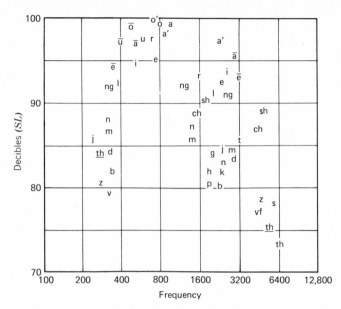

Fig. 6.5 *Frequency and intensity characteristics of the fundamental speech sounds. Those sounds having more than one principal frequency component appear at more than one location on the figure. [Source: Harvey Fletcher, Speech and Hearing (revised ed.), copyright © 1952, D. Van Nostrand Company, Company, Inc.]*

Fig. 6.6 *Distribution of sound energy by frequency of continuous speech averaged over a period of time. Most of the speech energy occurs in frequencies below 1000 Hz. (From J. Licklider & G. Miller in Handbook of Experimental Psychology, edited by S. S. Stevens, Wiley, New York, 1951, p. 1042. Reprinted by permission of the publisher.)*

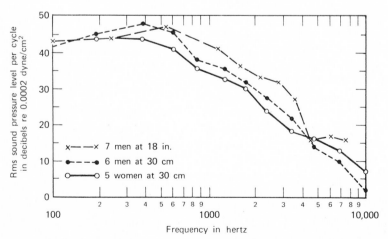

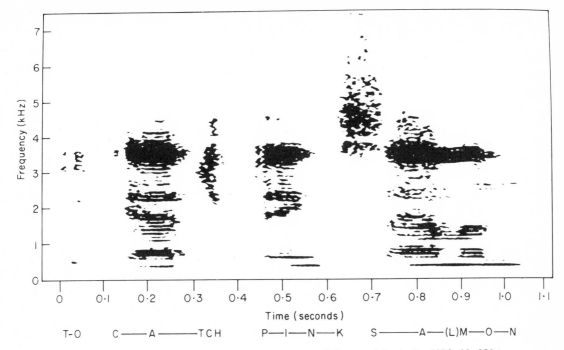

Fig. 6.7 *Spectrogram of the utterance: "to catch pink salmon." (Source: Mattingly, 1972, 60, 328.)*

sonants may be grouped into *stop* consonants or *plosive* sounds that are short sounds that cannot be held; such sounds are *b, p, t, d, k, g*. Sounds of consonants produced in the mouth by letting air escape through constriction between lips and teeth are called *aspirate* or *fricative* sounds—*th, sh, ch, h, z, s, f, v*. Sounds like *w, y, l, r, m,* and *n*, called *semivowels,* represent sounds that fall between the recognized consonants and vowels. Vowels are louder than consonants though some consonants are much louder than others. The energy in vowel sounds is almost entirely in the frequencies below 3000 Hz whereas that energy in a *ch* or *s* sound lies above 3000 Hz.

Another category of speech sounds, composed of vowels and consonants, is the *phoneme,* which is the smallest sound unit of a language that serves to distinguish one utterance from another (see Table 6.1). Phonemes classify sounds more on the basis of their physically distinguish-

ing features than on their vocal means of production. The English language uses about 40 phonemes, whereas some languages use as few as 20 and some use as many as 60 (Bergeijk, Pierce, & David, 1960).

Speech sounds do not consist of pure or even simple tones. Indeed, to account for the discrimination between the various vowels and consonants or phonemes on the basis of their physical sound waves turns out to be quite difficult. Most speech sounds represent a complex pattern of intensities and frequencies over time. A record that indicates the changes in the intensity and frequency pattern of utterances over time is called a sound *spectrogram.* A characteristic spectrogram is shown by Figure 6.7. Time is plotted along the abscissa, frequency on the ordinate, and the darkness of the record indicates intensity. The concentrations of acoustic energy that appear in the display as dark bars are called *formants.*

Table 6.1
THE PHONEMES OF GENERAL AMERICAN
ENGLISH[a]

Vowels	Consonants	
ee as in h*ea*t	*t* as in *t*ee	*s* as in *s*ee
I as in h*i*t	*p* as in *p*ea	*sh* as in *sh*ell
e as in h*ea*d	*k* as in *k*ey	*h* as in *h*e
ae as in h*a*d	*b* as in *b*ee	*v* as in *v*iew
ah as in f*a*ther	*d* as in *d*awn	*th* as in *th*en
aw as in c*a*ll	*g* as in *g*o	*z* as in *z*oo
U as in p*u*t	*m* as in *m*e	*zh* as in ga*r*age
oo as in c*oo*l	*n* as in *n*o	*l* as in *l*aw
ʌ as in t*o*n	*ng* as in si*ng*	*r* as in *r*ed
uh as in th*e*	*f* as in *f*ee	*y* as in *y*ou
er as in b*ir*d	*θ* as in *th*in	*w* as in *w*e
oi as in t*oi*l		
au as in sh*ou*t		
ei as in t*a*ke		
ou as in t*o*ne		
ai as in m*igh*t		

[a] General American is the dialect of English spoken in mid-western and western areas of the United States. Certain phonemes of other regional dialects (e.g. Southern) can be different. The phonemes of General American English include 16 vowels and 22 consonants as shown above.
Source: Denes & Pinson, 1973, p. 15.

SPEECH PERCEPTION WITH SOUND DISTORTION

Frequency Cutoffs

Speech perception is more than the recognition and identification of a sequence of differential excitations of the inner ear. The perception of a stream of sounds as a related sequence of words requires the operation of a complex central integrative mechanism. That speech perception involves considerably more than mere sound reception is indicated by the ability to perceive meaningful speech when the flow of acoustic energy is dis-

torted, say, when ranges of frequencies are eliminated.

In one study, whole bands of frequencies were completely removed from the speech of men and women. When frequencies above 1900 Hz were filtered out from speech, about 70% of the words were intelligible. Furthermore, the same result was obtained with the elimination of all sounds below 1900 Hz (French & Steinberg, 1947; see also Licklider & Miller, 1951, pp. 1052–1058). This is shown in Figure 6.8. In other words, as much of the total intelligibility is carried by frequencies below 1900 Hz as is carried by frequencies above 1900 Hz. There is a tradeoff in information retained and removed: Eliminating the high frequencies affects the perception of consonants more than vowels, whereas filtering out the low frequencies affects vowels more than consonants. Thus, neither all the high or low frequency speech components are necessary for a reasonable degree of intelligibility.

Fig. 6.8 *Intelligibility of Filtered Speech. Curves show number of words correctly understood when all frequencies above a given point are removed (leaving low frequencies only) or all frequencies below a given point are removed (leaving high frequencies only). (Source: Boring, Langfeld, & Weld, 1949, p. 349; derived from N. R. French and J. C. Steinberg, J. Acous. Soc. Amer., 1947, 19, 90–119.)*

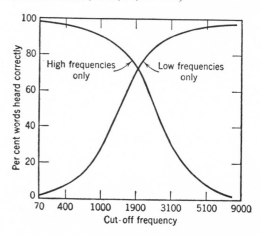

Amplitude Clipping

A form of amplitude distortion called *peak clipping* is one that cuts off the high amplitude parts of the speech waves (see Figure 6.9). The findings from a number of experiments on peak clipping agree that although peak clipping degrades the quality and naturalness of speech, a surprisingly large portion of the speech wave can be eliminated before intelligibility is affected. The solid line of Figure 6.10 shows the resistance to the effects of peak clipping. More than 95% of monosyllabic words are heard correctly even after a 24 *db* peak clipping (leaving only one-sixteenth of the original speech wave). The opposite of peak clipping is *center clipping,* in which the center part of the speech wave is eliminated. As shown in Figure 6.10, center clipping has a drastic effect on word intelligibility. The reason that peak clipping and center clipping differ on word perception to the extent that they do is that the center part of the speech wave contains the consonant sounds. As Licklider and Miller (1951) point out: "Only a small percentage of our vocal energy goes into consonants, but that small portion conveys a disproportionate amount of information" (p. 1058).

Fig. 6.9 *Diagram A is a schematic representation of the waveform of the word "Joe." B shows what is left after 6 db peak clipping, that is, after reduction to one-half the original peak-to-peak amplitude. C. illustrates 20 db peak clipping. (Source J. Licklider & G. Miller, Handbook of Experimental Psychology, Edited by S. S. Stevens, Wiley; New York, 1951, p. 1058. Reprinted by permission of the publisher.)*

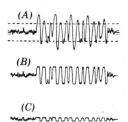

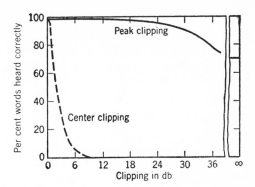

Fig. 6.10 *The effects of peak clipping and center clipping upon intelligibility. Peak clipping has little effect on intelligibility whereas center clipping renders the speech sound almost unintelligible. (From J. Licklider & G. Miller, Handbook of Experimental Psychology, edited by S. S. Stevens, Wiley, New York, 1951, p. 1058. Reprinted by permission of the publisher.)*

Context

The meaningful perception of the incoming pattern of stimulation is dependent on expectations as to what the stimulation should consist of. That is, a form of extra information is provided by the context in which sounds are heard. The importance of verbal context for speech perception is obvious in the following example (Warren, 1970; see also Warren and Warren, 1970): A missing speech sound (phoneme), represented by the blank space in the following spoken sentence, was replaced by a loud cough. "It was found that the ( )eel was on the orange." The blank before the word fragment "( )eel" can be determined by the context provided by the last word in the sentence—namely the listener hears the word "peel." Other words that could complete the sentence and alter the context are "axle" and "shoe." Each would indicate a different speech sound for the preceding word fragment, that is, "wheel" and "heel" respectively. Thus phonemic restoration conforms to the context provided. Notice that the perception of the missing sound was aided by words that appeared *after* the

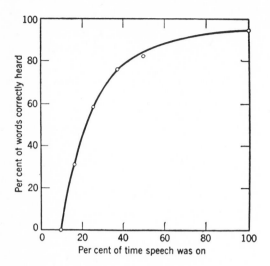

Fig. 6.11 *Intelligibility of Blanked Speech. Speech was turned on and off nine times per second. Quite short bursts of speech are enough to give good intelligibility. (Source: Boring, Langfeld, & Weld, 1948, p. 349; after G. A. Miller, Psychol. Bull., 1947, 44, 120. Copyright © 1947 by the American Psychological Association. Reprinted by permission.)*

cough. This indicates that the listener must be storing incomplete information until the necessary context is established. Interestingly, the missing sound was "heard" clearly although perception of where the cough occurred was poor. When a silent gap rather than a cough replaced the missing phoneme, the gap could be located.

Speech Blanking

A similar result occurs when sections of the flow of speech are eliminated by periodically turning the speech on and off by mechanical means. When conversation was blanked out for 50% of the time, speech quality was altered but only 15% of the words were lost (Miller, 1947). The general trend for blanking proportions is shown in Figure 6.11. Thus, under certain conditions speech perception is quite good even though the auditory systems hears the speech only half the time (see also Licklider & Miller, 1951, p. 1063–1064).

A THEORY OF SPEECH PERCEPTION

One of the major difficulties facing an understanding of speech perception is explaining how we perceive the sequence of sounds comprising the spoken message as distinct, well-articulated words when in fact there is little present in the physical stimulation to properly segment or bind the verbal message into words. It is likely that this phenomenon is a consequence of the listener's response to the input as speech. A stranger to a language perceives this immediately. A truly foreign language is heard as a rapid and continuous stream of utterances and for the naïve listener it is impossible to identify discrete words based only on their sounds.

One explanation for the perception of word boundaries is that the perceptual system must know what the word is before it can be properly segmented and perceptually bounded as a distinct word. According to one group of researchers, the perception of spoken language occurs as a result of a subtle form of articulation mimicry or covert speech performed prior to speech recognition. This has formed the basis of a theory whose key assumption is, ". . . that the sounds of speech are somehow perceived by reference to the ways we generate them" (Liberman, Cooper, Harris, MacNeilage, & Studdert-Kennedy, 1967, p. 70). It is a motor theory in that listeners are held to make use of their knowledge of the articulatory gestures that are ordinarily involved in the production of speech. In other words, an integral part of the process of speech recognition is speech production—the hearer is also a speaker.

According to Lieberman (1968):

The listeners "decode" the input speech signal by using their knowledge of the constraints that are imposed by the human articulatory "output" apparatus. In a sense we have proposed a "motor" theory of speech perception since we have suggested that there is a close relationship between the inherent properties of the speech output mechanism and the perceptual recognition routine. (P. 162)

It is further contended that because speech perception is so quick and so well established the requirement of actual motor responses is rendered minimal or nonexistent. The central nervous system, using feedback from previous experiences along with the basic knowledge of the grammar of the language, may function to eliminate the need for actual motor responses. The basic argument is that in the process of speech perception the brain in some way is able to make use of the results of associations with prior articulatory movements without recourse to actual articulation. Liberman et al. (1967) assume: "... that somewhere in the speaker's central nervous system there exist signals which stand in a one-to-one relation to the phonemes of the language" (p. 77).

Perhaps as with other sorts of human activities there is more than one method by which speech perception can be achieved. In any event it should be clear that the understanding of speech perception extends well beyond the boundaries of only the facts of acoustic reception in the ear.

ANIMAL COMMUNICATION

Although it is generally agreed that linguistic behavior is afforded only to humans, we should note that the sounds produced by many infrahuman animals, ranging from insects to primates, including fish, amphibia, and birds, may be used for the purpose of a form of intraspecies information exchange.

For the most part communicative behavior patterns are highly characteristic for the species, both in their production and in the sorts of information they convey. Insects such as the cicada and crickets (especially the male), for example, use signals to convey information as to courting and other mating-related activities and for maintaining contact with each other. Birds use sound signals—calls or songs—for such diverse activities as nesting, territorial defense, the establishment and maintenance of pair bonds, and even for parental recognition. By howling, wolves communicate information of their identify, their location, and perhaps something of their emotional state (Theberge, 1971). Primates also exchange acoustic signals in an informative way. Perhaps the most closely studied infrahuman group has been the rhesus monkey. Rowell (1962, pp. 93–94, excerpted in Marler & Hamilton, 1966, p. 469) has described nine calls or cries produced by the rhesus that express some aspect of the animal's condition. Table 6.2 describes them and shows the types of situations in which they occur (for discussions of animals' communication see e.g., Marler & Hamilton, 1966, Chapter 12).

It is of interest to consider the evolution of language from the general perspective of animal communication. It is held that the principal factor in the development of language is the unusual intellect that is uniquely man's, that is, language reflects the human intellect and accordingly is afforded only to man (see Lenneberg, 1967). Furthermore it has been argued that the vocal tract of man evolved from something like that of a chimpanzee (e.g., Lieberman & Crelin, 1971; Lieberman, Crelin & Klatt, 1972). Thus, the attainment of human language must be viewed as the product of a long evolutionary process that involved changes in anatomical structure through mutation, successive variation, and natural selection, which enhanced vocal communication. Extending this morphological transition to speech production and perception, we may ask how does the uniquely human form of communication come to be encoded in vocal articulatory gestures, that is, speech? According to Mattingly (1972) an analysis of facial gestures, particularly the repertory of facial grimaces of the chimpanzee, provides the basis of a speculation:

If such a grimace—for example the protruding and rounding of the lips—is accompanied by vocal-cord vibration, an

Table 6.2
RHESUS CALLS[a]

Roar	Long, fairly loud noise	Made by a very confident animal, when threatening another of inferior rank
Pant-threat	Like a roar, but divided into "syllables"	Made by a less confident animal, who wants support in making an attack
Bark	Like the single bark of a dog	Made by a threatening animal who is insuffiently aggressive to move forward
Growl	Like a bark, but quieter, shriller, and broken into short sound units	Given by a mildly alarmed animal
Shrill-bark	Not described	Alarm call, probably given to predators in the wild
Screech	An abrupt pitch change, up then down	Made when threatening a higher-ranked animal, and when excited and slightly alarmed
Geckering screech	Like a screech, but broken into syllables	Made when threatened by another animal
Scream	Shorter than the screech and without a rise and fall	Made when losing a fight while being bitten
Squeak	Short, very high pitched noises	Made by a defeated and exhausted animal at the end of a fight

[a] Source: In Marler and Hamilton, 1966, p. 469, after Rowell, 1962, pp. 93–94. Reprinted by permission of the publisher.

acoustic event characteristic of lip-rounding—a drop in the frequency of all formants—will be heard. Thus, . . . there was a potential acoustic cue corresponding to an overt articulatory gesture. Since most of us lip-read when face to face with another speaker, especially in a noisy environment, it appears that we still relate the overt labial articulation to its acoustic coding. Primitive man, on the other hand, may have used the acoustic cue when darkness or distance made face-to-face contact impossible. Similarly, he could relate visible jaw movement to its acoustic correlate. . . . Once having developed this limited ability to interpret acoustic cues in articulatory terms, it would not seem unreasonable that this ability could be generalized to include covert as well as overt articulators. Thus, speech might be regarded as a way of making invisible faces. (P. 336)

This chapter has focused principally on the informational aspects of acoustic energy, such as object detection, and localization and speech perception.

First we introduced the notion of brain asymmetry and hearing. It was noted that the neural message originating in the right ear is predominantly registered on the left hemisphere of the auditory brain, and the message from the left ear is principally registered on the right hemisphere of the brain. Furthermore, a number of studies indicate that the auditory cortex of the left hemisphere of the brain predominates in the perception of language-related stimulation and in sequential, analytic processing in general, whereas the right hemisphere is dominant in the reception of such forms of stimulation as pure tones and music.

The phenomena of auditory space perception—the locating and identification of sounds in space—were discussed for both monaural and binaural hearing. Monaural hearing can enable the evaluation of a sound-emitting object's relative distance; this is based mainly on the intensity of the sound source. However, for the precise localization of an object, binaural hearing is necessary. The cues afforded by binaural hearing are the time and intensity differences between the stimuli reaching each ear. That is, a sound closer to one ear reaches it sooner and with greater intensity than it does to the other ear. A number of phenomena relevant to sound location were discussed, such as the Doppler shift, stereophonic listening, and echolocation. The concepts discussed in auditory space perception were brought to bear on the striking ability of bats and the human blind to avoid obstacles.

The role that the auditory system plays in human speech communication was outlined. The physical characteristics of the sounds used in speech were identified and the perception of speech under a number of conditions of distortion was discussed; these were frequency cut-offs, amplitude clipping, phoneme omissions, and speech blanking. Finally, the evolution of language communication was briefly discussed within the context of animal communication. It was suggested that the attainment of human language is the product of a long evolutionary process.

Somesthesis I: Kinesthesis and Cutaneous Sense   7

This chapter and the one following are concerned with the two main topics that are collectively labeled *somesthesis: kinesthetic* sensitivity, which refers to spatial position and movement information occurring from mechanical stimulation of the mobile joints and muscles and *cutaneous* sensitivity, or skin sensitivity to touch or pressure, temperature, and pain. In the present context kinesthesis and the cutaneous sense are considered subsystems whose complex functional interactions provide information about the environment immediately adjacent to an organism. The mechanisms and phenomena of kinesthesis are described first, followed by the cutaneous sense of pressure or touch. In the next chapter, the cutaneous senses of temperature and pain are discussed.

KINESTHESIS

Kinesthesis (from the Greek *kineo,* "to move") refers to the reception of body-part position and movement—information about the posture, location, and movement in space of the limbs and other mobile parts of the jointed skeleton (e.g., fingers, wrist, limbs, head, trunk,

vertebrate column). Movement and position stimulation occurs at the joints of bones that possess linkages as shown in Figure 7.1. The mechanoreceptors for this information are *Pacinian corpuscles,* which lie in the mobile joints of the skeletal system. The receptors are stimulated by contact between the parts of the joint surfaces. Thus, stimulation occurs with changes in the angles at which the bones are held. In a sense, these corpuscles are subcutaneous pressure receptors.

Another potential source of information that may contribute to the perception of body-part location or kinesthesis results from innervation of muscles (e.g., Goodwin, McCloskey, and Matthews, 1972). Muscles and their attached tendons are well supplied with sensory nerves that respond to changes in tension when the muscle fiber is stretched or contracted. Stimulation of the appropriate receptors may produce patterns of excitation that lead to the perception of strain, such as that occurring when weight is supported. However, for kinesthesis the contribution of information from the muscles appears minor. Perception of limb location is probably not registered by muscle tension because information of limb posture or movement would require the registration of the length of the muscle. Muscle receptors register only stretch and strain information,

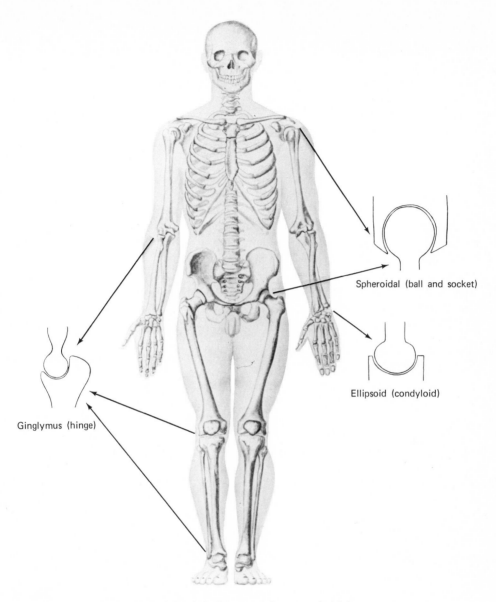

Spheroidal (ball and socket)

Ellipsoid (condyloid)

Ginglymus (hinge)

Anterior view of the skeletal system and some typical joints

Fig. 7.1 *Some of the possible movements between bones are indicated by the joints. In the hinge joint a spool-like surface of one bone fits into a half-moon surface in the other bone. Only a single plane of motion (bending) is permitted, usually flexion-extension. Examples are the elbow and knee joints. In the ball-and-socket joint a ball-like surface fits into a cup-like depression on the other bone. All planes of motion are permitted—it can bend and turn. The shoulder and hip joints are of this type. In the case of the condyloid joint an egg-shaped surface on one bone fits into a similar shape surface on the other. This joint permits side-to-side and back-and-forth motions. An example is the wrist joint. Other kinds of joints also occur within the skeletal system. In general, the angles to which the bones are moved are continuously registered by Pacinian corpuscles at the joints and provide the input for kinesthesis. (From Human Anatomy and Physiology, by J. Crouch & J. R. McClintic, Wiley, 1971, pp. 144 and 155. Reprinted by permission of the publisher.)*

neither of which yields information as to its length.

Further support for kinesthesis as mediated primarily by the joints is given in cases of clinical abnormalities. In certain rare nerve disorders, joint sensitivity may be left intact although input from the muscle receptors is abolished. This has also been produced experimentally by anesthetizing the muscles with cocaine (Goldscheider: cited in Geldard, 1972, p. 378). In such instances the perception of bodily movement is little affected, indicating that the joints play the major role in such perceptual acts. Further confirmation for this comes from an opposite sort of pathology in which certain bone disorders destroy joint receptivity without affecting the receptors of the muscles and tendons. In such cases the perception of correct limb position is rendered impossible. It appears, then, that the sensory inputs from tendons and muscles make their primary perceptual contribution in the detection of strain or effort rather than limb position or movement, that is, a feeling of strain added to the total kinesthetic effect when there is resistance to limb movement.

The detection of motion of the joints has been studied with movement of only one joint at a time. It should be noted that ordinarily it is not a single joint that moves. Frequently it is the relation between joints that registers information to the organism—what J. J. Gibson (1966) terms a *pose* of the body (p. 118). According to Geldard's (1972) review of the literature on the matter, of nine body joints tested in 1889 by Goldscheider for the threshold (minimum detected angular displacement) for passive movement, it was found that the shoulder was most sensitive to movement, closely followed by the wrist and knuckle of the index finger, and the ankle was the least sensitive. Furthermore, active voluntary movement produced a slightly greater sensitivity than did passive involuntary movement (Boring, 1942; Corso, 1967). This corresponds to some of the early findings in psychophysics by Weber that a smaller difference between two weights can be detected if they are actively lifted (involving kines-

thesis) than when they are merely placed on the skin.

Although kinesthetic stimulation does not result in a distinct perceptual experience such as hearing a sound (perhaps not even to the point of immediate awareness except when the need arises), the kinesthetic system continually provides a source of important information. Without any difficulty we know the position, posture, and the direction of the movement of our limbs in space. We scratch an itch we cannot see; we safely walk down a flight of stairs without directly gazing at our feet; and, in general, we may accurately touch any part of our body in the dark. In the laboratory, experiments have shown that man is capable of accurately pointing with his limbs without using vision (e.g., Cohen, L.A., 1958; Wood, 1969). When an individual is instructed to point with a hand-held rod to the gravitational vertical or horizontal, his average error is only a few degrees (Gibson, 1966, p. 118). The ability of the receptors at the joints to supply quantitative information about angles and distances is seen when a person accurately uses the distance between his two palms to mark off length no matter if the eyes are opened or closed. The main receptors for this particular action reside in the shoulder joint. Similarly, the gap spanned by the index finger and its opposable thumb is accurately used to mark off width or short distances. Here the receptors are in the knuckle and wrist joints. These abilities have been accurately demonstrated in the laboratory (e.g., Wertheimer, Michael, 1954; Teghtsoonian & Teghtsoonian, 1970). No doubt it is this activity that is referred to when we say we can measure an object or compare two objects on the basis of "touch."

THE SKIN AND CUTANEOUS EXPERIENCE

The skin of man, viewed as a sensory organ, is remarkable. It is by far the largest organ, form-

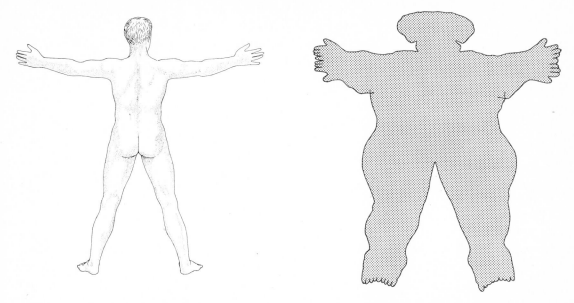

Fig. 7.2 *Total surface area of the skin, which seems surprisingly large in contrast to the outline of a human figure (left), is calculated by adding the areas of a series of cylinders constructed from an average of leg, arm, and torso circumferences. (From "The Skin," by W. Montagna, Scientific American, 1959, 11, pp. 58–59. Copyright © 1959 by Scientific American, Inc. All rights reserved.)*

ing an integument or covering for the entire body. A man 6 feet (1.83 meters) tall, of average weight and body build has about 3000 square inches (1.93 square meters) of skin area (see Figure 7.2). The skin is also the most versatile sensory organ of the body, serving as a flexible shield against many forms of foreign agents and mechanical injury. It holds in vital body fluids. It serves to ward off the harmful light waves (ultraviolet and infrared radiation) of the sun, and when appropriate, it stabilizes body temperature in birds and mammals, either cooling the body or retarding heat loss. It also has a role in regulating the pressure and direction of the blood flow. Finally, the skin has nerve endings embedded within it that can be stimulated in a variety of ways to mediate different sensations. The experiential result of skin stimulation is termed *cutaneous sensitivity.* Four basic qualities or sensations of cutaneous stimulation have been identified as

mediated by adequate stimulation of the skin: pressure or touch, cold, warmth, and pain.

Externally viewed, the skin appears as a highly variegated surface, manifesting distinct surface qualities and extensions—hairs, feathers, scales, creases, colorations, thicknesses—in different regions. However, the skin is not a single structural unit but is composed of layers. These layers, along with the sensory nerve endings, are identified and shown in cross section in the composite drawing of the skin in Figure 7.3. Although it is held that the nerve endings found in the skin are the receptors for cutaneous experience, it has not been clearly established that stimulation of a particular type of receptor exclusively initiates a certain cutaneous experience.

The sensations of pressure, cold and warmth, and pain have been based on subjects' responses rather than on the identification of anatomically distinct fibers. That is, evidence for the

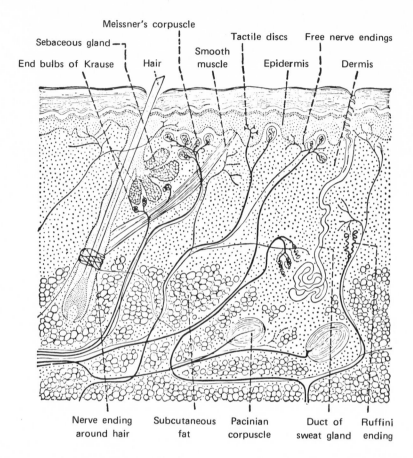

Sebaceous gland
Meissner's corpuscle
Tactile discs   Free nerve endings
End bulbs of Krause   Hair   Smooth   Epidermis   Dermis
                                    muscle

Nerve ending   Subcutaneous   Pacinian   Duct of   Ruffini
around hair   fat   corpuscle   sweat gland   ending

Fig. 7.3 *Composite diagram of the skin in cross section. The chief layers—epidermis, dermis, and subcutaneous tissue—are shown, as are also a hair follicle, the smooth muscle which erects the hair, and several kinds of nerve endings. In the epidermis are to be found tactile discs and free nerve endings; in the dermis are Meissner corpuscles, Krause end bulbs, Ruffini endings, and (around the base of the hair) free terminations. The subcutaneous tissue is chiefly fatty and vascular but contains Pacinian corpuscles, the largest of the specialized endings. (Source: Fundamentals of Neurology, by E. Gardner, W. B. Saunders, 1947. Reprinted by permission of the author and publisher.)*

existence of distinct cutaneous sensations is accessible only through introspective report. We will, however, examine some of the perceptual phenomena associated with cutaneous experiences and defer the issue of describing the underlying receptors subserving them for a later section.

Distribution of Cutaneous Sensitivity

Cutaneous information is registered by mechanical stimulation of the surface of the body.

In man this information is received predominantly from the skin, particularly of certain appendages. In lower animals cutaneous information is not only picked up directly by the skin but also by other external surface structures such as hairs, nails, claws, hooves, horns, vibrissae (whiskers), and antennae—structures that separate an organism from its immediate environment.

As we noted, the primary classes of information that are given by the skin are pressure or touch (sometimes called contact, tactual or tactile stimulation), temperature (cold and warmth), and pain. If we drew a grid on a part of the skin of a blindfolded subject and systematically explored the squares of that grid in turn with a heated rod and a cold rod, a hair, and a needle point, it is likely that our subject would report the cutaneous experiences of warmth, cold, pressure, and pain, respectively. A plot of the distribution of sensitive "spots" would provide us with a map of cutaneous sensitivity. In mapping all the spots for which temperature, pain, and pressure are represented, we find that regions of the skin are not uniformly sensitive to all stimuli. Some areas may be sensitive to slight contact only, some to temperature only. In other words, there is a distribution of distinct areas sensitive to different kinds of stimuli.

Pressure and Touch

A good part of the outer surface of the skin structure responds to the pressure or touch of the environment. In man, the guiding and exploratory parts of the body—the fingers, the hands, parts of the mouth, and the tip of the tongue—are most sensitive to those mechanical encounters with the environment that provide pressure or touch stimulation. Less sensitive areas, with fewer pressure spots, are the legs, arms, and trunk, areas where less important mechanical events occur. It is sometimes held that the underlying receptors for pressure are *free nerve endings* (called "*basket cells*", in hairy regions of the skin) and *Meissner corpuscles* (in hairless skin regions); however, the evidence in support of this is not substantial.

The adequate stimulus for touch or pressure is a mechanical deformation of the skin, that is, a change of shape or pressure differential. Uniformly distributed pressure or continuous gradations of pressure are not deforming, hence not mechanically stimulating. Consider the situation posed by Geldard (1972, p. 290) in which a finger is immersed in a heavy liquid such as

mercury, where the pressure deep in the liquid is greater than at the surface (see Figure 7.4). There is a continuous gradient of pressure from the surface on downward; hence, this gradient is not a deforming one and is an ineffective stimulus. The pressure is felt only at the boundary—the *discontinuity*—between liquid and air—and it is this discontinuity that provides the adequate stimulus. In general, discontinuities are the important stimulus events for the organism, not continuous gradations.

Thresholds for Pressure

Under certain conditions of stimulation, displacements of the skin less than 0.001 mm (0.00004 in) are sufficient to elicit a pressure sensation (Verillo, 1975, p. 178). However, the sensitivity to pressure stimulation varies not only with the strength of the mechanical stimulus applied but also with the region of the skin stimulated. Using nylon filaments, whose force could be precisely calibrated in milligrams, Weinstein (1968) tested various body parts for threshold levels of pressure or touch. The results for the right and left sides of the body, shown in Figure 7.5, indicate that the face is the most pressure-sensitive part of the

Fig. 7.4 *A finger immersed in mercury. Although the pressure deep in the liquid is much greater than that at the surface, only the discontinuity produced at the boundary between liquid and air is perceived. (Source: Gibson, J. J., 1966, p. 105.)*

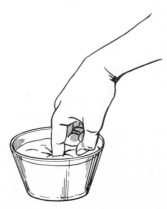

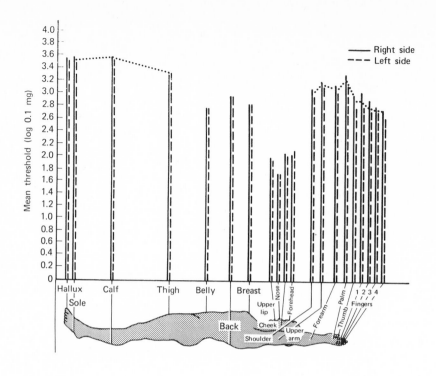

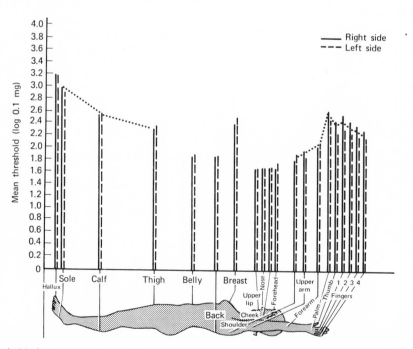

Fig. 7.5 *Thresholds for pressure. The ordinate represents the force necessary for perception at the threshold. Top figure is for males, bottom figure is for females. (Source: Weinstein, 1968, pp. 200–201. Reprinted by permission of the author and publisher.)*

body. The trunk is next, followed by the fingers and arms. The least sensitive body parts for pressure are found in the lower extremities. Males and females show about the same trend in sensitivity, but in general, women manifest lower thresholds, that is, they appear more sensitive to touch than males.

Point Localization for Pressure

It is possible to localize pressure sensations on the region of the skin where stimulation is applied; however, this ability largely varies with the region of the body stimulated. For example, stimulation applied to the finger tip or the tip of

Fig. 7.6 *The ordinate represents the distance between the body point stimulated and the subjects' perception of where stimulation occurred. (Source: Weinstein, 1968, p. 204. Reprinted by permission of the author and publisher.)*

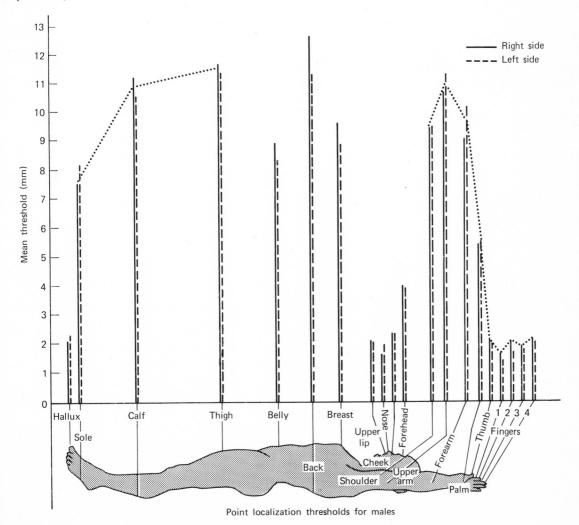

Point localization thresholds for males

the tongue is well localized (the average error is of the order of a millimeter). In contrast, stimulation of the upper arm, thigh or back produces an error of localization of more than a centimeter. Generally, the more mobile the skin regions stimulated (e.g., hands, feet, mouth), the more accurate is the point localization (see Figure 7.6).

Cortical representation plays a role in the point localization differences for various body regions. The skin is topographically projected and arranged in the sensory cortex. In other words, underlying nerve fibers from each part of the body surface of the skin are represented in a particular part of the sensory cortex. Some areas of the skin, such as those of the fingers, lips, and tongue, are more densely supplied with nerve fibers, hence they are more easily innervated, are more sensitive than others, and are correspondingly represented by larger areas of the sensory cortex. This is shown by the sensory *homunculus* (a topographic representation of the relative amount of brain devoted to various parts of the body) of Figure 7.7. Clearly, accuracy of localization at various skin sites is highly correlated with the amount of cortical representation devoted to the skin receptors of that body region.

Fig. 7.7 *A sensory homunculus. Projection of human body regions on the sensory cortex. The length of each line represents the proportion of the sensory cortex devoted to the body part indicated by the adjacent label. The caricatures of the body parts are drawn in about the same proportion as the lines. (Source: after Penfield and Rasmussen, The Cerebral Cortex of Man, New York, Macmillan, 1950.)*

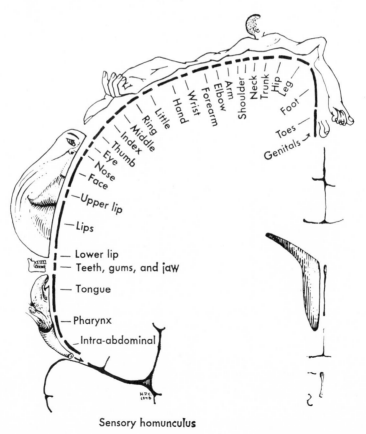

Sensory homunculus

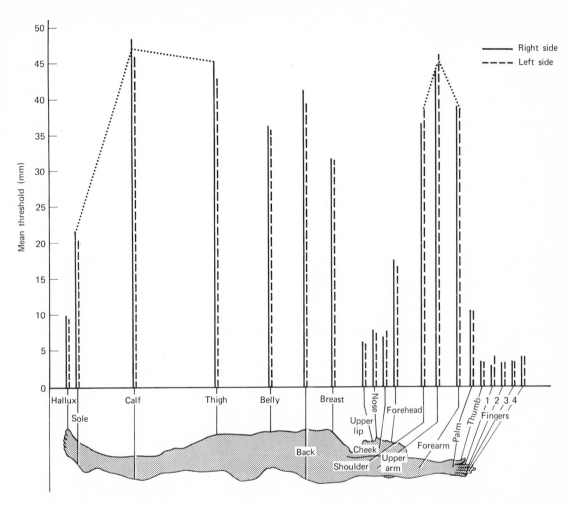

Fig. 7.8 *Two-point thresholds. The ordinate represents the minimum distance between two stimuli necessary for the perception of two distinct stimuli. (Source: Weinstein, 1968, p. 202. Reprinted by permission of the author and publisher.)*

Two-point Threshold

Another important measure of the localizing capability of the skin is called the *two-point threshold*. If a single region of the skin surface is stimulated by two stimuli that produce a unitary sensation and they are systematically moved apart, there is a separation in distance of the two stimuli that simultaneously gives rise to two distinct impressions of touch. The least distance between the two stimuli that is perceived is the two-point threshold. Some average values for two-point thresholds are shown in Figure 7.8. The numbers plotted on the ordinate represent the least distance between two simultaneously applied stimuli required for an impression of two discrete stimuli to be perceived. Like the localization of a single stimulus, the more mobile the region stimulated, the lower the two-point threshold. Similar to two-point determinations is the capacity of the skin for discriminating between objects on the basis of their size (Vierck & Jones, 1969).

Adaptation to Pressure

The result of continued pressure stimulation may be a decrease or even a complete elimination of its sensory experience: Pressure sensibility undergoes adaptation. As with thresholds, the temporal course of adaptation varies with a number of factors, particularly the size and intensity and skin area contacted. The time taken for the sensation produced by a weight resting on the skin to completely disappear is directly proportional to the intensity of this stimulus and inversely proportional to the skin area contacted (Geldard, 1972, p. 299). The sensation, however, can be quickly restored by a brief movement of the stimulus or some other form of abrupt change in the stimulation to a given skin area. A continuous change in stimulation, of course, is what normally occurs when the perceiver actively touches surfaces and objects.

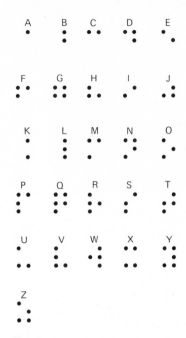

Fig. 7.9 *The Braille Alphabet. Various combinations of from one to six dots are used to represent letters and short words. (Source: Mueller & Rudolph, 1966, p. 14. Reprinted by permission of Time-Life Books, Inc.)*

COMPLEX TOUCH PHENOMENA

Reading with the Skin

We have noted that the fingers are quite sensitive to point localization and two-point discriminations. It is not surprising, then, that some sort of complex information extraction of a communicative form can occur from active touch stimulation. One example is the well-known Braille system devised by Louis Braille in the nineteenth century. The Braille alphabet is actually a reading system composed of raised dots on a surface that can be "read" by the skin, usually the tips of the fingers. As shown in Figure 7.9, various combinations of dots are used to represent letters and

words. By moving the finger over the raised surface of Braille, an experienced blind reader can read at the rate of 50 words per minute (Mueller & Rudolph, 1966). More recent is an electronic reading aid called the Opticon, which converts the visual image of a printed character directly into a tactual one for the fingertip. Users are able to read these tactual images at a rate of 60 words per minute (Bliss, 1971).

Communication of letters and words by touch is not limited to the skin of the fingers. If a letter is slowly traced on the back of the hand, it is not difficult to recognize the letter. It is known that it is possible to make discriminations between stimuli that vary in pressure intensity, temporal length of the stimulation (duration), rate at which successive impacts are delivered to the skin (frequency), and loci of skin sites stimulated (Geldard, 1960). By placing small contact vibrators that could be varied in these dimensions on the chests of subjects, Geldard (1966; 1968*b*) devised a language for use on the skin called *Vibratese*. It was constructed as follows: three levels of intensity (weak, medium, and strong) at three durations (0.1, 0.3, and 0.5 seconds) were delivered to five different locations on the chest, resulting in 45 separate signals. Each letter of the alphabet was assigned a signal that was its own combination of duration, intensity, and location. The most frequently occurring language elements were assigned shorter durations enabling users of the system to proceed at a rapid pace. Geldard reported that the Vibratese alphabet could be mastered in only a few hours, and eventually whole words and meaningful sentences were perceived. One subject successfully received signals at a rate of about twice that of proficient Morse code reception. (Military standards for the proficient Morse code receiver are 18 words per minute.) Reception of Vibratese was limited by the speed of the sending equipment.

Subsequent research focused on increasing the potential input of printed characters by using vibrators scattered over the body, two on each arm and leg and one on the abdomen. The main features of the system, which is called the *Optohapt* system, is shown in Figure 7.10. Basically, the Optohapt converts printed material into touch stimulation. The material to be read, which is also printed by the special typewriter shown in the figure, is scanned by an electronic circuit composed of photocells and relays; these, in turn, control a series of vibrators located on the body whose activation provides the meaningful touch stimulation. As shown in Figure 7.11, distinctive time-space patterns of vibratory bursts were assigned an alphabetic coding. The stimuli chosen for the alphabet were punctuation marks, numerals, literary and business symbols, and

Fig. 7.10 *The optohapt system involves an optical scanning device that converts the printed text to electrical impulses and eventually to vibratory bursts at the vibrator sites, as shown in the upper right figure. (Source: Geldard, 1966, p. 379. Reprinted with permission of the author and publisher.)*

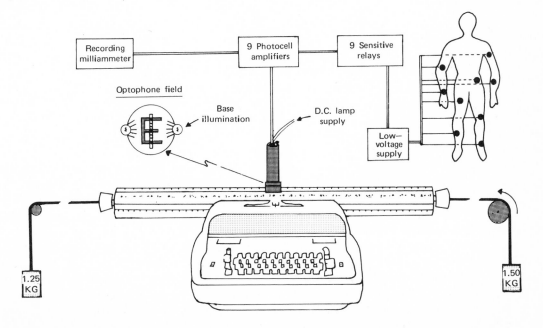

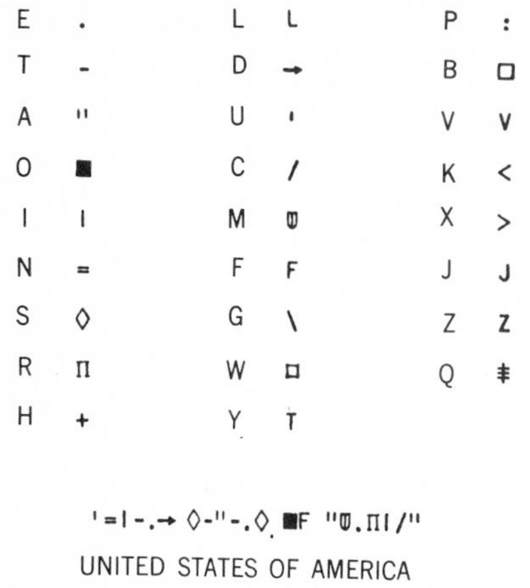

E	.	L	L	P	:
T	-	D	→	B	□
A	''	U	'	V	v
O	■	C	/	K	<
I	I	M	ᴍ	X	>
N	=	F	F	J	J
S	◊	G	\	Z	z
R	Π	W	□	Q	‡
H	+	Y	T		

' = I -. → ◊ - '' -. ◊ ■F ''ᴍ.ΠI /''

UNITED STATES OF AMERICA

Fig. 7.11 *Optohapt alphabet. The symbols, listed to the right of the alphabet, can be rapidly sent to and "read" by the skin. (Source: Geldard, 1968b, p. 318. Reprinted by permission of the author and publisher.)*

certain letters of the alphabet—characters chosen for their ease of discriminability. According to Geldard, an optimal presentation speed is at a rate of 70 characters per minute. The essential mode of operation of the Optohapt is to represent the symbol directly on the skin surface; the letter "V," for example, produces a rapid sweep from the topmost vibrator to the bottom one, and then reverses the sequence. It is as if the Optohapt "writes" on the skin surface with the vibrators in, as Geldard (1968a) puts it, "body English."

Pressure Phosphenes

Other means of producing an alphabetic coding from touch stimulation have been attempted. One possibility has its basis in *pressure phosphenes,* the subjective lights and images resulting from pressure stimulation of the eye. Typically, phosphenes are produced by applying pressure on the closed eyelid (Oster, 1970). Although they may appear to be completely random, in fact many of their characteristics such as their duration and location in the visual field can be controlled. Furthermore, the production of phosphenes does not require that pressure be ap-

plied directly to the external anatomy of the eye. It is possible to stimulate the visual area of the brain directly to produce phosphenes (Brindley & Lewin, 1968; Dobelle, Mladejovsky, & Girvin, 1974). Thus, the experience of phosphenes is available to persons who do not possess an intact visual system. One potential function of cortically produced phosphenes is for developing a visual prosthetic device. It may be possible by directly stimulating the brain to produce meaningful images. They would not necessarily be topographically similar to alphabet characters but as in the case of the symbols for the Optohapt, subjects could learn to associate a particular pattern of phosphenes with certain letters.

Seeing with the Skin

Another possibility for a means of cutaneous communication is to use the skin surface as a direct channel for pictorial material. A group of researchers (White, Saunders, Scadden, Bach-y-Rita, & Collins, 1970; Collins, 1971a) have developed a *vision substitution system* with the purpose of converting a visual image into an isomorphic cutaneous display. The apparatus for this is shown in Figure 7.12. It consists of a tripod mounted television camera—the "eye" of the system—that is connected to a 20×20 matrix of 400 vibrators mounted on the back of a stationary dental chair (see Figure 7.13). The vibrators cover an area about 25 cm square. The video image is electronically transformed so that a vibrator is active when its locus is within an illuminated region of the camera field. The subject seated in the chair with his back against the vibrators is appropriately stimulated when the camera picks up an image. Thus, when a subject moves the television camera across a scene, patterns of light intensity in the visual field are reproduced in successions of tactual impressions on the skin surface of the back.

The results from presentation of this relatively coarse tactual image are remarkable. Subjects, both blind and blindfolded normally-sighted, were able to perceive some simple

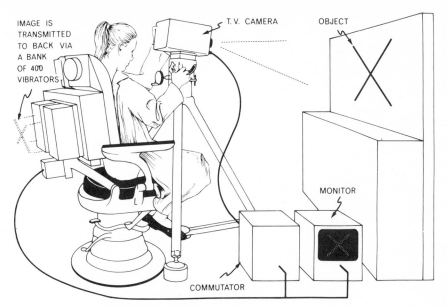

Fig. 7.12 *Schematic drawing of the vision substitution system. (Source: White, Saunders, Scadden, Bach-y-Rita, & Collins, 1970, p. 23. Reprinted by permission of the publisher).*

displays very soon after they had been introduced to the system. For example, they could describe the motion of a vertical stripe as it was moved from side to side or in a propeller motion, imitating the movement by appropriate hand gestures. They could discriminate between a stationary vertical and horizontal stripe and could indicate the orientation of a curved or diagonal line. Simple geometric shapes—a circle, a triangle, and a square—were accurately identified when subjects were allowed to scan the figures by moving the television camera and were given immediate correction after a wrong response. With sufficient experience, a collection of 25 complex items (e.g., coffee cup, telephone, stuffed animal) were identifiable. Furthermore, experienced subjects were also able to identify the objects and describe their arrangements on a table when the objects were viewed by the camera from slightly above (an angle of 20° off the horizontal). The fact that some objects at the rear were partially occluded by those in front suggests that some of the depth and distance information of the visual scene is provided in the corresponding cutaneous image.

One such cue for the location of an object in depth was its vertical position on the cutaneous display—the farther back its location on the table top, the higher up on the display. A second cue for tactually perceiving depth is based on the inverse relationship between the projected size and distance of an object. The change in the image size normally projected or the eye as the object distance is varied also occurred on the skin surface in this arrangement. One of the subjects was a blind psychologist who has taught this relationship (i.e., an inverse relation between the projected size of an object and its physical distance from an observer) to his classes for several years, but obviously he had never directly perceived it. His experience of the increase in the size of a tactual image, as an object was brought closer and closer to the camera and a decrease in image size as object distance from the camera was increased, produced in him a sort of insightful perceptual realization about the relation between projected size and physical distance—"a genuine 'aha' experience."

Some variables are critical. It appears to be

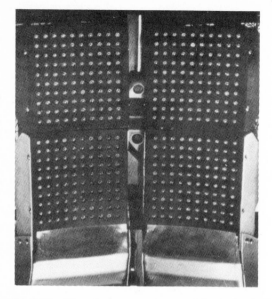

Fig. 7.13 *The vibrator array mounted in the back of the chair. (Source: White et al., 1970, p. 26. Reprinted by permission of the publisher.)*

particularly important that the television camera not be kept in a fixed position and that the subject actively control the movement of the camera. It appears that enabling subjects to perform self-generated explorations of figures by sweeping the camera over the display results in the kind of successive changes in the activity of the vibrators that are necessary for meaningful tactual images to be perceived.

According to the authors, subsequent development of the visual substitution system will be toward portability and increasing the amount of information received. As the authors comment, ". . . the limitations of this system are as yet more attributable to the poverty of the display than to taxing the information-handling capacities of the epidermis" (White et al., 1970, p. 27).

This chapter has focused on kinesthesis and on an introduction to cutaneous sensitivity. Kinesthesis refers to position and movement in-

formation registered from mechanical stimulation of the mobile parts of the jointed skeleton. It was noted that the receptors at the joints, Pacinian corpuscles, provide information about the position, posture, and direction of the jointed limbs in space.

Next the skin or cutaneous sense of touch or pressure was described. It was noted that the sensation of touch is registered by mechanical stimulation of the surface of the skin. However, there are regions of the skin not equally sensitive to touch stimulation. Some regions are more sensitive to either thermal or pain stimulation; in short, there is a distribution of distinct areas sensitive to different kinds of cutaneous stimuli. However, there is no substantial evidence that each area is served by an identifiable and/or a distinct receptor.

The adequate stimulus for touch or pressure is a deformation of the skin or a pressure differential between one part of the skin and another. Uniform or continuous gradations of pressure are not effective forms of stimulation.

In terms of absolute threshold values for pressure, the face, followed by the trunk, fingers, and arms are the most pressure-sensitive parts of the body. With regard to localizing the point on the skin where the pressure stimulus is applied, it is generally the case that the more mobile the skin region stimulated (i.e., the hands, mouth) the better the point localization. This also applies to a two-point threshold, which refers to the minimal distance between two stimuli applied to the skin giving rise to two distinct impressions of touch.

Finally a number of instances of complex touch phenomena were described: Braille system, Vibratese, pressure phosphenes, and the vision substitution system. It was noted that from the application of complex patterns of pressure on the skin it is possible to convert a visual image into a meaningful cutaneous experience that is isomorphic with the visual image.

In the next chapter we continue our discussion of the cutaneous modalities, introducing the temperature and pain senses.

8

Somesthesis II: Temperature and Pain

The primary emphasis in this chapter will be on temperature and pain reception. Although they refer to independent cutaneous modalities, they both differ from pressure in that their effective stimulation involves more than mechanical events.

TEMPERATURE

The sensation resulting from the temperature of a surface that is in contact with the skin is registered by a form of cutaneous stimulation although its mechanism is far from clear. Thermal sensitivity is irregularly distributed in spots over the skin surface. Exploration with warm or cold stimuli reveals that some spots are especially sensitive to warmth, other more numerous spots are more sensitive to cold stimulation (Figure 8.1). As shown in Figure 8.1, the sensitivity of a given thermal spot may vary markedly over time. Like touch, the number of thermally sensitive spots depends on the intensity of the stimulus applied. Part of the experience of thermal variability may be due to temperature shifts within the skin itself; that is, to normal heat interchanges occurring at the site of nerve stimulation. The skin tissue is continually undergoing thermal varia-

tions owing to heat radiation, conduction, and convection, as from moisture evaporation and dilation or constriction of the blood vessels of the subcutaneous tissue. In general, however, the body surface remains in a relatively stable thermal equilibrium with its immediate surroundings. Over the clothed areas of the body and the face, the skin temperature is close to 35° C, on the hands and arms at about 33° C, and of course, under the tongue at 37° C (98.6° F). Where blood flow is sluggish, as in the case of the ear lobe, the temperature may be significantly lower (20° C). However, the temperature of the skin per se as we shall see is not a good predictor of thermal experience.

Thermal Adaptation

Thermal sensations from the skin undergo adaptation. Initial exposure to a moderately cold or warm environment, as in the case of a swimming pool or bath, may initially result in very cold or hot experience, but eventually the thermal sensations will diminish and the water will feel slightly cool or warm. Prolonged warm or cold stimulation is likely to reduce the thermal sensitivity (raise the threshold values) for warmth and coldness, respectively. Although this is

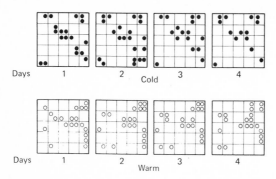

Days   1   2   3   4
Cold

Days   1   2   3   4
Warm

Fig. 8.1 *Successive mappings of cold and warm spots. The same region (1 sq cm) of the upper arm was mapped with a 1 mm-diameter cylinder for thermal spots on four different days. Observe that the distribution of spots shifted somewhat from mapping to mapping, but considerable stability of spots is also apparent. (Source: Dallenbach, 1927, 39, 418.)*

readily demonstrated for both warm and cold stimulation, perceived cold follows skin temperature to a greater extent than does warmth (Marks & Stevens, 1972). Moreover, both warm and cold sensitivities are simultaneously affected by warm or cold stimulation. Adaptation to a hot stimulus also produces a lowering of the threshold for cold. Similarly, prolonged cold stimulation reduces the threshold for warmth, so that lower than normal temperatures are sufficient to produce a sensation of warmth.

PHYSIOLOGICAL ZERO A unique aspect of complete adaptation to thermal stimulation is that the thermal quality of the adapting stimulus is not experienced. The narrow range of temperatures to which a response of neither warm nor cold occurs—a neutral zone of complete thermal adaptation or thermal indifference—is called *physiological zero*. The size of the neutral zone varies with a number of factors but it can be as small as 0.01° C or as large as 8° C. A change in temperature from physiological zero is required to produce a thermal experience whose quality varies with the direction of the temperature change. Normally, physiological zero corresponds

to the skin temperature of 33° C. The skin temperature for effecting physiological zero, however, can undergo variation. The demonstration attributed to John Locke in 1690 is appropriate here. If prior immersion of one hand is in a 40° C basin of water, the other in a 20° C basin and then both hands are shifted to a 33° C basin of water, the water in the 33° C basin will now feel distinctly cold to the hand that was in the warm water and warm to the hand originally in the cold water. Physiological zero has shifted as a consequence of adaptation. This relationship of the adapted skin temperature to the temperature of a new thermal environment, as schematized in Figure 8.2, also demonstrates that the skin does not furnish accurate temperature information. As indicated, the same physical temperature can feel cold to one hand and warm to the other. Thus, thermal experience occurs as a result of the *relation* of the temperature of the skin surface to its surroundings rather than from physical temperature itself.

In general, the more extreme the temperature, the longer the time required for adaptation. However, complete thermal adaptation occurs only within a restricted range of temperatures. Extremes of temperature do not completely adapt. Immersion of the hands, for example, in very cold

Fig. 8.2a *Each hand is placed in a separate basin of water and is thermally adapted to a different temperature.*

Left hand   Right hand

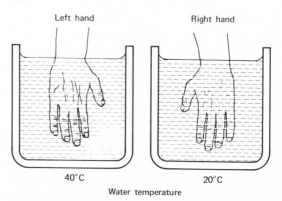

40°C   20°C

Water temperature

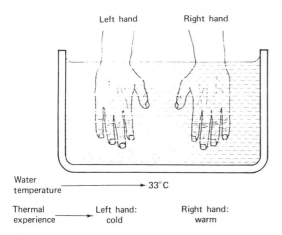

Left hand   Right hand

Water
temperature ——————————→ 33° C

Thermal
experience ————→ Left hand: Right hand:
                    cold   warm

Fig. 8.2b *Effects of thermal adaptation. When both hands are then placed in the 33° C water, the hand previously adapted to warm water feels cold, and the hand previously adapted to cold water feels warm. These effects of adaptation point out that the skin is not a good indicator of physical temperature.*

or very warm water will produce persistent cold and warm sensations. The temperature range for thermal indifference, within which total elimination of thermal sensation occurs, is generally put at 16° C to 42° C. However, these limits have been shown to vary with the method of measurement and perhaps with the bodily region stimulated. In one study using the skin of the forearm, a very narrow range of thermal indifference was observed—between 29° C and 37° C (Kenshalo & Scott, 1966). It was found that temperatures between these rather moderate extremes reached physiological zero relatively rapidly. Temperatures below or above these values did not undergo complete adaptation but continued to elicit the experience of coldness or warmth.

Temperature Discrimination

Differential sensitivity determinations for temperature (minimal discriminable changes in temperature, ΔT) are quite difficult to obtain, due in large part to problems of experimental procedures. In general, minimal discriminable

differences in temperature—the difference threshold—vary with the conditions under which they are measured. Some of these are the region of the skin surface stimulated, the previous thermal state to which the skin is adapted (physiological zero), the rate of thermal change, and the size of the region stimulated. These are further affected by the fact that adaptation to coldness or warmth influences the ΔT for warmth or coldness, respectively. However, some general statements on difference threshold can be offered. When the rate of thermal change (addition or withdrawal of heat) is small, larger deviations from skin temperature are required to produce a discriminable difference than if the temperature change occurs rapidly. Furthermore, the sensitivity to thermal change increases with increases in the size of the exposed skin surface. Thus, the palm of the hand in contact with the surface of an object provides a better impression of the temperature of an object than does the fingertips. The notion that general thermal experience is more accurate when larger regions of the skin are stimulated (temperature held constant) has been termed *spatial summation,* and it implies that the activation of individual temperature receptors sum together to augment the intensity of the thermal experience (see Kenshalo and Gallegos, 1967; Kenshalo, 1970).

Paradoxical Thermal Sensations

It has been reported that spots sensitive to cold will, under certain conditions, result in a cold impression although stimulated with a hot stimulus (45° C). This phenomenon, termed *paradoxical cold,* is of course, paradoxical in that a stimulus of fairly high temperature produces a cold sensation. Related to this is the psychological experience of "heat." If a stimulus in the neighborhood of 45° C or greater is applied to a small region of the skin surface that is sensitive to both warm and cold stimulation, the experience of "heat" occurs. Warm spots are appropriately activated by the warm stimulus and cold spots are simultaneously and paradoxically activated. The assumption is that the warm and cold sensations fuse and produce an overall sensation of intense heat.

It is possible to simulate heat experience by simultaneously applying warm and cold stimulation to neighboring warm and cold spots on the skin. One approach is to use the "heat grill" sketched in Figure 8.3. Each set of tubes represents markedly different thermal ranges (the cold coil at, say, 20° C and the warm coil at 40° C). The thermal impression from touching the heat grill with a region of the arm containing both warm and cold spots is of intense heat, enough so that the limb is quickly withdrawn

Fig. 8.3 *The "heat" grill. Cold water circulates through one coil, warm water circulates through the other coil. If a skin area is placed firmly against the grill, the experience of "heat" results, although neither of the coils is "hot." (Based on Psychology: Man in Perspective, by A. Buss, Wiley, New York, 1973, p. 176. Reprinted by permission of the publisher.)*

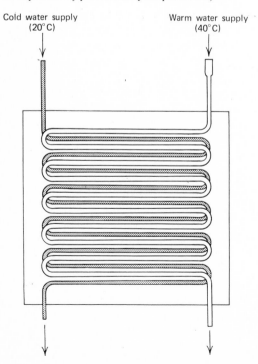

Cold water supply (20°C)   Warm water supply (40°C)

from the grill as if to avoid a burn though the grill is not physically hot.

Keep in mind that we are describing thermal sensations and impressions and as such, it is debatable whether heat is a separate and uniquely different perception occurring from the fusion of warmth and cold, or whether it is experienced as intense warmth with the addition of a slight quickly adapting stinging sensation. Although the phenomenon of paradoxical cold and the cutaneous experience of heat has theoretical implications for understanding thermal perception, a fully acceptable explanation for their occurrence is not available.

THEORIES OF THERMAL PERCEPTION

There are two main contending theories for explaining thermal sensitivity. The *specific receptor* theory assumes that specific and distinct receptors exist for warmth and cold. That is, there exists a positive correlation between physiological specificity and psychological specificity. Although this theory has had many important supporters, it is generally attributed to Max von Frey (1852–1932). He argued that two separate types of receptors, *Krause end bulbs* and *Ruffini cylinders,* mediate the sensations of cold and warmth, respectively. Support for this contention comes from a number of sources that show that certain structural and functional differences exist between the effecting of warm and cold experiences. Application of warm or cold stimuli results in different latencies of thermal response. That is, a cold sensation occurs sooner after stimulation than is the case for a warm sensation. Further evidence was shown in Figure 8.1, which describes certain spots of the skin sensitive to only one or the other thermal extreme. The number of warm and cold spots appears to vary independently of each other, producing variable temperature sensitivities throughout the body. In research using cats, types of receptor fibers that are differentially responsive to temperature increases and decreases have been identified (Henzel & Zotterman, 1951). Further evidence for receptor specificity comes from the fact that different thermal sensations can be actuated by different chemicals. Cold sensations are produced by menthol, whereas carbon dioxide, under certain conditions, will produce warmth.

Although it is possible that specific receptors such as Krause end bulbs and Ruffini cylinders are especially sensitive to temperature stimulation it is unlikely that they are the only receptors. Thermal experiences occur from regions of the skin where these receptors occur very sparsely or do not occur at all. For example, cold sensations occur from appropriate stimulation of hairy regions of the body, but there is very little evidence that there are any Krause end bulbs. It has often been cited (and often contested) that the range of cutaneous sensations—pressure, warmth, coldness, and pain—occurs from appropriate stimulation of the cornea of the eye, a structure containing only free nerve endings (see Lele & Weddell, 1956). Finally, the histological evidence supporting morphological distinction in cutaneous sensory receptors has been questioned in a number of expert quarters (e.g., Dallenbach, 1927; Milner, P., 1970; Kenshalo, 1971). We will return to the general issue of receptor specificity in a later section.

A second formulation, the *vascular theory* of thermal sensation proposed by Nafe and Kenshalo (Nafe, 1934; Kenshalo & Nafe, 1962) does not hold that specific nerve fibers in the skin are directly sensitive to warming or cooling or that there are separate systems for the two thermal impressions. Rather, a single mechanism for thermal sensibility is proposed: Both warm and cold sensations are mediated by activity of the neurovascular system. It is argued that specific thermal sensations are a matter of the characteristics of the nonneural vascular tissue in which sensory nerve endings are imbedded. More specifically, thermal sensations occur from constriction

and dilation of the smooth muscle walls of the blood vessels of the skin. The smooth muscles of the vascular system contract when cooled and relax when warmed. The direct responses of smooth muscle tissue producing size changes of the vessels initiate activity in the sensory nerve endings that are connected to the muscle walls, resulting in a thermal experience.

There are shortcomings in the vascular theory. For example, there is some evidence that temperature sensitivity is not significantly affected by the experimental prevention of vasodilation on a region of the forearm (Dawson, 1964). Furthermore, the vascular theory cannot account for the relative distribution of warm and cold spots. Warm spots frequently exist in separate skin areas from cold spots. If indeed there is only one mechanism underlying both warm and cold thermal experiences, then they should not manifest such divergent distributions on the skin. In general, the vast range of qualitative and quantitative differences between the sensations of warmth and coldness questions the basic assumption of a single mechanism subserving both. The acceptance of the activity of the blood vessels serving a primary role for thermal experience remains tentative (see Geldard, 1972, pp. 370–374, for a review). In general, neither the specific receptor theory nor the vascular theory is adequate to account for all the findings—and the issue of explaining thermal experience is unresolved.

PAIN

It is obvious that toward the extremes of temperature—freezing and boiling—thermal experience merges with pain. This is an adaptive association because intense thermal stimulation can produce tissue damage. As painful stimuli are unequivocally reacted to, this fusion serves to protect the organism against harmful and perhaps even lethal thermal extremes. This points out that a significant benefit from the reception of pain is warning of potential biological harm.

Although tissue damage is neither a necessary nor a sufficient condition for the experience of pain, as a trend, most forms of pain-producing stimuli are potentially damaging: intense thermal, acoustic, photic and electrical stimulation, under certain conditions, can result in serious bodily harm. There are exceptions, of course, but in the general case, from an evolutionary point of view, the perception of pain offers an important biological advantage for the survival of the organism. Failure to perceive pain is extremely maladaptive. Reports of self-inflicted injury due to pathological pain insensitivity (i.e., lacking a pain sense) have included serious injuries of the skin, flesh and bones, burns from hot surfaces and liquids, and even chewing off the tip of the tongue (e.g., Cohen, Kipnes, Kunkle, & Kubzansky, 1955).

Though we know that pain may be evoked by many sorts of stimuli, the exact characteristics of the stimuli that excite the receptor cells are not determined. An early hypothesis for pain perception was that sensory receptors for pain are not specialized to react to a simple form of energy. Since pain is an accompaniment of most intense forms of stimulation, it is produced by *overstimulation* of any cutaneous receptor. However, overstimulation in itself is insufficient to account for the production of pain because pain can occur without intense stimulation and pain may not necessarily occur with it.

Another alternative is to assume that pain is a unique perceptual experience resulting from the excitation of a specialized receptor—a *nociceptor* (a receptor whose effective stimulation produces injury to the body and whose sensations are unpleasant)—that can be triggered by a wide range of stimuli. This is supported by the fact that, using mapping techniques, there are regions or spots of the skin the stimulation of which yields only the sensation of pain. Of interest is that pain spots are more numerous than pressure and

thermal spots, and their distribution appears to be quite diffuse. Further evidence for pain as a separate sense modality comes from measurements taken when the skin is made insensitive by the use of morphine and codeine. Such drugs render the skin insensitive to pain but have little effect on the other cutaneous systems (Candland, 1968). Also the thresholds for pain and touch have been shown to differ on a number of quantitative dimensions (Gibson, 1968).

The identification of a specialized receptor for pain has been a problem for the researcher. Based on the fact that free nerve endings are ubiquitously distributed throughout the skin as well as in much of the internal anatomy, muscles, tendons, joints, and connective tissue of the viscera, they are often the proposed candidate for the nociceptor.

The Qualities of Pain

It is possible to distinguish pain from most other sensory experiences and even to distinguish between classes of pain. Skin pain produced by brief physical encounters with the skin may be characterized as "sharp" or "bright." They are well localized, immediately responded to, and they are experienced as being quite different from so-called "dull" pain originating from deep within the body (the chest and abdomen), which may produce other bodily reactions (e.g., sweating, palpitations) and in general are poorly localized (Békésy, 1971).

At times pain originating from internal organs may appear to occur from another region of the body, usually the surface of the skin. Such phenomena are called *referred pain*. For example, the intense pain arising from the heart associated with *angina pectoris* appears to come from the chest wall and a skin region lying on the inner surface of the upper arm (Kenshalo, 1971, p. 161; see also Rosenthal, 1968).

Under certain circumstances, the phenomenon of *double pain* may result. That is, two kinds of pain, "sharp" and "dull" occuring from the same stimulation, may be distinguished. The sharp pain is rapidly aroused and is gradually followed by a more persistent dull pain. Another experiential dichotomy is between "pricking" pain, a pain produced by a very brief skin surface contact, and "burning" pain, where the pain-producing stimulus is of greater duration. The list of pains can be further extended to include irritations. For example, *itch,* produced clinically by mechanical and chemical means, is considered a low-grade pain (Geldard, 1972).

We noted that pain spots are widely distributed throughout the body. An idea of the distribution, obtained by systematically exploring various bodily regions with a pointed instrument with a constant force, is shown in Table 8.1. Near the top of the list should be added two structures highly sensitive to pain, the cornea of the eye and the tympanic membrane. As Geldard (1972) points out, "The most exquisite pain in the body can originate from these sources" (p. 326).

Pain Thresholds

Because of marked individual differences in pain experience, general statements as to the amount of stimulus application necessary to produce a pain response as well as to assess differential sensitivity are difficult to make. This difficulty is compounded by the fact that pain can be elicited by very different stimuli and thus they may not uniformly produce the same pain quality. Also the same stimulus at different intensities can produce different painful experiences. Furthermore, if tissue damage occurs, subsidiary effects such as inflammation and swelling provide a further complexity in evaluating the pain experience.

It is generally agreed that when the skin is mechanically stimulated the appropriate stimulus for pain is the lengthwise stretching of the skin. This is supported by the observations that injury to the skin, such as cutting, will be painful if, in

Table 8.1

DISTRIBUTION OF PAIN SENSITIVITY OBTAINED BY
SYSTEMATICALLY EXPLORING VARIOUS REGIONS OF THE BODY
WITH A SPINE-TIPPED HAIR[a]

Skin Region	Pain "Points"/cm^2
Back of knee (popliteal fossa)	232
Neck region (jugular fossa)	228
Bend of elbow (cubital fossa)	224
Shoulder blade (interscapular region)	212
Volar side of forearm	203
Back of hand	188
Forehead	184
Buttocks	180
Eyelid	172
Scalp	144
Radial surface, middle finger	95
Ball of thumb	60
Sole of foot	48
Tip of nose	44

[a] From *The Human Senses,* by F. A. Geldard, Wiley, New York, 1972, p. 325. Reprinted by permission of the publisher.

the process, the skin is stretched. If cutting is done on skin that is rendered immobile, no pain is experienced.

The threshold for pain has been shown to be influenced by stimulation of the auditory system—a phenomenon called *audio analgesia*. It was reported that for a significant number of dental patients pain from drilling and tooth extraction was completely eliminated when sound was appropriately presented to the patient by headphones (Gardner, Licklider, & Weisz, 1960). The experimental situation was that the patient heard stereophonic music and a masking ("hissing") noise whose intensity level he had to adjust in order to mask the pain. The basic instructions were to increase the noise level when pain was first felt, until relief occurred. Sound stimulation delivered in this manner has served as the single effective analgesic for several thousand dental operations.

Subsequent research on audio analgesia has been unfavorable to the view that intense masking noise *alone* directly suppresses pain or elevates the pain threshold (Camp, Martin, & Chapman, 1962; Carlin, Ward, Gershon, & Ingraham, 1962). Whether audio analgesia is effective due to distraction of the pain, to the suggestion that pain will be lessened, to anxiety reduction by having subjects exercise some control over the testing situation, or to a pain inhibitory physiological mechanism is unresolved.

Pain thresholds may be affected not only by the amount of painful stimulation but by how that stimulation is distributed. Messing and Campbell (1971) demonstrated with rats that when electric shock (presumably painful stimulation) was divided over two anatomically distinct and widely separated loci (neck *and* tail) the avoidance response was less than when the same amount of electric shock was applied to a single anatomical region (neck *or* tail), that is, ". . . with stimuli applied to a single locus, the resulting pain is greater than when equal shock intensities are applied to separate anatomical loci" (p. 227).

There are subjective factors that also affect pain perception: suggestibility, attitude, expectation, distraction and attention, anxiety and motivational variables have profound effects on pain perception. Thus, an injury sustained in battle or competitive sports may not elicit the same degree of pain as a similar wound experienced in a more tranquil setting.

Pain Adaptation

Most people who have suffered prolonged conditions of pain—toothache, headache, burn—concur that the pain seems to extend indefinitely—that is, it does not adapt. Moreover, from an evolutionary point of view, it could be argued that the sensation of pain should not undergo adaptation for then it would not have survival value. However, a profound biological benefit of pain is seen in the initial effect of pain. So long as the initial stimulation is perceived and reacted to there is really no need for continued stimulation. Hence adaptability is not maladaptive. Indeed, because of the very nature of pain experience, it usually effects an immediate response. Furthermore, in those cases where pain does not appear to adapt it is not clear if the stimulus and receptor conditions at the region of injury are held constant. Most painful conditions occur with continuously varying conditions at the site of injury, ". . . chiefly rhythmic ones based on circulatory events" (Geldard, 1972, p. 327). Thus, pain may not *appear* to undergo adaptation because different regions are continually being stimulated.

The evidence strongly favors the notion that pain does adapt. Within limits, depending on the stimulus conditions, the skin adapts to the pain of thermal extremes. Complete pain adaptation, for example, occurs within 5 min when the hand is immersed in 0° C water. The rate of adaptation varies with the amount of skin involved, because with a smaller area adaptation occurs sooner. Similarly, the pain occurring from temperatures up to about 47° C may be adapted to also, although the pain from temperatures above this, which are in the range of tissue damage, are nonadapting (Kenshalo, 1971; Hardy, Stolwijk, & Hoffman, 1968). In general, the smaller the region to which the painful heat stimulation is applied, the more likely is adaptation to occur.

Pain induced by mechanical stimulation is adapted to not because of neural fatigue due to continual stimulation but because of a lack of effective stimulation. The pain produced by insertion of a needle soon adapts, but recurs when the needle is withdrawn. It is the tissue movement that is the painful stimulation, and a lack of stimulation creates the condition for adaptation.

Adaptation to pain provides further evidence in support of the view that pain is a distinct and separate sense rather than a secondary sensation resulting from overstimulation of one of the cutaneous receptor mechanisms. For example, in the course of pain adaptation to, say, intensely applied cold stimulation, the feeling of pain gradually subsides leaving only a cool feeling. In general, residual effects, specific to the stimuli applied, replace the pain. These are the results that would be expected if pain is a distinct cutaneous modality; that is, it adapts independently of the other skin senses.

THEORIES OF PAIN

In the discussions above, we have noted two classes of pain theories. *Specificity* theory proposes that pain is a distinct and separate sensory modality with its own set of specific peripheral pain receptors in the body—free nerve endings—that project to a central pain center (usually the thalamus). *Pattern* theory, in contrast, ignores physiological specialization and assumes that general stimulus intensity or the summation of neural impulses by a central mechanism are the critical determinants of pain. In one version it is argued that the pattern of

stimulation for pain is produced by intense stimulation of nonspecific peripheral receptors (e.g., Nafe, 1934). A third theory has been proposed that is consonant with the notion of a class of specific peripheral pain receptors and a form of patterning and central summation of nerve impulses.

Consistent with the contention of specific peripheral pain receptors, Melzack and Wall (1965; see also Melzack, 1973) have described a *gate control theory* of pain reception that focuses on afferent nerve impulse transmission from the skin to the spinal cord. It is a theory that assumes a competitive interaction between two different kinds of nerve fibers reaching the first central transmission (T) cells of the spinal cord. The theory further assumes that there exists a neurological gate control system at the top of the spinal cord that modulates or "gates" the amount of nerve impulse transmission from peripheral fibers of the skin to the T cells and that pain results when the output of the T cells reaches or exceeds a critical level. Several structures play a role in determining what transmission there will be from the central T cells. The actual gate control system is primarily affected by the inhibitory effect on T cell stimulation of the *substantia gelatinosa*, a structure composed of small densely packed cells that form a functional unit extending the length of the spinal cord. The factors involved in the transmission of impulses from peripheral nerves to T cells in the spinal cord are schematically diagramed in Figure 8.4. Crucial to the theory is the kind of fibers making connection to the *substantia gelatinosa*. Pain is carried by at least two different types of nerve fibers: Large diameter, myelinated (sheathed), rapidly conducting fibers (L fibers in the figure) convey "sharp" pain as well as other sensory events; and small diameter, unmyelinated, slow conducting fibers (S fibers in the figure) convey "burning" pain. Both types of fibers have branches going to the *substantia gelatinosa*. As shown in the figure, the L fibers excite the *substantia gelatinosa*, which in turn blocks the effect of L fibers on the T cells.

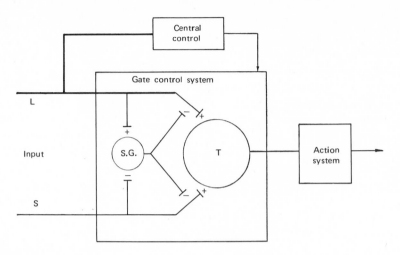

Fig. 8.4 *Schematic diagram of the gate-control theory of pain mechanisms: L, the large-diameter fibers: S, the small-diameter fibers. The fibers project to the substantia gelatinosa (SG) and first central transmission (T) cells. The inhibitory effect exerted by SG on the afferent fiber terminals is increased by activity in L fibers and decreased by activity in S fibers. The central control trigger is represented by a line running from the large-fiber system to the central control mechanisms; these mechanisms, in turn, project back to the gate control system. +, Excitation: −, inhibition. (Source: Melzack & Walls, 1965, Science, 150, 975, November 1965. Copyright © 1965 by the American Association for the Advancement of Science. Reprinted by permission of the publisher and the first author.)*

That is, although nerve impulses in large fibers are extremely effective in initially activating T cells, their later effect is reduced in that L fibers act to inhibit themselves by a feedback mechanism. Large fibers also act to block the small diameter fiber inputs by way of the *substantia gelatinosa*—in short, by stimulating the *substantia gelatinosa* they close the theorized gate. In contrast, S fibers inhibit the *substantia gelatinosa* so that they can excite the T cells of the sensory pathways. That is, they hold the gate in a relatively open position. At levels of high stimulation that accompany injury, bursts of S fiber input will reduce the inhibitory effect of the *substantia gelatinosa* and stimulate the T cells at a high rate, which results in pain. Thus, if a gentle stimulation is applied to the skin, the afferent volley will contain large fiber impulses that will partially close the gate. As the stimulus intensity is increased, more receptor units are

recruited and the resultant positive and negative effects in the large and small fibers will tend to counteract each other—the inhibitory effect of the *substantia gelatinosa* is negated—with the net result of increased stimulation of the T cells. Furthermore, when stimulation is prolonged the large fibers adapt, producing a relative increase in small fiber activity—the gate is opened further. Thus, the total number of active fibers and the relative balance of activity in large and small fibers at the point of the spinal gate determines the excitatory effects at the T cells. When the arriving impulses reach a critical level, there is a firing of the T cells that in turn activates the neural mechanisms of a postulated central decoding system. This system is assumed to be sensitive to the firing frequency of the T cells in that when the frequency is low, the stimulation is interpreted as nonpainful, but a high frequency is interpreted as pain. This theory explains pain as a result of an increase in the activity of *S* fibers or a decrease in activity of *L* fibers (see also Casey, 1973).

Notice that the theory also provides for the cognitive-motivational-emotional dimension of pain. The central control in the figure is the mechanism whereby activities subserving general excitement or emotion, attention, attitude, and prior experiences exert control over the afferent sensory input and modulate pain reception through the gate control system (see Melzack & Casey, 1968).

Although direct physiological verification is lacking, there is empirical support for this theory. One testable implication for this theory is that pain relief should be achieved by decreasing the input of the small fibers and increasing the input of the larger fibers. The latter was essentially performed by Livingston (1948) who observed that *causalgia* (a severe and prolonged burning pain produced by lesion to a peripheral nerve bundle) could be effectively controlled by therapy such as bathing the injured region in gently moving water followed by massage—both of which serve to increase the input in the large fiber system. More recently, Wall and Sweet (1967) applied low intensity electrical pulses— experienced as "tingling"—to patients with chronic cutaneous pain. These stimuli produced impulses only in large diameter fibers because these have the lowest electrical threshold. Pressure applied during the electrical stimulation failed to evoke pain. Four of eight patients with peripheral nerve diseases experienced relief of their pain for more than half an hour after electrical stimulation for 2 min. In addition, Satran and Goldstein (1973) demonstrated that the application of cutaneous electrical stimulation to normal adult male subjects raised temporarily (up to 20 min) the threshold for pain elicited by electric shock.

The gate control theory also provides for speculations of the basis of *phantom limb pain*— apparent pain in an amputated limb. Although usually phantom limb pain tends to decrease and eventually disappear, there are cases where the pain intensifies over time. It is difficult to account for such pain because the peripheral pain receptors are removed along with the limbs. However, Melzack (1970) has noted that when a limb is amputated, about half of the cut nerve fibers that still remain in the stump die. The rest regenerate and grow into stump tissue, and these fibers are usually of small diameter and slow conducting. Thus, the full range of fiber sizes is missing. Most critical and relevant to our present discussion is that a lack of large diameter fibers means that there is a corresponding lack of inhibitory effect in the sensory pathway from the spinal cord to the brain. That is, the spinal gate is opened and in some cases, pain is the result.

Mention must also be made of the striking and profound anesthetic effects produced by the traditional Oriental therapy for the general treatment of disease and control of pain, *acupuncture* (from the Latin, *acus* for "needle" and *pungere,* "to sting"). We are not here concerned with the merits of acupuncture for the treatment of disease but with its application to pain. In most cases needles, set in movement ("twirled") and often heated, are inserted at various bodily loci. The potential needle sites are charted precisely and vary with the ailment. Although Western medicine has been cautious in accepting acupuncture as valid, it is under careful scrutiny and the reporting thus far has been mainly, though not exclusively, positive (see Brown, P. E., 1972; Taub, 1972; Cheng, 1973; Clark & Yang, 1974). Precisely how acupuncture works to eliminate pain is still a matter of conjecture. However, the gate control theory is a reasonable candidate. The sensory input appears to be a critical factor. Perhaps twirling and heating the needle produce a stream of nonpainful sensations that stimulate the large diameter fibers (*L*) of the sensory nerves, which close the hypothesized gate in the spinal cord. Accordingly, the needles, by selectively and continuously stimulating the large diameter nerve fibers, initiate the inhibitory influence of the *substantia gelatinosa* and hence block pain inpulses that travel along the small diameter nerve fibers. This of course does not explain the full range of anesthetic effects produced by acupuncture, for example, inserting needles in the arm to allow painless dental extractions. However, it has been speculated that perhaps there is a second gate in the thalamus of the brain that prevents pain from reaching the cerebral cortex from above or below the spinal cord. Obviously, we are at the very beginnings of understanding this unusual means of pain control.

DERMAL OPTICAL PERCEPTION

Claims have been made about man's possession of a form of eyeless vision called *dermal optical perception* in which light is assumed to be sensed through the skin (Youtz, 1964; Pick, 1964). The proponents contend that certain persons are able to discriminate and identify material on the basis of its color by the use of only the fingertips. However, on the whole the claims outweigh the evidence. Moreover, many important physical controls have not been taken and alternative explanations cannot be ruled out (Gardner, M., 1966). One alternative proposal to the possession of a dermal light-sensitive mechanism is use of a refined temperature sense enabling the perception of very slight differences in temperature (Youtz, 1964).

It should be pointed out that the notion of light sensors distributed along the skin is conceivable. It has been noted that a dermal light reaction occurs in many phyla of metazoa and some aquatic and amphibian animals (Steven, 1963). An electrical response by the skin to an intense flash of light has been reported with the frog and some species of small mammals (Becker & Cone, 1966). One well-controlled study provides some positive evidence that human observers can discriminate light from darkness with the hands and arms (Steinberg, D. D., 1966).

DOCTRINE OF SPECIFIC NERVE ENERGIES

A very important issue whose relevance to cutaneous reception has been intentionally skirted throughout our discussion until the basic skin senses had been introduced concerns the relationship between distinct cutaneous sensations and distinct underlying receptors of the skin. In 1826 Johannes Mueller (see Dennis, 1948) published what was to become a very influential treatise, known as the *Doctrine of Specific Nerve Energies*. The doctrine, in brief, states that the *quality* of the sensation elicited by a stimulus depends primarily on the nerve excited and secondarily on the stimulus itself. Moreover, the sensation is the same regardless of where along its length the sensory nerve is stimulated. Accordingly, specific sensations are a matter of the activation of *specific* nerve fibers.

> *The nerve of each sense seems to be capable of one determinate kind of sensation only, and not of those proper to the other organs of sense; hence one nerve of sense cannot take the place and perform the function of another sense. (Mueller, J., 1838: from Dennis, 1948, P. 165)*

Thus, for example, excitations of the optic nerve by abnormal mechanical means such as a blow, produces the sensation of light and color. Similarly, cold sensations occur from stimulation of a cold spot regardless of the nature of the stimulus. This reasoning led to the assumption of a direct link between the peripheral sensory organs and specific cortical neurons. That is, the site of specificity was located at the cortical termination of the sensory nerve. Applied to our present discussion, Mueller's doctrine suggests that each region of the skin is provided with a number of sensory nerve endings, each particularly responsive to a different type of stimulation, each linked to a specific neural terminus in the sensory cortex, and each yielding a specific cutaneous sensation—pressure, temperature, or pain. Accordingly, the different skin sensations arise because each sensory nerve has its own characteristic structure, type of activity, and neural connections to the sensory cortex. In short, morphologically different neural structures signal different sensory events. As we have noted earlier, this led to attempts to identify the types of receptor endings associated with the four main cutaneous sensations, and some positive relations were reported (von Frey: see Kenshalo, 1971, pp. 118–122). However, these have not stood the test of repeated investigations. The example, noted earlier, of the cornea of the eye is relevant here. Stimulation of the cornea can cause sensations of pressure, warmth, cold, and pain, although histological analysis reveals only free nerve endings. Structurally distinct receptors specific to different cutaneous sensations have not been unequivocally reported. Indeed, the concept of four primary cutaneous modalities, each bearing a one-to-one correspondence to the physical dimensions of the stimulus and to a specific skin receptor, goes well beyond the findings. In general, specifiable sensations may occur specific to the stimulus, but the underlying receptors do not necessarily manifest a similar specialization.

The contemporary view is that specialized endings are not necessary for the detection of different sensory qualities. Furthermore, the notion of distinct nerve fibers extending from the peripheral cutaneous receptors of the skin to the specific receiving regions of the brain is not consistent with modern concepts of neurophysiology. Kenshalo (1971) has succinctly commented on this matter:

> The activity of peripheral sensory nerve fibers passes through several synapses on its way to the brain. At each synapse, the patterns of activity undergo temporal and spatial modifications. When they finally arrive at the brain, they bear little resemblance to the patterns of activity that started at the peripheral receptors. (P. 122)

Acceptance of Mueller's Doctrine of Specific Nerve Energies denies the informative role played by the cutaneous system since tacitly assumed in the doctrine is that impulses in sensory nerves cannot specify the characteristics of the stimuli that excite the sensory receptors. That is, we cannot be directly aware of external objects; rather, the input information is merely that certain receptors have been excited. Accordingly, the causes—the environmental events—of the excitations of our nerves are not given by the stimulation. However, the fact is that information about objects and events of the external world is given in cutaneous stimulation. Indeed, in the general case, it is the *source* of the stimulation that is perceived, not the state of the skin. Perhaps as J. J. Gibson (1966) states:

> Information about the cause of arousal may not get into a nervous system through a single receptor, but it may well get into the nervous system through a combination of receptors. We may sometimes be "aware of the state of a nerve," as Müller put it, but we are more likely to be aware of patterns and transformations of input that specify the causes of arousal quite independently of the specific nerves that are firing. (P. 38)

Viewed this way, Mueller's doctrine of specific receptors for each cutaneous modality becomes irrelevant. Thus far, there is no clear evidence that a specialized receptor serves a special skin sense, and in general, the precise process underlying cutaneous reception is far from understood.

THE HAPTIC SYSTEM

The combined input from the skin and from the joints provides the basis of a perceptual channel called the *haptic* system (from the Greek "to lay hold of"). According to J. J. Gibson (1966), who has most recently identified and stressed the importance of this channel, the haptic system ". . . is an apparatus by which the individual gets information about the environment and his body. He feels an object relative to the body and the body relative to an object. It is the perceptual system by which animals and men are literally in touch with the environment" (p. 97).

Haptic perception normally results from many sorts of contacts between the environment and the organism's body. Indeed, most voluntary encounters produce both joint and skin stimulation. For example, when we perform the common act of identifying an object by handling it, we obtain information about the position of our joints and about skin contact concurrently. Anatomically distinct receptors act in conjunction to produce a unitary experience. Furthermore, the nerve pathways for the cutaneous sense and kinesthesis are very similar, are both projected to the same area of the somethetic cortex, and as a matter of experimental convenience they have usually been investigated together (Milner, P., 1970). In brief, kinesthetic and cutaneous inputs combine to act as a single functional perceptual system.

It is not passively applied cutaneous and kinesthetic stimulation that provides and registers the necessary information for haptic perception but "active touch," concurrent cutaneous and kinesthetic stimulation that results from self-produced exploratory and purposive environmental encounters by the body (Gibson, J. J., 1962, 1966; see also Krueger, 1970). One product of this obtained coincident stimulation is the perception of spatial features of objects and surfaces. No doubt it is the gathering of such stimulation that we actually refer to when we say we "touch" something with our fingers or hands.

Active touch need not be restricted to the appendages. As we noted earlier with the vision substitution system, the surface of the back may be quite informative if stimulation is obtained rather than imposed. Interestingly, the capacity to

hold liquid samples in the mouth has been accompanied by the ability to judge the relative bulk of the sample (Gregson & Matterson, 1967); that is, the mouth is also a haptic receptor.

In concluding this section, it should be added that in natural, nonlaboratory conditions we extract a richer input and perceive a good bit more than indicated by our earlier discussion. We cannot here give a complete inventory of haptic capacities, but it is obvious that various combinations and syntheses of spatial, intensive, and temporal patterns of obtained skin and joint stimulation reveal many characteristics of objects that go well beyond those of pressure or temperature: for example, we can identify hardness or softness, density, size, outline and shape, texture and consistency, and certain more elusive subjective qualities such as a tickle (due to a pattern of pressure stimulation) or oiliness, wetness and dampness (which is held to be due to both pressure and cold stimulation). No matter how one classifies the input from the skin and joints, clearly it constitutes a very elaborate and informative means of environmental interaction.

In this chapter we have continued our discussion of somesthesis focusing on the cutaneous senses of temperature and pain. Sensations of temperature—warmth or coldness—result from skin contact with thermal stimuli; however, the thermal experience occurs as a result of the relation of the temperature of the skin surface to that of its surroundings rather than from the physical temperature of the surroundings alone. That is, skin temperature itself is not a good indicator of thermal experience. Within limits, if the thermal environment is held invariant, the sensory experience of either warmth or coldness diminishes until complete adaptation of thermal sensation results. The temperature range of stimuli to which a response of neither warmth nor coldness occurs is called physiological zero.

There are a number of theories of thermal sensitivity. One holds that there are specific and distinct receptors for warm and cold sensations.

However, histological and other forms of evidence do not support this notion. A vascular theory contends that there is single mechanism mediated by the activity of the neurovascular system. It holds that thermal sensations result from the constriction and dilation of the smooth muscle walls of the blood vessels of the skin; the smooth muscles of the vascular system constrict when cooled and relax when warmed. The sensory nerves imbedded in the vascular tissue register the size changes of the blood vessels of the skin (dilation or constriction), which gives rise to the thermal experience. Inadequacies of this theory were also noted. In general, the issue of explaining the temperature sense is unresolved.

The sensation of pain may be invoked by many kinds of stimulation. One explanation of pain reception is that since pain is an accompaniment of most intense forms of stimulation, it is thereby produced by overstimulation of any cutaneous sensory receptor. An alternative is to posit the existence of a nociceptor, a specific receptor that can be activated by a wide range of stimuli and that produces the painful sensation. The receptors proposed for this are the free nerve endings. A third theory, the spinal gate theory, contends that pain is the result of the relative afferent nerve impulse transmission from the skin to the spinal cord. Fast-conducting, large-diameter fibers in the sensory nerves running from the skin to the central nervous system close the "gate" in the pain-signaling system and thus reduce the degree of pain received; slow-conducting, small-diameter fibers open the spinal gate and increase the pain signals reaching the brain. Some empirical studies lend tentative support to this theory. In addition, a number of phenomena related to pain sensitivity were discussed: the qualities of pain, thresholds, auditory analgesia, pain adaptation, and acupuncture.

A brief section on Mueller's Law of Specific Nerve Energies was presented. The doctrine, which has had a great influence on the study of sensation, states that the sensation produced by a stimulus depends primarily on the nerve excited, not on the stimulus itself. That is, specific sensations are a matter of the activation of specific nerve fibers. This notion led to attempts to identify four receptor types associated with the four main cutaneous sensations; however, it was noted that this is not consistent with the known facts of sense-receptor morphology or neurophysiology.

In the last section we noted that the combined inputs from the skin and joints—cutaneous and kinesthetic information—provide a modality or perceptual channel called the haptic system. This is a system by which the individual normally obtains information about the adjacent environment. Indeed, it is actively obtained coincident stimulation from the skin and joints that enables the perception of spatial features of objects and surfaces.

9

The Chemical Sensory System I: Taste

Our focus in this chapter and the following one will be on the chemical senses: taste (gustation) and smell (olfaction). Unlike the sensory systems discussed in preceding chapters, both taste and smell depend on receptors that are normally stimulated by chemical substances. Accordingly, the receptors are termed *chemoreceptors*. Aside from the fact that the taste and smell systems are both activated by chemical stimuli, they are also functionally related. In man, the interdependence of smell and taste in the case of food ingestion can be easily demonstrated. If the input for smell is reduced or eliminated by blockage of the air passages of the nostrils, as sometimes happens during a "cold" (in which an overproduction of mucous results in a congestion of the olfactory sensory cells), or by holding the nostrils closed, two different food substances may taste quite similar. For example, under these circumstances, a bite of raw potato does not taste very different from a bite of apple. This indicates that many taste qualities assigned to food are in fact due to their odors. Meat is an instance of this; most of its sensory qualities are olfactory. According to Moncrieff (1951) *anosmic* individuals (lacking a sense of smell) cannot distinguish between meats by taste experience alone. This suggests a diet aid for certain individuals—a reduction in the odor of foods that renders them somewhat "tasteless"

may result in a decrease in their appeal, therefore perhaps a decrease in consumption.

Moreover, it is neither necessary nor even possible to make a distinction between taste and smell for all animals. There is evidence that many forms of aquatic life can detect the presence of chemical substances in their immediate environments. Fish possess a pit resembling a nose lined with chemoreceptors, as well as taste receptors scattered over the surface of the body and mouth. In water the ability to detect the presence of chemical substances is not easily separated into smell and taste, since both give information about chemical substances in a surrounding medium. Perhaps when life emerged from the sea in the form of amphibia, a general chemoreceptive system separated into two anatomically distinct but functionally united mechanisms to take into account the chemical information occurring in two different environmental media. According to Glass (1967), taste has evolutionary priority, preceding smell. Smell developed as a means of extracting chemical information from air—"taste at a distance"—typically occurring as a by-product of breathing and sniffing. It is an active process enabling the detection of events at a distance by means of their odors. In fact, the close relationship between breathing and smelling suggests that a channel of information is continually open and explains the high degree of alertness that many organisms show to the presence of odors. In contrast, the capacity to detect information from liquids became limited to the mouth and tongue; the mouth, being somewhat internalized, retained a liquid base of saliva and moist mucosa. In addition to its set of receptors for perceiving chemical solutions, the mouth also possesses the capacity for perceiving haptic information such as relative location, bulk, texture, and temperature of substances.

As suggested by J. J. Gibson (1966) and others, functionally taste and smell together may be considered a food-seeking and sampling system, consisting of numerous dietary activities—seeking, testing, and selecting or rejecting the food or drink. Of course, smell precedes taste in this process. As Moncrieff (1951) puts it: "Smell is the distance receptor for food and taste gives the food the final check, approving it, or disapproving, such disapproval being the forerunner of disgust" (p. 58). However, for certain environmental events, taste and smell may be independently employed. Smell may be used for the reception of nonnutritive information such as detecting the presence of predator or prey or for sexual activities, whereas taste aids in the regulation of the intake of nutrients and the avoidance of toxic substances. That is, taste enables an organism to "sample" substances prior to ingestion. For example, taste alone is responsible for certain kinds of dietary preferences, as in the case of the salt-deprived rat, which, when confronted with a series of foods, chooses the salt (Richter, 1942).

THE CHEMICAL STIMULUS AND TASTE EXPERIENCE

The potential stimulus for taste must be a dissolved or sapid (soluble) substance. Normally, in order to be tasted, a substance must go into solution on coming in contact with saliva. On the basis of human experience, four basic or primary tastes have been distinguished: sweet, sour, salty, and bitter.

The existence for man of four primary taste qualities, though widely agreed on, has been consistently questioned and remains a controversial issue. The commonly accepted model of the four basic tastes proposed by Henning in 1916 is shown in geometric form in Figure 9.1. Although there have been models with as many as 12 basic tastes, recent research has provided reliable evidence for only a fifth taste—alkaline. Using subjects' similarity judgments and ratings of 19 gustatory stimuli, S. S. Schiffman and Erickson (1971) found that the stimuli could be ordered into five groups: salty, sour, bitter, sweet, and an alkaline group (the latter as typified by NaOH and Na_2CO_3). In addition Susan Schiffman (1974a; Schiffman, S. S. & Dackis, 1975) has reported some evidence for the existence of a sulfurous and fatty taste. However, until there is a great deal of empirical substantiation, the vast literature on taste is likely to recognize the existence of only four primaries.

There has been a good deal of speculation as to the relative significance to the organism of these primary tastes. According to Moncrieff

Fig. 9.1 *Hennings's taste tetrahedron. The figure is an equilateral tetrahedron with the presumed four principal tastes located at the four corners. Intermediate tastes consisting of mixtures of any two primary tastes are located on the edges, and tastes produced by three primary tastes are located on the surfaces of the geometric form. (From The Human Senses, by F. A. Geldard, Wiley, New York, 1972, p. 505. Reprinted by permission of the publisher.)*

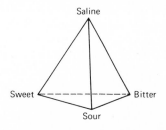

(1951), saltiness and sourness are more basic owing to the evolutionary development of taste from aquatic life: "As we are descended from sea-inhabiting invertebrates we should expect the salt taste to be the most primitive, followed by the acid taste, which would function chiefly as a warning. These two tastes are more concerned with environment and safety than with food. Later, when bitter and sweet tastes made their appearance they were concerned with nutrition" (Moncrieff, 1951, p. 131). Salt is obviously basic to sea life, whereas sourness may indicate the presence of foul water. Sweet tastes, so acceptable to many species, usually accompany substances that have food value (see Nordsiek, 1972). Bitter tastes may signal the potential ingestion of noxious or toxic substances.

As far as specifying the chemical stimulus for taste experience, it is generally noted that sour primarily results from acid compounds and the intensity of the sour taste appears to depend on the concentration of hydrogen ions. However, with hydrogen-ion concentration equated, an organic acid tastes more sour than an inorganic one. Moreover, not all acids taste sour (e.g., amino acids and sulphonic acids are sweet), and

chemical substances other than acids may also taste sour. Salts generally, but not always, taste salty; for example, cesium chloride is bitter. Bitter tastes occur from alkaloids such as strychnine and quinine, but other chemical substances such as potassium iodine and magnisium sulfate also taste bitter. Sweet tastes, generally resulting from nutrients, are associated with organic substances such as carbohydrates and amino acids, but at low concentrations the nonnutritional synthetic, saccharin, and beryllium salts also taste sweet. In addition two proteins, found in some tropical fruits, contain no carbohydrates, yet taste intensely sweet (Cagen, 1973).

Adding to the complexity of specifying the adequate stimulus is the fact that for some inorganic salts taste quality changes with concentration. For example, the compound LiCl tastes sweet at low concentrations, and changes to sour and salty as the concentration increases (Dzendolet & Meiselman, 1967). Two other examples are given in Table 9.1.

There are too many exceptions to account directly and exactly for all taste on the basis of chemical composition. The fact is that no definitive rules relating taste experience to the chemical

Table 9.1
THE TASTE OF SALTS AT DIFFERENT CONCENTRATIONS[a]

Molar Concentration[b]	NaCl	KCl
0.009	no taste	sweet
0.010	weak sweet	strong sweet
0.02	sweet	sweet, perhaps bitter
0.03	sweet	bitter
0.04	salt, slightly sweet	bitter
0.05	salty	bitter, salty
0.1	salty	bitter, salty
0.2	pure salty	salty, bitter, sour
1.0	pure salty	salty, bitter, sour

[a] Source: Pfaffman, 1959b, Vol. 1, p. 516.
[b] Molar concentration, abbreviated as mol or M, represents the number of grams of solute divided by its molecular weight, per liter of total solution.

composition of substances have been constructed. It is even possible to produce a taste experience by injecting a chemical stimulus directly into the blood stream. For example, when injected, saccharin produces the taste experience of sweetness. Similarly, "Vitamin B₄" produces a peanut-like taste and sodium dehydrocholate, a bitter taste. Both taste and smell are aroused by the arsenical Neosalvarsan, as well as by camphor and oil of turpentine when these solutions are injected intravenously in the arm (cited in Geldard, 1972, p. 483).

Taste sensations produced by electrical stimulation are also possible. When the tongue is electrically stimulated by a steady direct current, a sour taste results. The taste experienced is dependent on the frequency and intensity of the current. Moreover, alternating and direct current may produce different tastes, (Pfaffman, 1959b).

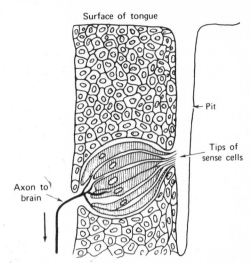

Fig. 9.2 *Semischematic structure of a taste bud. The tips of the sense cells extend into a pit. Clusters of taste buds form papillae. [Source: R. S. Woodworth, Psychology (4th Ed.) 1940, p. 507. Holt, Rinehart and Winston].*

ANATOMY OF TASTE RECEPTION

The basic receptor structures for taste, called *taste buds* (shown in Figure 9.2), are specialized receptor organs located in microscopically small pits and grooves of the mouth, soft palate, throat, pharynx, the inside of the cheeks, and particularly along the dorsal surface of the tongue. Taste buds, which number about 9000 in man, are generally found in clusters lying within small, but visible elevations on the tongue, called *papillae.* Several different types of papillae, distinguished by shape and location, have been identified: *fungiform, foliate, circumvallate,* and *filiform* (see Figure 9.3). The filiform papillae, primarily located in the center of the tongue, are the only ones presumed devoid of taste buds.

Taste receptors have a multiple nerve supply: The *chorda tympani* branch of the facial nerve serves the front part of the tongue, the *glossopharyngeal* nerve serves the back of the tongue, and the *Vagus* nerve, the deeper recesses of the throat, the pharynx, and larynx.

The cells comprising taste buds (from 40 to 60 cells each) terminate in finger-like projections called *microvilli,* which extend into taste pores and are in direct contact with chemical solutions applied to the surface of the tongue. Taste cells appear to have a short life and are renewed constantly. By "tagging" or labeling the dividing cells with radioactive material, Beidler (1963) has demonstrated that new cells continually move into the taste buds to become taste cells and that taste cells have a life of only several days. Indeed, the taste cell is one of the fastest aging cells in the body. As the taste cell ages, it moves from the edge of a taste bud toward the center. These findings suggest that differences in cell types within a taste bud actually represent different stages in development, degeneration, and migration of the taste cell. Of interest is the suggestion that the sensitivity of a taste cell varies with its age. Accordingly, with increasing age of the organism, taste cell replacement becomes slower and the sense of taste diminishes. According to one

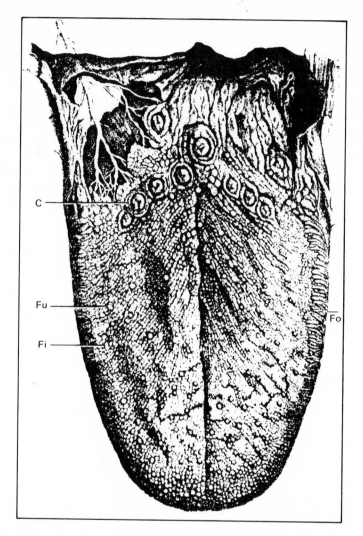

Fig. 9.3 *Distribution of papillae along dorsal surface of tongue: C, circumvallate; Fu, fungiform; Fi, filiform; Fo, foliate. (From the Human Senses, by F. A. Geldard, Wiley, New York, 1972, p. 488. Reprinted by permission of the publisher.)*

observation, the taste qualities of sweetness and saltiness appear to show the greatest decrease with age, and bitter and sour tastes are heightened (Schiffman, 1974b). However, it is maintained that the sense of smell declines much more rapidly than the sense of taste. "Hence, foods which are bitter but have a pleasant odor (e.g., green pepper—many other vegetables—chocolate) are experienced as just plain bitter by an aged person because the pleasant odor no longer contributes to the flavor" (Schiffman, S. S., 1975).

THRESHOLDS OF TASTE

A number of stimulus conditions affect both the absolute and differential thresholds of taste. Some of these are the chemical stimulus and its concentration, the location and size of the area of application, prior chemical condition of the mouth, prior dietary conditions, temperature of the chemical substance, species of animal tested, and various procedural variables of testing. As an example, consider temperature: Depending on the substance, hot or cold temperatures decrease sensitivity. Some of the effects of temperature on thresholds are given in Figure 9.4. The threshold for salt (NaCl) increases (sensitivity decreases) with a rise in temperature of the chemical stimulus from 17° C to 42° C. Thus, salted foods taste less salty when they are hot. A similar trend

exists for the bitter taste (quinine). Sweet (dulcin) thresholds are lowest at about 35° C and increase with either increases or decreases in the temperature of the test solution. Thus, a sweetened hot or cold beverage tastes sweeter when the liquid reaches about 35° C . A sour solution, HCl, appears unaffected by temperature changes over the range of 17° C to 42° C (data from Hahn: cited in Geldard, 1972, p. 492).

The chemical state of the mouth is also a critical threshold variable. Saliva has a complex chemical composition. It not only contains a weak solution of NaCl but has ionic constituents of chlorides, phosphates, sulphates, and carbonates as well as organic components of proteins, enzymes, and carbon dioxide (Geldard, 1972, p. 575). When the tongue is continually rinsed with distilled water, rendering the taste receptors relatively saliva-free, thresholds for NaCl are significantly decreased (McBurney & Pfaffman, 1963; O'Mahoney & Wingate, 1974).

Threshold value determinations are also influenced by the differing taste sensitivities in different regions of the tongue. That is, not all tongue regions are equally responsive to all chemical stimuli. As Figure 9.5a and Figure 9.5b show, sensitivity to bitterness is greatest at the back of the tongue, sweetness at the tip, sourness on the edges, and saltiness throughout the tongue surface but best toward the tip.

Locus specificity has led to the search for four types of taste receptors. Békésy (1964a, 1966) has argued that individual papillae have specialized functions and all cells within a given papilla produce the same taste when activated. His data come from the results of direct current electrical stimulation of single papillae. When individual papillae were stimulated with positive current, his subjects reported a single and specific taste. He also reported that the different papillae can be identified on the basis of their structure. However, due to the elaborate testing procedure required, the reports on such specificity of papillae are not conclusive and some nonsupportive

Fig. 9.4 *The effect of temperature on taste thresholds for sodium chloride, quinine sulphate, dulcin, and hydrochloric acid. The ordinate gives the threshold values in arbitrary units. Notice that the value of one unit on the ordinate differs for each of the four substances, as shown by the key in the figure. (Source: Pfaffman, 1951, p. 1153.)*

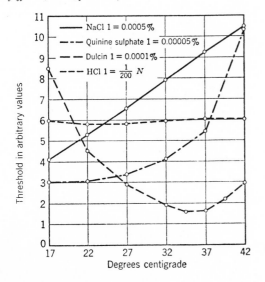

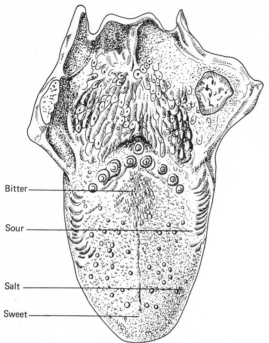

Bitter

Sour

Salt

Sweet

Fig. 9.5a *Distribution of taste sensitivity along the tongue. (From Psychology: Man in Perspective, by A. Buss, Wiley, New York, 1973, p. 179. Reprinted by permission of the publisher.)*

data have also been reported (Harper, Jay, & Erickson, 1966; McCutcheon & Saunders, 1972). Clearly, Mueller's doctrine of specific nerve energies has had an effect on the research and theory of gustation and olfaction (see Dzendolet, 1969); however, it is not clear whether papillae are highly specific to distinguishable tastes (See Pfaffman, 1974a,b.). As we will see in a later section, there is an alternative explanation to neural specificity for taste experience.

It should be clear from our brief discussion of the variables affecting thresholds that their measurement is a difficult and often unreliable matter. However, in spite of these problems, some threshold determinations for man have been made and are shown in Table 9.2.

Taste thresholds for some chemical solutions also vary considerably from taster to taster and for the same taster over time. Two such chemicals are vanillin and phenyl thiocarbamide (PTC). Variability of threshold values for PTC is of some interest because the threshold distribution is bimodal. That is, some individuals have significantly higher thresholds for PTC than do others. The relative lack of sensitivity to PTC is

Fig. 9.5b *Graphic depiction of the distribution of taste sensitivity of the tongue. Sensitivity is plotted as the reciprocal of the threshold. (Source: Boring, 1942, p. 452.)*

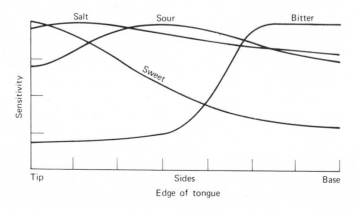

Table 9.2

ABSOLUTE TASTE THRESHOLDS FOR
REPRESENTATIVE STIMULI[a]

Substance	Median Threshold (Molar Concentration)[b]
Caffeine	.0007
Nicotine	.000019
Quinine sulphate	.000008
Citric acid	.0023
Acetic acid	.0018
Hydrochloric acid	.0009
Sodium iodide	.028
Sodium chloride	.01
Sodium fluoride	.005
Glucose	.08
Sucrose	.01
Sodium saccharin	.000023

[a] Source: Pfaffman, 1959b, Vol. 1, Tables 2 (p. 514), 4 (p. 517), 6 (p. 519), 8 (p. 521).
[b] Molar concentration represents the number of grams of solute divided by its molecular weight, per liter of total solution.

generally believed to be an inherited (recessive) characteristic, attributed in part to the constituents of the saliva.

A topic relevant to threshold determination is the psychophysical relationship between the physical concentration of the taste stimulus and the intensity of the taste experience. An indirect attempt at assessing this has been made by having subjects specify the perceived intensity of different concentrations of the four basic tastes in terms of a standard taste unit called the *gust* (Beebe-Center & Waddell, 1948). A gust is defined as the perceived intensity of a 1% sucrose solution. Thus, the perceived intensity of a solution providing any of the four tastes is expressed in gust units by comparing each solution with the intensity of a sucrose (sweet) standard. It is possible for subjects to choose a salty or bitter or sour solution that tastes half or twice as salty, bitter, or sour or is equal in perceived intensity to the sweetness of the standard solution. In general, the

concentration required to match a gust was lowest in a bitter solution, followed by sour and salt (for samples of quinine sulphate, tartaric acid, and sodium chloride, respectively).

When scaled by direct methods (i.e., magnitude estimation, see Chapter 2), stimulus concentration and taste intensity are related by a power function in which the exponent varies markedly with the particular solution scaled, 1.4 for NaCl, 0.8 for saccharin, and 1.3 for sucrose (e.g., Stevens, 1961b, 1972). Thus, the sweet taste of saccharin intensifies more slowly than does its stimulus concentration, whereas sucrose produces the reverse effect.

ADAPTATION

Prolonged exposure of the tongue to an invariant solution results in a decrease in or complete lack of sensitivity to the solution. This decrement in taste sensitivity, which we observed in the other sensory modalities, is due to *adaptation*. Complete adaptation is primarily a laboratory condition since, in the normal course of tasting, tongue and chewing movements result in continual stimulus change. The shifting of chemical substances over different regions of the tongue, stimulating different receptors at different times, precludes the conditions of constant stimulation necessary for gustatory adaptation. Adaptation phenomena for taste, however, are shown clearly with isolated papillae.

An interesting neural finding of taste adaptation for man is that during continuous stimulation the peripheral neural response of the *chorda tympani* appears to decline, paralleling the decrement in the taste sensation (Borg, Diamant, Oakley, Ström, & Zotterman, 1967).

The adaptation rate—the time required for the disappearance of the taste sensation—is principally, although not exclusively, a matter of the concentration of the adapting solution. The higher the concentration, the greater the time required for the completion of adaptation. Average time for various solutions and concentrations have been cited (Geldard, 1972, p. 513): for sour (tartaric acid), 1.5 min to 3 min; for sweet (sucrose), 1.0 to 5.0 min; for bitter (quinine hydrochloride), 1.5 to 2.5 min; and for salt, 20 sec to 2.0 min.

It should be clear that adaptation involves not only the loss of taste sensation but an increase in the threshold level. During adaptation the absolute threshold increases until it is higher than the concentration of the adapting solution. Thus, at this point adaptation is complete and no taste experience occurs. When the adapting solution is removed, thereby decreasing the adaptation process, the threshold falls back to its original value. The higher the concentration of the adapting solution, the greater is the time needed for the absolute threshold to reach a value exceeding the

adapting solution; correspondingly, the time required to regain the initial threshold value is somewhat increased. Figure 9.6a illustrates the relationship of concentration level to the temporal course of adaptation, and Figure 9.6b illustrates that adaptation is also dependent on the chemical nature of the solution producing it.

Taste adaptation is a dynamic rather than a static process in that there are various taste interactions and taste shifts that are induced by the adapting process. For example, after adaptation to NaCl is complete, concentrations lower than the adapting solution (subadapting concentrations) of salt tasted either bitter or sour (Bartoshuk, McBurney, & Pfaffman, 1964; Smith & McBurney, 1969). Moreover, the magnitude of the bitter or sour taste increased as the subadapting concentration decreased reaching a maximum at zero concentration; that is, the maximum sour

Fig. 9.6a *The course of adaptation and recovery for three concentrations of sodium chloride is shown for a 30 sec adaptation period and a 30 sec recovery period. The ordinate indicates the threshold concentrations. Each curve indicates the temporal course of shifts in threshold values for various intervals after adaptation or recovery had begun. The unadapted threshold is 0.24%. (Source: Pfaffman, 1951, p..1154; after Hahn, 1934. Reprinted with permission of the publisher.)*

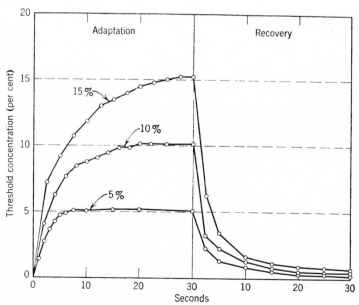

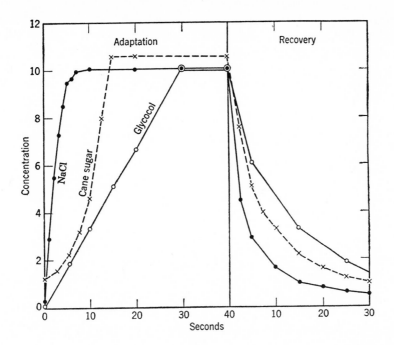

Fig. 9.6b *Adaptation and recovery curves for three substances. The NaCl curve is similar to that labeled 5% in 9.6a; the adapting solution of cane sugar had a concentration of 10%, and that of glycocol, 1%. The ordinate units are arbitrary; 10 units is equal to the adapting concentration. This makes all three curves more nearly comparable. The adaptation curve for NaCl is negatively accelerated; that for sugar, positively accelerated; and that for glycocol, linear. (Source: Pfaffman, 1951, p. 1155; modified from Hahn, Kuckulies, and Taeger, 1938. Reprinted by permission of the publisher.)*

or bitter taste was greatest when the subadapting solution became distilled water (McBurney, 1966).

These findings indicate that adaptation to certain chemical substances not only causes changes in the taste of other compounds that are tasted immediately following the adapting solution, but they show that adaptation can also impart a particular taste to water (e.g., Bartoshuk, 1968). Such effects have been termed *adaptation-produced potentiation*. McBurney and Shick (1971) have shown that each of the four primary tastes can be induced by adaptation to certain chemical solutions. For example, the effect of adaptation to bitter substances (e.g., caffeine) was to potentiate a sweet taste from water;

adaptation to sweet substances (sucrose, fructose, and saccharin) resulted in a sour and bitter taste from water; adaptation to salts potentiated sour, sweet, and some bitter water tastes; and sour (e.g., citric acid) adapting solutions produced sweet water tastes. Of 27 chemical compounds tested, only adaptation to urea (sour-bitter) produced a reliable salty taste from water.

In addition, the taste quality induced by water after adaptation to a chemical solution sums with the taste of another solution having the same quality. For example, adaptation to quinine hydrochloride (normally bitter) produces a sweet water taste. When adaptation to quinine hydrochloride is followed by the administration of a weak sucrose solution, the sucrose tastes sweeter than normal (McBurney, 1969). Similarly, when the tongue is sweet-adapted (producing a sour water taste), the taste intensity of a sour solution is increased.

TASTE INTERACTIONS

Numerous complex interactions among the primary taste qualities precludes any single set of combinatorial rules for predicting the product of taste mixtures. The result of combining two chemical solutions whose single components each appeals to a different taste is a complex psychophysiological event: The solutions do not function independently of each other, but, depending on the chemical substances, may show facilitative or inhibitory effects in combination. Condiments work on this principle, selectively inhibiting and augmenting taste qualities.

The literature on taste mixtures is both equivocal and sparse. According to one study (cited in Geldard, 1972, pp. 509–511), bitterness (represented by caffeine) does not affect saltiness or sweetness but enhances sourness. Saltiness does not affect bitterness, but reduces sweetness at high concentrations and enhances sourness at high and low, but not moderate, concentrations. Sucrose reduces bitterness and sourness but has little effect on saltiness. Sourness (citric acid) is a general enhancer; it has a moderate enhancing effect on saltiness and sweetness and a marked enhancement on bitterness.

Békésy (1964b) has argued that not all taste qualities can interact. In his experiment, the two sides of the tongue were simultaneously stimulated, each side with a different taste stimulus. To the four primary tastes, Békésy added the cutaneous sensations of warmth and cold to produce six stimuli. When all combination pairs of these six stimuli were presented over a series of trials, two general results occurred. For some combinations, a single fused taste sensation occur-

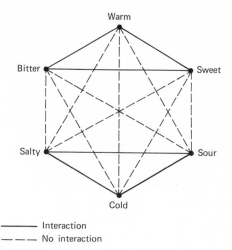

Fig. 9.7 *Schematic representation of the six stimuli that can be experienced on the tongue. Stimuli connected by solid lines can interact; those joined by dashed lines cannot. (Source: Békésy, Science 1964, 145, 835, August 1964. Copyright © 1964 by the American Association for the Advancement of Science.)*

red in the middle of the tongue; for other combinations, two distinctive spatially separated taste sensations resulted. The results are schematized in Figure 9.7. Warmth, bitterness and sweetness interact to yield fused sensations, as do cold, sourness and saltiness. However, there is no interaction of taste stimuli between these groups. Thus, for example, when appropriately applied, sweetness and sourness or bitterness and saltiness are experienced as separate sensations, lying on opposite sides of the tongue. According to Békésy, these findings suggest that two different types of receptors may be responsible for taste experience—in short, a "duplexity" theory of taste.

TASTE MODIFIERS

Additional interactions affecting taste experience occur with some drugs and chemical compounds that have different effects on the four basic tastes. That is, there are substances that differentially suppress some taste qualities and enhance others. One such drug that enhances the palatability of food is monosodium glutamate (MSG), a chemical commercially sold under several trade names (e.g., Áccent). It is presumed to act not by imparting its own taste but by modifying the taste receptors to accentuate the taste character of food, hence serving as a taste stimulant. By itself, MSG elicits all four primary tastes, principally saltiness and sweetness, and gives off little or no odor. Mosel and Kantrowitz (1952) studied the effect of MSG on the absolute thresholds of the primary tastes. Essentially they measured the absolute threshold of sweet, salty, sour, and bitter solutions before and after exposure to MSG. Their results show that thresholds for saltiness and sweetness were unaffected whereas for sourness and especially for bitterness, sensitivity was greatly increased. However, when present in relatively high concentrations, well above threshold levels, MSG has been held to accentuate sweet and salty tastes in food.

The leaves of the Indian plant, *Gymnesma sylvestre,* have been shown to suppress sweetness, without affecting the response to salty, acid, or bitter substances. For example, sugar loses its taste and feels like sand after chewing the plant leaves. The effect is attributed to gymnemic acid in the form of potassium gymnemate (KG) found in the plant leaves (Bartoshuk, Dateo, Vandenbelt, Butterick, & Long, 1969). Warren and Pfaffman (1959) observed threshold increase of sucrose and saccharin after exposure to either an aqueous extract of the leaves or purified potassium gymnemic acid. That is, after exposure to potassium gymnemate the sweetness of both test solutions decreased. Electrophysiological investigation showed that gymnemic acid acts peripherally by blocking the *chorda tympani* response to sugar and saccharin (cited in Bartoshuk et al., 1969).

Another chemical that differentially affects taste experience is *Synsepalum dulcificum* or *Richardella dulcifica,* most commonly called "miraculin," a fruit plant indigenous to tropical West Africa. The plant produces olive-shaped berries, 1 to 2 cm long—so called "miracle fruit"—that turn red when ripe. The striking effect of the fruit is that while tasteless itself, exposure of the tongue to the thin layer of fruit pulp for at least three minutes causes any sour substance to taste sweet and this effect can last for several hours. Miraculin somehow converts a sour taste into a sweet one without impairing the bitter, salt, or sweet response. It is likely that miraculin decreases the response to acid rather than increasing the sweet taste because on tasting dilute solutions of acids after the application of miraculin, neither the acid nor a sweet taste is perceptible (Henning, Brouwer, Van Der Wel, & Francke, 1969). However stable the phenomenon, the mechanism of the action of taste modification remains unclear. Dzendolet (1969) argues that miraculin blocks the receptor sites for sourness (see also Halpern, 1967; Henning et al., 1969) whereas Kurihara, Kurihara, & Beidler, (1969) contend that the effect of miraculin is brought about by the addition of a sweet taste.

MSG, *Gymnesma sylvestre,* and miraculin produce their effects by selectively affecting other tastes: Sweet and sour tastes are modified by *Gymnesma sylvestre* and miraculin respectively. In contrast, exposure of the tongue to an artichoke (*Cynara scolymus*) can make water taste sweet (Bartoshuk, Lee, & Scarpellino, 1972). Exposure of the tongue to the extract from one-fourth of an artichoke heart (10 ml of a 2.75% solution of artichoke extract) makes water taste as sweet as a solution of 2 teaspoons of sucrose in 6 oz of water, and the duration of the effect may exceed 4 min. This taste-modifying phenomenon appears to be caused by two artichoke components, chlorogenic acid and cynarin. According to the authors, the sweetness induced by the artichoke is not due to mixing of a sweet-tasting additive with the substance to be tasted, but is produced by temporarily altering the tongue so that a normally gustatory-neutral substance tastes sweet. As it has been written, the artichoke is a vegetable "of which there is more after it has been eaten."

NEURAL RECORDING

Electrophysiological methods have enabled the study of gustatory nerve-impulse traffic. When, for example, a microelectrode is inserted into a single taste cell and a taste solution is flowed over the tongue, a measurable change in frequency discharge occurs. Applying various chemical substances to the cell reveals that, in general, a single cell is responsive to more than one specific solution. Some cells respond to a broad range of stimuli, whereas other cells may respond to relatively few. Also evident is that different cells show different sensitivities to the same stimuli (Kimura & Beidler, 1961; see also Beidler & Gross, 1971).

A similar lack of specificity has been observed in single nerve fiber recordings from the cat's *chorda tympani*. In general they show that fibers are not specific to different chemical solutions but that most fibers respond to more than a single taste stimulus. The afferent recordings of single cell and nerve fiber stimulation show little evidence of neural specificity for taste stimuli.

A general lack of specificity of peripheral neural units poses important problems to understanding taste experiences. Pfaffman (1959*b*, 1964) has proposed an "afferent code" for taste. He argues that taste is based on the relative activity across a population of fibers. As Figure 9.8 shows, individual fibers do fire to more than one taste stimulus, but they do not all have the same pattern of firing. That is, there is considerable diversity in fiber sensitivity to taste stimulation. That each fiber has its own profile suggests

that taste quality, rather than being coded by a single fiber or set of specific fibers, is a matter of the pattern developed across a great number of fibers: "Differential sensitivity rather than specificity, patterned discharges rather than a mosaic of sensitivities . . ." (Pfaffman, 1959*a*, p. 231). Given a lack of neural specificity, a reasonable speculation is that at least part of the coding of taste occurs in the pathways to the brain or in the brain itself.

A critical question about the recordings of neural activity is what relation these discharge patterns have to the different taste qualities, that is, to the actual tastes experienced. Erickson (1963) developed a very interesting behavioral test to investigate across-fiber patterning. He recorded the firings of a number of individual *chorda tympani* fibers in response to different salts. Figure 9.9 shows the neural activity of 13 individual taste fibers when stimulated by three different salt solutions: sodium chloride (NaCl), potassium chloride (KCl) and ammonium chloride (NH_4Cl). Clearly, stimulation with ammonium chloride and potassium chloride produces quite similar across-fiber patterns in rates of firing. In contrast, the neural firing pattern of sodium chloride is quite different. In order to decide whether these neural similarities and differences relate to actual taste sensations a behavioral test based on taste generalization was used. That is, the question asked is: Do ammonium and potassium chlorides taste similar to each other, and does sodium chloride differ from both? Rats were trained to avoid one of the salts by shocking them when they ingested a solution of it. When they showed an avoidance of this test solution, they were tested with the other solutions. This was done for all three salts. One group was shocked for drinking ammonium chloride, one for potassium chloride, and one for sodium chloride. When tested with the two salts for which they were not shocked, the rats showed a significant generalization to the salt most similar in neural pattern response to the salt for which they were shocked. Thus, rats that had been trained initially

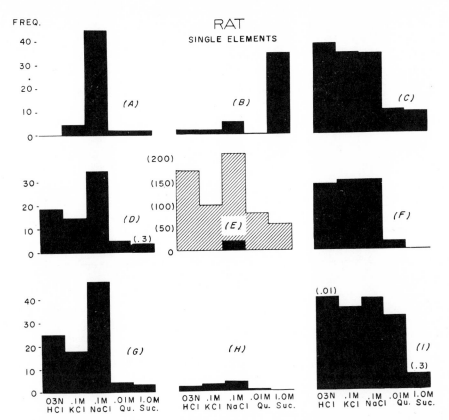

Fig. 9.8 *The pattern of taste responses in nine different single sensory nerve fibers of the rat. The solid bar graphs give the frequency of response in impulses per second for different taste stimuli (indicated along the abscissa). The crosshatched bar graph shows the relative response of the total nerve (integrated response) to these same solutions. Figures in parentheses give magnitudes in arbitrary units. (Sucrose of 0.3 M is used as test solution in elements D and I and 0.01 HCL in element I.) (Source: Pfaffman, 1955, 18, 433. Reprinted by permission of the author.)*

to avoid ammonium chloride avoided the potassium chloride significantly more than they avoided the sodium chloride. Likewise, rats that had learned to avoid potassium chloride avoided the ammonium chloride much more than they did the sodium chloride. Finally, rats trained to avoid sodium chloride showed relatively little avoidance of either ammonium chloride or potassium chloride.

To summarize the results of the behavioral tests, responses learned to KCl generalized to NH₄Cl and vice versa.

Responses learned to either KCl or NH₄Cl generalized much less to NaCl and vice versa. It appears that, for the rat, KCl and NH₄Cl taste more nearly alike than either do to NaCl. Therefore, in addition to concluding that there are many fiber types in gustation, one may conclude that the neural message for gustatory quality is a pattern made up of the amount of neural activity across many neural elements. (Erickson, 1963, P. 213)

Thus, according to Erickson's analysis, different

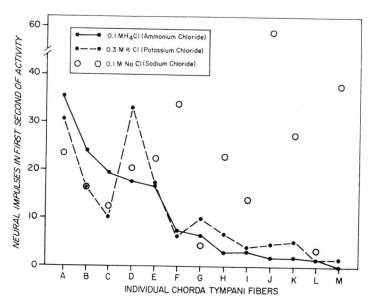

Fig. 9.9   *The neural response of 13 chorda tympani fibers of a rat's tongue to three salts. The fibers are arranged in order of responsiveness to ammonium chloride. It is clear from the neural across-fiber patterning in firing rates that the potassium chloride pattern is similar to that of the ammonium chloride, and both patterns differ from the sodium chloride pattern. (Reprinted with permission from R. P. Erickson, "Sensory neural patterns and gustation,' Olfaction and Taste, edited by Y. Zotterman, 1963, Pergamon Press.)*

firing patterns across taste fibers account for different sensations. This general result has also been demonstrated with the avoidance reaction given off by lithium chloride (LiCl) (Nachman, 1963). That these findings are relatively independent of species is shown by the essential replication of this study with opossums (Marshall, 1968).

Notice should be taken of the recent position held by Pfaffman (e.g., 1974a,b) on this matter. He contends that when one examines a large population of single fibers and samples more widely in species and in different receptor fields of the tongue area, there appears to be clusters that are most responsive to salty, sour, sweet or bitter solutions. He suggests:

> . . . *in mammals, multiple sensitivity to taste stimuli clusters around certain modalities . . . as revealed by the quality of their 'best' stimulus. Two-thirds of our sample of taste*

units fall readily into one of the four classic taste categories with a peak at one basic taste stimulus. 'Side bands' around such peaks produce a certain degree of multiple sensitivity. One-third of the responsive fibers, however, cannot be classified by a single 'best stimulus' but appear to have broad multiple sensitivity. . . . Processing gustatory information by relatively specific classes of receptors . . . and across fiber patterning are not incompatible principles. Both may operate concurrently to extend the variety and range of discrimination (Pfaffman, 1975).

TASTE PREFERENCES AND TASTE WORLDS

Most of our discussion has focused on the taste qualities that are pertinent to human experience. This is a reflection of the available literature, which, in turn, is due principally to interest and relative ease of study. However, taste experience among lower animals, when studied, is somewhat different. Clearly, under many conditions gustatory stimuli are motivating and can elicit behavior—acquisition or avoidance activity—from an organism. Although for man, sweet and salty solutions are positive "approach-type" stimuli and bitter substances are negative "avoidance-type" stimuli, this is not the case for all species. All animals do not react similarly to a given chemical solution. Generally, the chicken and the cat are indifferent to the sweet stimuli that are readily accepted by most species (Zotterman, 1961; Kare & Ficken, 1963). Sodium chloride preference is also species-specific. Whereas the cat and rabbit show a preference for NaCl, the hamster shows aversion (Carpenter, 1956). Species preferences also differ markedly for sweet solutions. For example, man reacts positively to the two nonnutritive sweeteners, dulcin and saccharin, yet in one study, rats showed a preference for only saccharin, and squirrel monkeys preferred only dulcin (Fisher, Pfaffman, & Brown, 1965).

There appears to be no clear line of evolutionary development for taste receptors. Species differ in the type, locus, and number of taste buds. Table 9.3 presents the average number of taste buds for a group of animals. However, there is no obvious relationship between the number of tastebuds and the taste experiences of the animals. Animals with many gustatory receptors do not necessarily taste more, nor are they more sensitive than those possessing fewer receptors.

The literature on food preferences of animals is quite complex, often equivocal and sometimes contradictory. However, the findings indicate that the four basic taste qualities assigned to human sensory experience are not appropriate for all animals. Indeed, the species' uniquenesses in taste preferences have many corresponding nutritional and metabolic determinants. We can reasonably conclude that there are "separate taste worlds for

Table 9.3
THE AVERAGE NUMBER OF TASTE BUDS FOR VARIOUS ANIMALS[a]

Chicken	24
Pigeon	37
Bullfinch	46
Starling	200
Duck	200
Parrot	350
Snake	0
Kitten	473
Bat	800
Human	9,000
Pig and Goat	15,000
Rabbit	17,000
Calf	25,000
Catfish	100,000

[a] Source: Kare & Ficken, 1963, Reprinted with permission from *Olfaction and Taste,* edited by Y. Zotterman, 1963, Pergamon Press.

each species" (Kare and Ficken, 1963, p. 296), and that the taste system of a particular species is adapted to the species' own unique metabolic requirements (Maller, 1967).

Taste Preference and Deprivation

There are many instances of compensatory taste appetites or cravings that arise from a state of physiological need. A dramatic intake of NaCl follows adrenalectomy (which produces a marked salt deficiency) or controlled dietary restriction of NaCl in the laboratory rat (e.g., Richter, 1939, 1942; Nachman, 1962). Salt-deprived rats show an increased intake at all concentrations, including weak solutions at a concentration level below that normally taken by intact animals (see Pfaffman, 1963; Wolf, 1969). A compensatory preference has also been shown for ruminants (Bell, F. R., 1963). Similarly, thiamine-deficient rats show a strong preference for alternative diets as opposed to the experimentally deficient diet (Rodgers & Rozin, 1966; Zahorik & Maier, 1969). In general, a deficit induced by food deprivation may amplify the role of taste in the control of food intake (Jacobs, H. L., 1967).

Origins of Taste Preferences

Although it is reasonable to assume that for many animals sweet and perhaps salty solutions are positive and bitter ones are aversive—suggesting a relationship between taste, nutrients, and poisons—the origin of taste preference is not agreed on. However, for some animals, preferences appear sufficiently early to suggest a biological genesis. Thus, human infants of one to three days of age discriminated a solution of sugar from water and showed a distinct preference for the former (Desor, Maller, & Turner, 1973). H. L. Jacobs (1964) found that the maximum acceptability of sweet solutions for rats was reached seven to nine days after birth. Whether broad taste preferences are primarily biologically determined cannot be decided on; however, in man the acceptability of certain foods is partially determined by education and custom. Specific seasonings, spices, and condiments have a basic ethnic origin and their use is culturally linked. That is, we cultivate or acquire a "taste" for certain foods. Who would risk sampling ". . . the coagulated secretion of the modified skin-glands of a cow after it had undergone bacterial decomposition" (Matthews & Knight, 1963, p. 205)? Those who do, have sampled cheese. Some cultures and ethnic groups savor food considered inedible by other groups (e.g., brains, insects, octopus tentacles). Certainly, the palatability of some bitter solutions, such as alcoholic beverages, coffee and tea, may be acquired. It may be that the foods given us at certain critical times in our formative years determine, in part, many of the foods we subsequently prefer (Greene, Desor, & Maller, 1975).

We have assumed that a significant functional role of the taste system is to regulate the ingestion of nutrients and the rejection of toxic solutions. Although this may be acceptable for animals in the wild, the biological advantage of the taste system for man must be tempered. A pertinent caveat has been expressed by Glass (1967):

> *Man himself, the most domesticated of mammals, seems to stand at a fresh crossroad in the evolution of the regulation of eating. Satiety is no longer a sufficient guard against overeating, and hunger is no longer a sufficient bulwark against dietary insufficiencies. Man has provided himself with too many foods unknown in the natural environment, too many natural goods appealing to his appetite but unbalanced or deleterious when consumed in great quantity. Even milk and milk products, as adult foods, come under grave suspicion. Man is too adaptable in diet, in spite of his cultural conservatism in matters of food and appetite, to pick and choose safely on the basis of flavor and appetite as guides to nutrition. (P. vi)*

Functionally, taste and smell together may be considered a food-seeking and sampling system. However, in this chapter we have principally focused on the sense of taste.

The receptors for taste—taste buds—are activated by chemical substances that are sapid; that is, they go into solution upon coming in contact with saliva. On the basis of human experience four primary tastes have been distinguished: salt, sour, sweet, and bitter. However, the extact chemical stimuli for unequivocally activating these qualities have not been identified.

Thresholds for taste vary with the taste quality investigated and are subject to many of the experimental conditions of testing, such as the chemical concentration, the locus and area of application, prior chemical state of the tongue or mouth, and the temperature of the solution. For example, the thresholds for salty and bitter tastes increase with a rise in temperature, whereas the threshold for sweet taste is lowest at 35° C and increases with either an increase or decrease in temperature from this value. Additionally, the tongue regions are not equally responsive to all chemical stimuli. Sensitivity to bitter solutions is greater at the base of the tongue, sweet at the tip, sour along the sides, and salt over much of the tongue surface but best toward the tip. However, differential locus sensitivity has not led to corresponding taste buds or papillae (groups of taste buds) specificity.

Taste experience undergoes adaptation (relative lack of sensitivity) when the tongue is subject to prolonged exposure to an invariant solution. A number of factors affect adaptation, especially the concentration of the adapting solution. Moreover, the adaptation of one taste quality affects the taste of certain chemical solutions that are sampled immediately following the adapting solution. Adaptation can also impart a particular taste to water—an effect called adaptation-produced potentiation. For example, adaptation to caffeine (bitter) appears to potentiate a sweet taste from water.

The effects of taste modifiers such as MSG, gymnemic acid (a sweet suppressant) and the so-called miracle fruit (a sweet enhancer) was discussed. In addition, it was noted that exposure of the tongue to the extract from one-quarter of an artichoke heart makes water taste as sweet as a solution of two teaspoons of sucrose in six ounces of water.

The lack of specificity of taste nerve fibers to different chemical solutions has given rise to the proposal of an afferent code for taste quality. As described by Pfaffman, taste is based on the relative activity across a population of fibers. This corresponds to the observation that individual taste fibers do fire to more than one taste stimulus, but they do not manifest the same pattern of firing. That is, each fiber has its own firing profile suggesting that taste quality, rather than coded by a single fiber or set of specific fibers, is due to the firing pattern developed across a number of fibers. Some evidence for this notion was summarized.

Finally, taste preferences and their origin were discussed. It was noted that different species have quite different taste preferences, which are likely adapted to the species' nutritional and metabolic requirements. Clearly, in the case of man the acceptability and palatability of certain foods is, in part, due to education and custom.

The Chemical Sensory System II: Smell

10

Functionally, the sense of smell or olfaction (or *osmics*: the science of odors) serves in the reception of information from chemical events that transpire at a distance as well as nearby. Notice the dog's ability to track both air and ground scents. In many lower animals, the sense of smell may be quite necessary for an efficient orientation to their environment. This is especially true for nocturnal animals or those that dwell in poorly lit environments, since their locomotion is dependent on a source of nonvisual information. Animals possessing a keen sense of smell are called *macrosmatic,* animals lacking it are *microsmatic.* For many animals, smell plays an important role in sexual selection and mating. Some predators hunt their prey and some prey avoid their predators by smell. There are instances where animals utilize the emission and pickup of odors for their survival to a dramatic degree. For example, the female gypsy moth emits a scent that, with proper wind conditions, can attract the male moth from miles away (Wilson, 1963; see also Beroza & Knipling, 1972). The inky secretion discharged by a frightened octopus or squid serves not only to decrease an attacker's vision but to dull the olfactory sensitivity of pursuing predator fish (Milne & Milne, 1967). Olfaction is of lesser importance to avian and arboreal species than to terrestrial and aquatic species. It is totally absent in some animals, such as the porpoise and perhaps the whale, who as lung-breathing aquatic mammals, cannot use their nose under water to receive odors (Altman, 1966). (Animals totally lacking a sense of smell are called *anosmatic.*) As we noted earlier (Chapter 6), in these animals the sense of hearing has evolved to a degree that perhaps serves to compensate for their lack of an adequate smell sense.

Though the importance of smell for man—hardly necessary for survival—is much less than for most other animals, in combination with taste it can aid in food selection (e.g., detection of spoiled food), maintenance of a clean environment, and in the case of certain odors, smell may provide some pleasant esthetic sensations (e.g., the scent of food and of flowers).

THE ADEQUATE CHEMICAL STIMULUS AND ODORS

The potential stimulus for the smell system must be a volatile or readily vaporizable substance. Accordingly, solids and liquids must pass into a gaseous state. Volatility, however, is necessary but not sufficient for stimulation of the smell system since many substances—water, for example—are volatile yet odorless. Potentially odorous substances must also be water and limpoid (fatty) soluble in order to penetrate the watery film and limpoid layer that covers the olfactory receptors.

In general, the normal chemical stimuli for olfaction are organic rather than inorganic substances. For the most part they are mixtures of chemical compounds: environmental odors emitted by vegetative life (fruits and flowers), decaying matter (flesh and feces), and scent-producing glands of animals. In brief, the natural odors occur as signals for the recognition and location of nutrients, predators, and mates.

Under usual conditions, none of the elements occurring free in nature is odorous in its atomic state. However, when heated to the evaporization point, elementary arsenic yields a garlicky odor. In addition, six of the elements are odorous in a combined state. Four of the elements—fluorine, chlorine, bromine, and iodine, the halogens—are odorous when they form diatomic molecules only (F_2, Cl_2, Br_2, and I_2, respectively). These all share a chlorine-like smell and are poisonous and acutely irritating. The remaining odorous elements produce their effect in a polyatomic state: yellow phosphorous (P_4) smells garlicky, and oxygen as ozone (O_3) smells like either garlic or chlorine (Moncrieff, 1951). Of interest is that these seven odorous elements occur in the high valence group of the periodic table: phosphorous and arsenic in group 5, oxygen in group 6, and the halogens in group 7. The suggestion that the high state of valency has an effect on odor production, though appealing, is mitigated by the fact that other elements in the high valence group are not odorous.

Unlike taste qualities, the basic smell attributes are far from agreed on. Many classifications of odors have been made on the basis of subjective experience, but a general problem encountered in this task is isolating the basic or primary odors whose mixtures yield the many thousands of possible complex odors. One attempt to establish a classification of odors is based on a geometrical construction—Henning's "smell prism"—shown in Figure 10.1. The triangular prism is supposed to be hollow with six primary odors—fragrant, putrid, ethereal, burned, resinous, and spicy—occupying the corners. Along the surfaces and edges lie the intermediate odors that are blends of several primaries (see Figure 10.2). Henning's classification was based on the odorant descriptions of six experienced subjects whose results were in fairly close agreement. Other classifications have used fewer or greater numbers of basic odors. The Crocker-Henderson system offers four: burnt, fragrant, acid, and caprylic (goaty). A sevenfold categorization devised by the eighteenth century Swedish botanist, Linneaus, as an aid in the classification of plants, was subsequently extended by Zwaardemaker in 1895 (see Moncrieff, 1951, p. 221) to give a ninefold arrangement of odors: ethereal (e.g., fruits), aromatic (spices), fragrant (flowers), ambrosial (musk), alliaceous (chlorine), empyreumatic (roast coffee), caprilic or hircine (cheese), repulsive (bedbugs, French marigolds), and nauseating (decaying meat, feces).

Fig. 10.1 *Henning's smell prism. (Source: R. S. Woodworth, Experimental Psychology, 1938, p. 487, Holt, Rinehart and Winston.)*

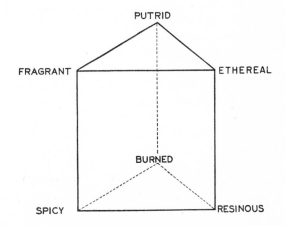

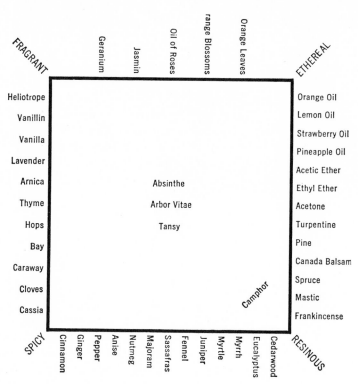

Fig. 10.2 *A face of Henning's smell prism. The odors lying along any edge resemble only the odors located at the two corners bounding that edge, and are more like the corner to which they lie nearer. (Source: R. S. Woodworth, Experimental Psychology, 1938, p. 486, Holt, Rinehart and Winston.)*

In the main, none of these classifications has met with widespread acceptance. A more recent scheme involving a sevenfold classification attempts to establish direct links between the chemical composition of substances and perceived odors. It is called the *stereochemical* (or *steric*) *theory of odors,* and it is a modern version of earlier theorizing (Amoore, Johnston, & Rubin, 1964). According to the authors, their precursors are Lucretius, the first century (B.C.) Roman Epicurean poet, and more recently Moncrieff, in 1951. The development of the theory is as follows: Based on the terms most frequently used to describe the odors of organic compounds, the seven odors, shown in Table 10.1, were identified as probable primaries. Using the techniques of stereochemistry, from which it is possible to

construct a three-dimensional model of the molecule of any chemical compound from its structural formula, it was noted that all the models for molecules of compounds that shared a similar odor had similar geometric properties, that is, they were all of about the same shape and diameter. For example, all chemicals with a camphoraceous molecule were roughly spherical in shape and had a diameter of approximately 7 Å units (Å, an angstrom is ten-millionth of a millimeter). This was shown with a degree of success for five of the seven primaries, as shown in Figure 10.3. The molecules responsible for pungent and putrid are of various shapes and sizes. However, the electric charge of the molecules is held responsible for their odors. Accordingly, the pungent class of odors is composed of compounds

Table 10.1
PRIMARY ODORS WITH CHEMICAL AND FAMILIAR EXAMPLES[a]

Primary Odor	Chemical Example	Familiar Example
Camphoraceous	Hexachloroethane, Camphor	Moth repellent
Musky	Butylbenzene	Musk, civetone
Floral	Ethyl Carbinol	Rose, lavender
Minty	Menthol	Peppermint
Ethereal	Diethyl ether	Cleaning fluid
Pungent	Formic acid	Vinegar, roasted coffee
Putrid	Butyl Mercaptan, Hydrogen sulfide	Rotten egg

[a] Based on Amoore, 1964.

whose molecules, due to a deficiency of electrons (electrophilic), have a positive charge and a strong affinity for electrons. Putrid odors are produced by molecules with an excess of electrons (nucleophilic), which are strongly attracted by the nuclei of adjacent atoms.

The next step involved the assumption that there are different receptor sites or ultramicroscopic slots in the nerve fiber membrane, each with a distinctive size and shape. From a stereochemical analysis it is possible to synthesize and modify molecules of certain shapes. According to the proponents of the stereochemical theory, it is also possible to predict odors of the resultant molecules on the basis of their geometric properties. Within limits judgments of odor similarity relate reasonably well to molecular shape. It follows, then, that a change in the shape of a molecule changes its odor. It should be pointed out that the empirical or structural formula may differ markedly between molecules, but substances whose molecules have the same shape and size share the same odor. A complex odor is comprised of more than one primary odor in varying proportions. It occurs when molecules can fit into more than one receptor site. An example cited by the proponents of the stereochemical theory is almond-scented compounds, which fit into the presumed camphoraceous, floral, and pepperminty sites.

This theory is sometimes referred to as a "lock-and-key" theory: The key is the molecule with certain geometric properties; the lock is an assumed receptor site that accommodates molecules with the geometric properties of the key. Keys are specific to locks and both are specific to odors. In general, the theory has required a number of modifications (Amoore, 1965) and does not have wide acceptance. This is due largely to a lack of clear evidence of distinct and specific receptor sites as well as some disconfirmatory evidence. Thus S. S. Schiffman (1974*b*, 1974*c*) has reported that changes in certain molecules which do not alter its size and shape appreciably have a profound impact on smell quality. Moreover, she concluded that "There are no clear psychological groups or classes of stimuli, merely trends (p. 115)." We must thus conclude that the theory in its present form is incomplete.

ANATOMY OF THE OLFACTORY SYSTEM

Relatively little is known of the physiology of the olfactory process, owing to the inaccessibility of the receptors (see Figure 10.4). The entire odor-sensitive tissue region, called the *olfactory*

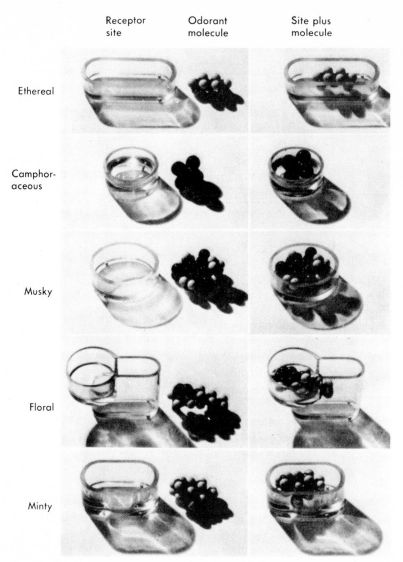

	Receptor site	Odorant molecule	Site plus molecule
Ethereal			
Camphor-aceous			
Musky			
Floral			
Minty			

Fig. 10.3 *Models of olfactory receptor sites and of molecules that "fit" them in the stereochemical theory of odor. (From Amoore, 1964.)*

epithelium or *olfactory mucosa,* occupies a total area of about one square inch. It is located on both sides of the nasal cavity which is divided by the nasal septum. The olfactory receptors are located in the mucous membrane high in each side of the nasal cavity (see Figure 10.5). They are relatively long, narrow, column-shaped cells, each less than a micron in diameter, surrounded by pigmented (yellowish-brown) supporting cells. There are estimated to be about 10,000,000 olfactory cells in man (Wenzel, 1973). On one end of the receptors, cilia project down into the fluid covering of the mucous membrane. Extending from the other end are nerve filaments comprising

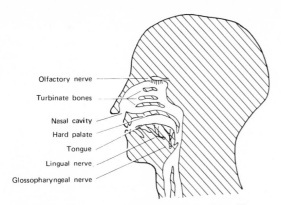

Olfactory nerve
Turbinate bones
Nasal cavity
Hard palate
Tongue
Lingual nerve
Glossopharyngeal nerve

Fig. 10.4 *The nasal passages. (From The Human Senses, by F. A. Geldard, Wiley, New York, 1972, p. 444. Reprinted by permission of the publisher.)*

olfactory nerve fibers, which connect to the olfactory bulb of the brain at a relay connection called the *glomerulus,* further connecting with other parts of the brain by olfactory tracts. The receptors thus serve the function of reception and conduction. Geldard (1972) points out that this duality of function is common in the relatively primitive nervous systems of lower vertebrates and here reflects the antiquity of the olfactory system in phylogenetic development.

In the olfactory bulb, a relatively large number of fibers converge on a single cell which in turn proceeds rather directly to the higher cortical regions. The activity of many cilia (six to 12) serving a single olfactory receptor cell, and further neural convergence in the olfactory brain, display a general funneling of neural response (and olfactory information), which contributes to the extreme sensitivity of the olfactory system. It is estimated that at the level of the olfactory bulb there is about a thousand-to-one reduction in the nerve fibers conveying sensory information to the brain.

When air is inspired, accompanying gaseous

Fig. 10.5 *Schematic anatomy of olfactory system. (Source: Krech & Crutchfield, 1958, p. 184. Reprinted by permission of the authors.)*

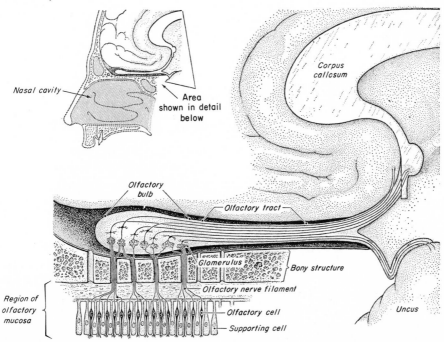

Nasal cavity
Area shown in detail below
Corpus callosum
Olfactory bulb
Olfactory tract
Glomerulus
Bony structure
Olfactory nerve filament
Region of olfactory mucosa
Olfactory cell
Supporting cell
Uncus

stimuli are carried to the olfactory epithelium by small eddy currents. The air stream is warmed and filtered as it passes three baffle-shaped *turbinate* bones in the upper part of the nose. The stimuli are dissolved in the olfactory epithelium by the fluid covering. This stimulates the cilia, and by means of some poorly understood biochemical process provokes the olfactory cells into neural activity. The more vigorous the inhalation, as in active sniffing, the more of the olfactory epithelium is bathed by the odorant and the greater is the stimulation. Odor stimulation may also occur during expiration, especially during eating.

ELECTRICAL ACTIVITY OF OLFACTORY RECEPTORS

It is assumed that electrical changes that occur at the surface of the olfactory epithelium within the olfactory nerves are a measure of the activity of olfactory sense cells and this, in turn, is specific to different odorants. The amplitude of these electrical responses increases proportionally to the intensity (logarithmic) and the duration of the stimulus. For intense olfactory stimuli the electrical response rises rapidly, peaks higher, and decays relatively slowly in contrast to weak stimuli. In short, the amount of neural activity increases with increases in the concentration of a given odorant.

Aside from the relationship between neural response and odorant concentration, there is evidence that some odorant differentiation occurs at the receptor level. Since there is a topographical representation of the olfactory epithelium in the olfactory bulb, it is possible that different odorants, owing to certain unspecified differences in their molecular properties, produce specific and distinctive spatial and temporal patterns of neural activity. Mozell (1964, 1966) recorded the neural traffic from the frog's olfactory nerve branch serv-

ing two widely disparate spatial loci of the olfactory epithelium. The result was that differences in the magnitude of the neural discharge from each epithelium location was specific to the odorants. For example, octane affected one location more than the other, whereas citral produced the reverse effect. A second neural difference was that the response latency of the discharge (onset) of the two nerve branches differed for different odorants.

Similarly, Gesteland, Lettvin, Pitts, and Rojas (1963), recording from the receptors of the frog's olfactory epithelium, noted selective patterns of neural response from the application of distinctive odorants. When tested with 25 different odorants, each receptor whose activity was recorded was responsive to only several, the magnitude of the response varying from odor to odor. Thus, although limited by the means of measuring neural response, there is evidence to assume that distinctive spatial and temporal patterns of discharge result for different odorants, that is, "... a time-space encoding of the mucosal analysis of incoming vapors" (Mozell, 1964).

THRESHOLDS

Absolute threshold determinations have been made for a number of odorant materials indicating that extremely low concentrations are sufficient. With respect to the concentration of molecules, it has been estimated that olfaction is the more sensitive of the chemical senses—10,000 times as sensitive as taste, according to Moncrieff (1951). A striking example of olfactory sensitivity is given by mercaptan: A concentration of 1 molecule of mercaptan per 50 trillion molecules of air is detected (note that a sniff of 20 cc volume at this concentration level would contain about 10 trillion molecules of mercaptan, Geldard, 1972, p. 448). Another dramatic example is given by skatol, which has an objectional fecal odor: A single milligram of skatol will produce an unpleasant odor in a hall 500 meters long by 100 meters wide and 50 meters high (Moncrieff, 1951, p. 101). Indeed, it is because the amounts of the odorous vapor required for the minimal detectible stimulus are so small that very complicated methods of threshold measurements must be employed.

Many threshold measures have been made using the *olfactometer,* devised by Zwaardmaker, a Dutch physiologist (see Figure 10.6). In its basic form, it consists of a glass tube that slips into the sleeve of a larger odorant tube. The other end of the glass tube is inserted in the subject's nostril. The greater the extent of the odorant tube exposed to the currents of air drawn through the tube by the subject's inspiration, the greater the concentration of odorous material reaching the receptors. Stimulation may be to one nostril, termed *monorhinic,* to two nostrils si-

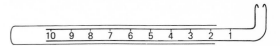

Fig. 10.6*b* *The amount of odor is determined and measured by the length in centimeters of the odor tube exposed to the current of air. There is also a double form of the device to permit dirhinic and dichorhinic stimulation.*

multaneously, called *dirhinic,* or with a different odor to each nostril, *dichorhinic.*

The olfactometer has been used to establish a standard odorant unit, the *olfactie,* defined as the length of odor tube in centimeters exposed at threshold. For example, one olfactie of India rubber equals 0.7 cm (Pfaffman, 1951). Currently there are a number of other more sophisticated methods for measuring odor detection levels. Perhaps the most elaborate of all methods of assessing olfactory sensitivity is the *olfactorium,* a glass double chamber that actually is an area where the odor environment is completely controlled. Prior to the administration of the odorant all residual body odor is removed from the subject by bathing. The vapor of the chamber consists of only the odorous chemicals and a known quantity of air at a controlled temperature and humidity (both of which can influence volatility).

In general, threshold measurements are significantly influenced by the methods and procedures used for introducing the odorant to the receptors (see Mozell, 1971, pp. 197–201). A listing of threshold concentrations for some representative odorants are given in Table 10.2. Using other techniques, different threshold values have been reported. No matter what the method, however, man is extremely sensitive to minute amounts of certain odorants. It has been noted that of the number of molecules entering the nostrils, only a small fraction actually make contact with the receptors owing to prior absorption. In normal inspiration only about 2% of the odorant molecules entering the nose reach the

Fig. 10.6*a* *Zwaardemaker's monorhinic olfactometer. The bent-up end of the tube is inserted into the nostril. The other end is fitted into the sleeve of a larger stimulus tube made of odorous material. As the subject sniffs, air is drawn through the odor-bearing larger tube and then through the smaller tube to the nostrils. (From C. Pfaffman, in Handbook of Experimental Psychology, edited by S. S. Stevens, Wiley, New York, 1951, p. 1163. Reprinted by permission of the publisher.)*

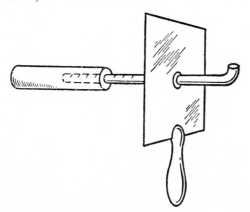

Table 10.2

SOME REPRESENTATIVE ODOR THRESHOLDS[a]

Substance	Odor	Threshold Concentrations[b]
Carbon tetrachloride	sweet	4.533
Methyl salicylate	wintergreen	.100
Amyl acetate	banana oil	.039
N-butyric acid	perspiration	.009
Benzene	kerosiney	.0088
Safrol	sassafras	.005
Ethyl acetate	fruity	.0036
Pyridine	burned	.00074
Hydrogen sulfide	rotten eggs	.00018
N-butyl sulfide	foul, sulfurous	.00009
Coumarin	new-mown hay	.00002
Citral	lemony	.000003
Ethyl mercaptan	decayed cabbage	.00000066
Trinitro-tertiary-butyl xylene	musk	.000000075

[a] Source: Wenger, Jones & Jones, 1956, Holt, Rinehart and Winston, p. 148.
[b] Milligrams per liter of air.

olfactory epithelium and by statistical calculation, from one to nine molecules, depending on the odorant, are required to excite a single receptor and at least 40 receptors must be excited to reach threshold (De Vries & Stuiver, 1961). Indeed, Mozell (1971) points out that the olfactory system can detect the presence of a smaller number of molecules than can most laboratory methods used for the same purpose.

Thresholds and Gender

Thresholds for certain odorants may be affected by the interaction of gender and hormonal variation of an individual. It has been reported that the absolute threshold for "exaltolide", a musk-like synthetic lactone odorant used as a fixative in perfume, varies in the human female according to the stage of the reproductive or menstrual cycle. In a series of studies by Le Magnen (cited in Vierling & Rock, 1967), it was noted that most

sexually mature women perceived the odor of a sample of exaltolide as intense whereas most immature females and males and mature males either barely perceived it or were insensitive to it. Examination of the perception of the males to exaltolide revealed that of those studied, half the males were anosmic to exaltolide and for the remaining men, their threshold was 1000 times greater than for that of sexually mature women. Subsequent research on the absolute threshold of exaltolide indicated that two peaks in olfactory sensitivity result: 17 days and eight days before the menses, just preceding the theoretical ovulatory phase and during the luteal phase, respectively (Vierling & Rock, 1967). These peak times are approximately when estrogen secretion levels peak, suggesting that the presence of estrogen influences the sensitivity to exaltolide. This is given additional support by the findings that women deprived of normal estrogen by ovariectomies had higher thresholds than normal females, but that restoration of the threshold to within a normal range followed the administration of a form of estrogen. It appears, then, that the hormonal status may exercise an effect on olfactory thresholds. We will return to the significance of the sensitivity to exaltolide in a later section.

Differential Thresholds

Unlike the strikingly low concentration levels required for the absolute threshold, the differential threshold values are quite high. That is, if the absolute sensitivity is high, differential sensitivity is not. According to one report, the concentration of an odorant must change by more than 25% in order for a change in its intensity to be perceived (Engen, 1970). The relative insensitivity to differences in intensities of odorants may be due in part to the anatomy of the receptors. That is, the pooling of information from stimulated fibers in the olfactory brain, which on one hand enables the perception of extremely small amounts of odorants, may likewise reduce the possibility of discriminating between concentration levels. Thus, there appears to be a lack of fine intensity discrimination in olfaction though it improves with practice (Engen & Pfaffman, 1959; Desor & Beauchamp, 1974).

The psychophysical relationship between the concentration of the physical odorant and its subjective intensity has been studied by using methods of magnitude estimation (see Chapter 2). This relation for a number of odorants has approximated a power function with typical exponents, varying between 0.40 and 0.60. Jones (1958a, 1958b) has reported that the exponents for butanol, ethyl acetate, cyclohexane, pyridine, heptane, octane, and benzene were 0.5 ± 0.1. Reese and Stevens (1960) cite an exponent of 0.55 for the natural odor of coffee. These findings mean that for olfaction, the perceived magnitude grows more slowly than the stimulus concentration.

ADAPTATION

Continued exposure to an odorant results in an increase in the threshold or a decline in sensitivity to that odorant: In short, continued odor stimulation results in *adaptation*. Figure 10.7 is a plot of one of the earliest quantitative studies on olfactory adaptation. Depending on the odorant and its concentration, with a sufficient exposure duration, odor experience tends to disappear. Olfactory adaptation is a common experience. The cooking odors initially experienced when first entering a kitchen are quite different after several minutes of exposure.

Fig. 10.7 *Olfactory adaptation curves. Increasing adaptation is measured by the increase of the olfactory threshold (in olfacties), shown by the ordinate. Each point represents increases in the absolute thresholds after various lengths of exposure to the odorant. The curves for the different odorants and concentration indicate that the rate of adaptation is determined by the specific character of the odorant and its concentration (indicated by each line). In general, increasing the adaptation time increases the threshold. (Source: Pfaffman, 1951, p. 1165; after Zwaardemaker. Reprinted with permission of the publisher.)*

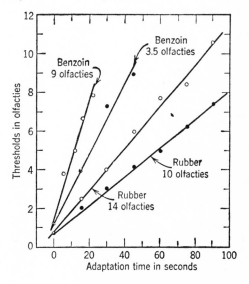

Although it can be advantageous to reduce the sensitivity to certain unpleasant odors, adaptation also has dangerous consequences. Miners once used canaries to detect the presence of lethal methane gas to which their own receptors had adapted before the presence of the gas was noted.

The relative absence of odorants (as with exposure to pure air) can result in increased olfactory sensitivity. In one study of nine odorants, as reported in Geldard (1972, p. 458), exposure to pure air resulted in a decreased threshold, depending on the odorant, ranging from about 9% (for pyridine) to 39% (artificial musk). The average threshold drop due to prior exposure to pure air was about 25%. However, like the effect of saliva on taste, our odor world is continually filled so that usually we are at least partially odor-adapted. Along with intensive changes, qualitative changes also result from continued exposure to certain odorants. Thus, the smell of nitrobenzol changes from a bitter almond odor to a tarry odor with continued exposure. Similarly, the odor of mercaptan, which initially is unpleasant, may soon acquire a pleasant ethereal quality (Pfaffman, 1951).

Olfactory adaptation is a selective phenomenon. Although its effect is greatest on the adapting stimulus, adaptation to one odorant may affect the threshold of another stimulus—an effect called *cross adaptation*. Some examples, shown in Figure 10.8, indicate that exposure to any one of the odorants—camphor, eucalyptol, or eugenol—elevates the threshold of the remaining odorants. In contrast, benzaldehyde shows little threshold shift effects and produces little threshold changes in the other three odorants.

ODOR MIXTURES

When two different odorants that do not react chemically are simultaneously administered, several results are possible. The two odorant components may continue to be identified, depending on their initial distinctiveness. However, the more similar the components, the greater is the tendency for the odorants to blend or fuse and yield a third unitary odor. Another possibility of odorant mixtures is *masking,* which typically appears when the concentration of one odor sufficiently surpasses that of the other—an effect that

Fig. 10.8 *The selective character of olfactory adaptation. The ordinate indicates the threshold rise in olfacties after adaptation by each of four substances: camphor (C), eucalyptol (Ec), eugenol (Eg), and benzaldehyde (B). Self-adaptation is indicated by the solid bar; threshold changes for the other substances are indicated by crosshatching. The threshold for each substance is most influenced by itself. The sensitivity to benzaldehyde is little affected by these substances and has little effect on their thresholds. (Source: Pfaffman, 1951, p. 1166. Reprinted with permission of the publisher.)*

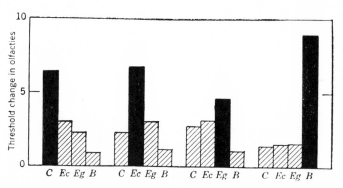

is often erroneously referred to as "deodorization." True deodorization occurs only when the odorous molecules are removed from the olfactory environment. This can be produced by submitting the contaminated air to adsorbants such as activated charcoal.

It has sometimes been reported that an additional interaction effect called *compensation* results from certain odor combinations. It refers to a mutual alteration between odorants—the cancellation or neutralization of odor sensation—by the simultaneous presentation of odorants. For example, the odor of paraffin or cedarwood is held to cancel the odor of India rubber. However, odor compensation has been demonstrated only under certain conditions (Köster, 1969), and the general status of odor neutralization remains controversial (Geldard, 1972). Of course, it is possible to eliminate odor quality by chemically producing anosmia. Thus, in weak solution, formalin (formaldehyde) vaporizes to cause temporary anosmia (Leukel, 1972).

body. What will be good for the body will usually be liked" (Moncrieff, 1966, p. 208). Thus, the odor of carrion, so repulsive to many animals, is attractive to the scavenger.

Moncrieff (1966) has performed an extensive investigation on the relationship of odor preferences to many human personality and constitutional variables that has resulted in a number of generalizations. Using a collection of 132 different odorants, some natural and others synthetic, Moncrieff found that those odorant materials that were best liked were from flowers and fruits and from substances derived from natural products. A second finding of interest to our present discussion is that odor preference is affected by concentration. Most chemicals yield pleasant odors when they are in dilution. In a number of instances the perception of a given odorant will vary from pleasant to unpleasant as its concentration is increased. Moncrieff (1966) has published a wealth of information on odor preferences, and the interested reader is urged to examine his monograph.

ODOR PREFERENCES

As we noted, all animals do not require or possess the same level of olfactory sensitivity, nor do they share the same spectrum of odor detectability. Because olfaction generally serves a biological function, it follows that, depending on species, the odors that are best perceived are those that are biologically relevant. J. J. Gibson (1966) comments on this point. "The evolution of perception by smell did not take the same course in all species, since what constitutes food for one does not always constitute food for another. Carnivores might be expected to detect the odor of meat better than the odor of clover, while herbivores would do the reverse" (p. 146).

Odor preference should similarly follow the adaptive trend of odor reception. Namely that, "Like or dislike of an odor, especially of food, is partly determined by the requirements of the

PSYCHOBIOLOGICAL FUNCTIONS OF OLFACTION: PHEROMONES

The olfactory system receives biologically useful information although its importance varies with animal groups. For many arthropod and infraprimate mammalian species, olfaction serves in important survival functions. It enables the perception of the sources of odors—food, sex object, predator—and it conveys information for the performance and perception of certain forms of behavior such as orientation, sexual activity, territory and trail marking, aggression, and species recognition. In certain animal species, olfaction also enables a form of chemical communication. One process by which this occurs involves the use of chemical communicants or signals called *pheromones* (from the Greek, *pherein,* "to carry," and *horman,* to "excite") (Marler and Hamilton,

1966). Pheromones are chemical substances secreted to the external environment and exchanged among members of the same species. Unlike hormones, which are secreted in the blood stream and regulate an organism's internal environment, pheromones are excreted by specialized glands of the skin or in the urine. These substances produce specific reactions in the behavior or physiology of receptive animals of the same species as the donor. The mode of influence of pheromones may take either of two general forms. "Releasers" produce an immediate and direct effect (e.g., the attraction of a bitch in heat). "Primers" act by producing a receptive state of physiological change such as affecting the estrus cycle. Olfactory sex pheromones have been identified for many insects, and synthetic variants are sometimes used for insect control. Pheromones are used in achieving aggregation in insects. Thus worker honey bees, on finding a source of food, release a scent (geraniol and citral) that attracts other bees (cited in Marler & Hamilton, 1966). This same species also makes use of chemical signals for colony recognition.

A number of studies have identified the existence of chemical excretions of the mouse that influence hormonal activity, the estrus cycle, and hence the reproductive physiology and behavior of other mice (e.g., Vandenbergh, Whitsett, & Lombardi, 1975). In addition, it has been reported that removal of the olfactory bulb abolishes not only the estrus cycle but eliminates maternal behavior in lactating mice (Gandelman, Zarrow, Denenberg, & Meyers, 1971). In a related study, olfactory bulb removal eliminated mating behavior in the male hamster (Murphy & Schneider, 1969). It appears that the ability to smell is a prerequisite for reproductive behavior in some mammalian species. Some of the pheromonal effects are quite stylized. For example, Michael and Keverne (1968) report that the pheromones excreted by the boar elicits an immobilization reflex on sows in estrus so that the sows stand rigid while mating.

There are also classes of pheromones that serve to signal the presence of danger—alarm pheromones. In one study (Valenta & Rigby, 1968), rats that had been trained to make a single response (bar press) were used. When an air sample taken from the vicinity of rats who were undergoing a stressful exposure (electric shock) was introduced into the test chamber of the trained rats, their responses were interrupted. No such effect occurred when air from unstressed rats was introduced. The indication is that rats who were shocked excreted a detectable chemical—the alarm pheromone—that disrupted the learned behavior of the trained rats. Similarly, Wasserman and Jensen (1969) have demonstrated that the odor trace of a rat undergoing experimental extinction can significantly disrupt the performance of nonextinguished rats (see Gleason & Reynierse, 1969 and Bronson, 1971 for a review of infrahuman pheromones).

The role of pheromones in microsmatic primates is not clear, but it has been noted that among the prosimians pheromones are used for territorial marking and sexual behavior. In higher primates there is evidence that the sexual activity of males and females is partially mediated by a sexual pheromone. In one study, experimentally anosmic male rhesus monkeys showed no interest in receptive females until normal olfactory function was restored (Michael & Keverne, 1968). In addition, males with normal olfaction were more sexually responsive to females that were administered estrogen than to females experimentally lacking this hormone. These findings suggest that a hormonal-dependent vaginal pheromone may affect primate sexual behavior. It should be noted that although pheromones may not play as dominant a role as visual or certain behavioral cues, or even be essential for primate breeding, their presence may confer an advantage in certain environments by identifying the sexually receptive females, thereby increasing the likelihood of fertile matings.

The existence of pheromones in man is not

certain, but there are suggestions. Perfumers make ample use of certain mammalian sex pheromones such as civetone (produced by the anal glandular pouch of the male and female civet, a nocturnal felid found in Africa and Asia) and musk (from the anal scent glands of the male musk deer), substances used principally as fixatives and extenders. Both pheromones are normally used by their donors for territory markings and as sex attractants. Apart from their practical function of extending the more valued components of commercial perfumes, the odors of sex pheromones of lower mammals appear to have some attraction for the human. We noted earlier than exaltolide evokes a threshold response in the human female that varies according to her reproductive cycle. In addition its musk-like odor is pleasant and attractive to females ("sweet" and "like perfume" were the most frequent comments in one study; Vierling & Rock, 1967). Of some relevance to our discussion is that a compound found in human urine also has a sharp musk-like odor, and the adult male secretes about twice as much as does the adult female (Vierling & Rock, 1967). The conjecture here, of course, is that exaltolide mimics a sexually relevant human pheromone. In addition, a female vaginal secretion of volatile fatty acids, similar to those possessing sex-attractant properties in other primate species, has been suggested as a possible human pheromone (Michael, Bonsall, & Warner, 1974).

There are other indications of pheromonal-type mechanisms operating at the human level. It has been reported that schizophrenics give off a peculiar and characteristic acidic odor in their sweat, and this substance has been identified (Smith, Thompson, & Koster, 1969).

McClintock (1971) has reported a study on women (all dormitory residents of a women's college) that indicates that the menstrual cycles of close friends and roommates fall into synchrony. The critical factor producing menstrual synchrony, according to McClintock, was that the in-

dividuals interact and remain in close proximity to one another. One explanation for her findings is that the mechanism underlying this menstrual synchrony phenomenon is pheromonal.

Whether normal genital secretions of a volatile nature, for both the human male and female, exert sex-attractant influences on humans is not known. If these odorants do play a role, the popularity of deodorants, especially the intimate types for the female genital region is rendered particularly unnatural (see Comfort, 1971).

Though knowledge of chemical communication systems is at a comparatively early stage and many questions remain to be answered, the burgeoning interest and literature on pheromones testifies to the important influence olfaction has on behavior.

In this chapter we have described the processes and phenomena of smell or olfaction. It was noted that although the sense of smell is not necessary for man's survival it does provide crucial biologically relevant information for many species.

The adequate stimulus for smell is a volatile substance that must also be water and limpoid soluble. Generally the normal chemical stimuli for the olfactory system are organic substances that are mixtures of chemical compounds.

The basic categories of odors are not agreed on. However, there are various classifications based on subjective experience. One scheme, called the stereochemical theory, emphasizes the geometric properties—size and shape—of the molecules comprising the odorant. This theory assumes that the molecules of certain sizes and shapes must fit into correspondingly shaped receptor sites of the olfactory membrane, much as a key fits in a lock. When substances of similar molecular construction (keys) stimulate the same receptor sites (locks), they produce similar olfactory qualities. This theory, as with others, is inconsistent with a number of empirical findings.

The anatomy of the olfactory systems was

outlined, and it was noted that the receptors serve the functions of reception and conduction. In general, the degree of neural activity increases with increases in the concentration of a given odorant.

Threshold measures indicate that extremely low concentrations are sufficient for detection. However, differential sensitivity is relatively poor; that is, the concentration of an odorant must change by a good deal in order for a change in its intensity to be perceived.

Phenomena relevant to olfaction, such as adaptation, masking, cross-adaptation, compensation and odor preferences were discussed.

Finally a means of chemical communication by way of pheromones was described. Pheromones are chemical substances secreted to the external environment and exchanged among members of the same species to produce behavioral or physiological reactions in the receptive animals. Pheromonal communication has been shown for a number of animal species including primates and there is some preliminary evidence for a possible human pheromone.

11

The Visual System

In many forms of life, vision is crucial for gaining spatial knowledge about the arrangement of objects and the presence of events in the environment. This knowledge depends on information such as shape and texture, size and distance, brightness, color, and movement. Vision is the dominant sensory system for man. This can be experimentally demonstrated when vision is put in conflict with another sensory modality. Rock and Victor (1964; see also Rock & Harris, 1967) examined the priority of vision over touch by providing an experimental situation in which a square was made to look like a rectangle whose sides appeared in the proportion of two to one (see Figure 11.1, *a & b*). When the subject both felt and saw the square through a distorting lens, which produced an optical compression of the width, the square was perceived as a rectangle. That is, the stimulus was perceived on the basis of the distorted visual input rather than the undistorted tactual one.

Because vision is so dominant a sense in man, it has been studied in great detail and more is known of it than the other senses. Accordingly, a major portion of the remainder of this book will be devoted to the visual modality.

THE PHYSICAL STIMULUS

The physical properties of the visual stimulus—radiant electromagnetic energy—are compatible with two apparently different conceptions of light. Based on the fact that radiant energy is propagated in a continuous wave form, we can describe it by its wavelength (or its inverse, frequency). Radiant energy also behaves as if it is emitted as discrete particles or quanta of energy. The quantum unit of photic energy is called a *photon*, and the intensity of a source may be given as the number of photon units emitted. According to contemporary physical theory, the apparent paradox that light possesses both wave and particle properties is resolved by the recognition that light is composed of specific particles of matter—photons—and that photon motion is best described by a wave equation (see Rubin & Walls, 1969). In brief, "... photons are the components of a light beam whereas the wave is a description of it" (Feinberg, 1968, p. 55). Indeed, the two are quantitatively related in that the shorter the wavelength, the greater the energy. Suffice it to say, visible light is generally described by its wavelength and its intensity.

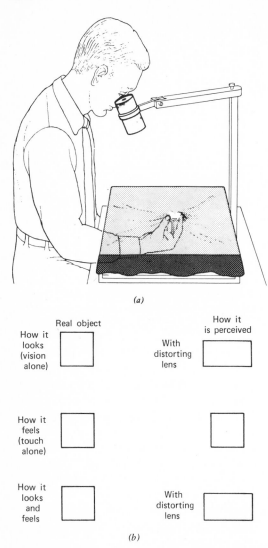

(a)

(b)

Fig. 11.1 *a. Experimental arrangement used to present the subject with contradictory information from vision and from touch. The apparatus included a reducing lens, a cloth over the subject's hand so that he would not deduce from the small appearance of his hand that he was looking through a reducing lens, and a square made of hard plastic. In the experiment depicted, the subject looked at the square and simultaneously grasped it. The lens optically produced a rectangle. The results for this and other conditions are schematized in Figure 11.1b (From Vision and Touch, by Rock, I., and Harris, C. S., in Scientific American, 1967, 216, 97. Copyright © 1967 by Scientific American, Inc. All rights reserved.)*

Color or *hue* is the psychological correlate to wavelength. The intensity of light refers to the amount of radiant energy, and its psychological correlate is *brightness*.

Wavelengths vary from trillionths of a meter to many kilometers in length (see Figure 11.2). However, the wave lengths of radiant energy of significance to the visual systems of most animal species occupy a relatively small region of the total electromagnetic spectrum. Under normal conditions for most vertebrates, visible radiation-light extends from about 380 nanometers (*nm*, billionths of a meter) to about 760 nm. This range constitutes only a narrow band, about one-seventieth of the total spectrum. Part of the reason for the evolution of the eyes' reception of only a limited portion of the spectrum may be due to the filtering of light energy by the ozone layer (15 miles above the earth) so that four-fifths of

Table 11.1
LUMINANCE VALUES FOR TYPICAL VISUAL STIMULI[a]

	Scale of luminance (millilamberts)	
	10^{10}	
Sun's surface at noon	10^{9}	Damaging
	10^{8}	
	10^{7}	
Tungsten filament	10^{6}	
	10^{5}	
White paper in sunlight	10^{4}	Photopic
	10^{3}	(color vision)
	10^{2}	
Comfortable reading	10	
	1	
	10^{-1}	
White paper in moonlight	10^{-2}	
	10^{-3}	Scotopic
White paper in starlight	10^{-4}	(colorless vision)
	10^{-5}	
Absolute threshold	10^{-6}	

[a] Source: L. A. Riggs, in *Vision and Visual Perception*, edited by C. H. Graham, Wiley, New York, 1965, p. 26. Reprinted by permission of the publisher.

In figure (b), labels read: Real object; How it is perceived. Rows: How it looks (vision alone) — With distorting lens. How it feels (touch alone). How it looks and feels — With distorting lens.

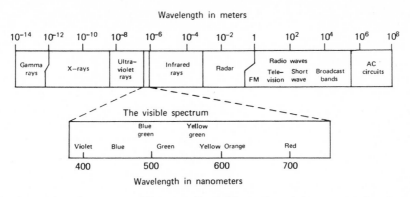

Fig. 11.2 *The electromagnetic spectrum. The normally visible portion of the spectrum is enlarged in the lower part of the figure. (Source: Geldard, 1972, p. 20; after Chapanis, Garner, and Morgan, 1949.)*

the solar energy reaching the terrain lies between 300 nm and 1100 nm (Geldard, 1972). In addition, as light enters water it undergoes absorption, scattering and, even at moderate depths, extinction. By one accounting, the short ultraviolet waves are almost extinguished in a few millimeters of water, the infrared waves are eliminated in about a meter, thereby leaving the narrow band of the visible spectrum shown in Figure 11.2 (Walls, 1963, p. 373). Thus, aquatic creatures whose vision is adapted to the available light spectrum and those terrestrial animals owing their origins to aquatic forms of life share a similar visible spectrum.

The measurement of the intensity dimension of a photic stimulus requires extremely complex procedures, and they are specified in a diverse array of units. However, only two aspects need concern us: the physical intensity of the radiant energy falling on a surface—the amount of *incident light,* and the intensity of the light reaching the eye from a surface—the amount of *reflected light.* The former is called *illuminance.* A common English unit of illuminance is the *foot-candle* (ft-c) defined as the illumination received on a surface 1 foot square located 1 foot from a standard candle. Another unit of illuminance, used initially in physiological optics to denote the illuminance of the retinal image, is the *troland.* The troland is defined as the illuminance

produced by one candle per square meter passing through a pupil opening of one square mm. However, because it is defined in terms of assumed characteristics of the eye, it is not often employed. A metric unit of illuminance is the *meter-candle* (m-c), defined as the illumination on a surface of one meter square located one meter from a standard candle. One meter-candle equals 0.0929 foot-candles. Notice that the farther away a surface rests from the light source, the less is the amount of light reaching it. Specifically, the intensity of the illumination of a surface varies inversely with the square of the distance between the light source and the illuminated surface.

Ordinarily we do not look directly at a light source: Most of the light that we see is reflected from surfaces. The intensity of the light reflected from an illuminated surface is termed *luminance.* An English unit of luminance is the *foot-lambert* (ft-L) defined as the total amount of light emitted in all directions from a perfectly reflecting and diffusing surface receiving one *foot-candle.* Another common unit of luminance is the *millilambert* (mL), which is equivalent to 0.929 ft-L. An often employed alternative unit of luminance is candles per square meter (c/m^2), which is equal to 0.3142 mL. Table 11.1 shows luminance levels for some typical sources of stimulation. Because the visual system can respond to a great range of luminance levels, logarithmic transformations are often encountered. As in the case of acoustic energy, the use of logarithms reduces an enormous range of values to a few. With a base 10, a luminance of 1 converts to a value of 0 in the log scale ($\log_{10} 1 = 0$). Similarly, a luminance of 10 converts to a value of 1, a luminance of 100 to a value of 2, and so on. Observe that a difference of one log unit reflects a tenfold difference in intensity.

Radiant energy is informative only when it is intercepted by matter. In the initial stage of vision, radiant energy must be transduced into a neurally acceptable form. That is, the physical energy acts on receptive tissue to produce impulses that convey sensory information. The kind of tissue that is responsive to photic energy is found in the simplest of organisms. Some organisms, such as the single-celled amoeba,

Fig. 11.3 *Examples of some primitive "eyes." (Source: Gregory, 1973, p. 24. Reprinted by permission of the author, publisher, and the Cranbook Institute of Science.)*

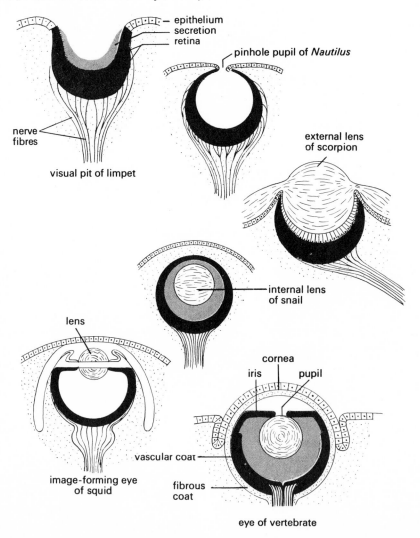

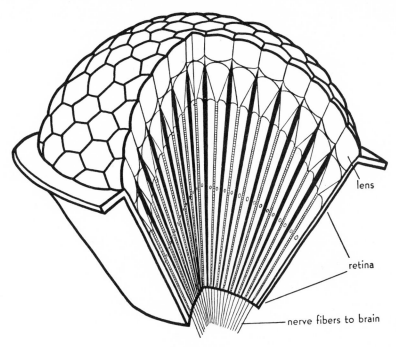

lens

retina

nerve fibers to brain

Fig. 11.4 *Three-dimensional cutaway view of compound eye of an arthropod. (Source: Buchsbaum, 1948, p. 246.)*

possess no specialized photoreceptors; rather, the entire body is light sensitive. However, most animals have a region on their body that is maximally sensitive to light. Of course, mere responsivity to light is quite a different matter from actually receiving an image. Indeed, many of the light-sensitive structures of lower forms of life act primarily to concentrate light upon a photosensitive pigment. That is, they serve as light-gathering rather than image-forming organs. It is from advanced stages of evolution that an *eikonogenic* or image-forming eye developed. The structural transition in light-sensitive organs from simple light gatherer to image former is suggested in Figure 11.3.

According to Wald (1959), only three of the major phyla have developed image-forming eyes: the arthropods (insects, crabs; see Figure 11.4), mollusks (squid, octopus), and vertebrates. Many different optical devices for forming an image have evolved within these phyla. For example, the cephalopod mollusk, Nautilus, has a pinhole eye (a small hole in an opaque surface forms an image on a surface behind it). The tiny arthropod, Copilia, has a lens and a single attached light receptor that moves back and forth scanning the image in a way similar to the method used by a TV camera.

All image-forming eyes have advantages and limitations. The pinhole eye provides an image in focus at all distances from the object viewed. However, it can admit only a small amount of light to its photosensitive tissue. The compound eye of arthropods (Figure 11.4) consists of a mosaic of tubular units, called *ommatidia,* that are clustered tightly together and arranged so that the outer surface forms a hemisphere. Each ommatidium registers only the light directly in front of it; this produces a single image constructed from an enormous number of separate signals. The compound eye is especially effective for detecting movement. However, this form of visual system is effective at only a very close object distance. In contrast, the vertebrate eye is quite effective in long-range viewing, but it cannot resolve images at the short distances at which the arthropod eye is effective.

ANATOMY OF THE VERTEBRATE EYE

The vertebrate eye is built on a single basic plan: From fish to mammal, all vertebrate eyes possess a photo-sensitive layer called a *retina,* and a lens whose optical properties are such that it focuses an image upon the retina. Figure 11.5 presents a cross-sectional slice of a human eye. We will first describe its major structural components and then discuss several important functional mechanisms. The eyeball, lying in a protective socket of the skull, is a globular structure, about 20 mm in diameter. The outer covering of the eyeball is a tough white opaque coat called the *sclera* (seen as the "white" of the eye).

The sclerotic covering at the front of the eye becomes the translucent membrane called the *cornea.* Light rays entering the cornea are refracted or bent by its surface. The cornea is approximately 11.6 mm in diameter, 0.8 mm thick at the center, and 1.0 mm thick at the periphery (Brown, 1965). A second layer of the eyeball called the *choroid* is attached to the sclera. It consists largely of blood vessels and provides a major source of nutrition for the eye. In addition, the choroid layer is heavily pigmented; this enables the absorption of most extraneous light entering the eye, thereby reducing reflections within the eyeball that might blur the image. However, some animals possess a retinal layer, called the *tapetum,* that reflects back some of the light entering the eye. It is the reflection of light from their retinae that accounts for the "eyeshine" that appears from the eyes of many familiar animals. What is occurring, say when we drive past a cat or dog at night, is that the animal's eyes are reflecting back some of the light of the car's headlights rather than absorbing the light as in the case of the human choroid layer. The function of the tapetum

Fig. 11.5 *Gross structure of the human eye. (From Color in Business, Science, and Industry, by D. B. Judd, Wiley, New York, 1952. Reprinted by permission of the publisher.)*

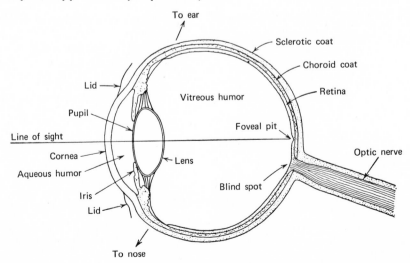

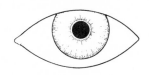

Fig. 11.6 *Optical similarity of diaphragm and iris of camera. Both adjust to the intensity of light.*

is not clear, though Walls (1963, pp. 228–246) suggests that it may play a role in acuity.

In the front of the eye the choroid is modified to form the *iris*. Behind the cornea, lying on the lens, the disk-like pigmented iris controls the amount of light entering the eye—a structural analogy to the diaphragm of a camera (see Figure 11.6). When lighting conditions are poor, the iris opens to increase the size of the *pupil*—the round black opening surrounded by the iris. The human pupil is circular but a variety of shapes exists for different species. Figure 11.7 shows the vertical slit pupil of a cat during constriction. Such a pupil allows an essentially nocturnal animal to hunt in bright day light (as in the case of the cat)

or to bask in the comfort of the sun (e.g., the crocodile) (Duke-Elder, 1958, p. 612).

In man the range of pupil size extends from 1.5 to over 9 mm in diameter (Goldwater, 1972). Pupil size is controlled by two opposing smooth muscles in the iris, the *sphincter* and the *dilator* (Figure 11.8). According to Brown (1965), the sphincter forms a ring of about 0.8 mm thick around the pupil and can shorten as much as 87% to constrict the pupil. The dilator consists of radial fibers in the iris.

The crystalline lens of the vertebrate eye divides it into two unequal chambers—a small one in front filled with watery fluid held under pressure, the *aqueous humor,* which helps to maintain the shape of the eye and provides the metabolic requirements of the cornea; and a larger chamber behind the lens filled with a jelly-like protein, the *vitreous humor.* These fluids, both transparent, aid in holding the lens in place and allow its housing to be flexible. A set of muscles, the *ciliary muscles,* attached to the lens by ligaments (the zonal fibers of Figure 11.8), controls its curvature, which varies depending on

Fig. 11.7 *The pupils of the cat in dilation (A), and in constriction showing the extremely narrow vertical slits (B). (Source: Duke-Elder, 1958, p. 613. Reprinted by permission of the publisher.)*

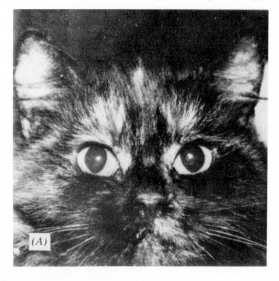 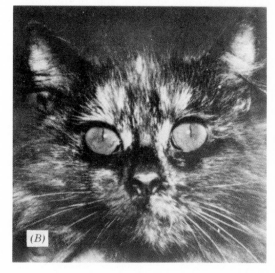

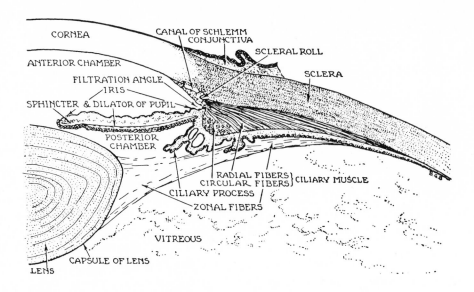

Fig. 11.8 *Detail of anterior segment of human eye, showing anatomy of structures affecting the pupillary response and curvature of the lens. (From J. L. Brown, in Vision an.` Visual Perception, edited by C. H. Graham, Wiley, New York, 1965, p. 44. Reprinted by permission of the publisher).*

the distance of the object focused. (We will discuss this mechanism in a separate section.) From a comparative viewpoint, lens size bears an interesting relation to the normal lighting conditions of an animal's habitat. Because large lenses can collect more light than smaller ones, nocturnal animals have evolved larger lenses relative to the size of their eyeballs than have day-active animals. Figure 11.9 points this out.

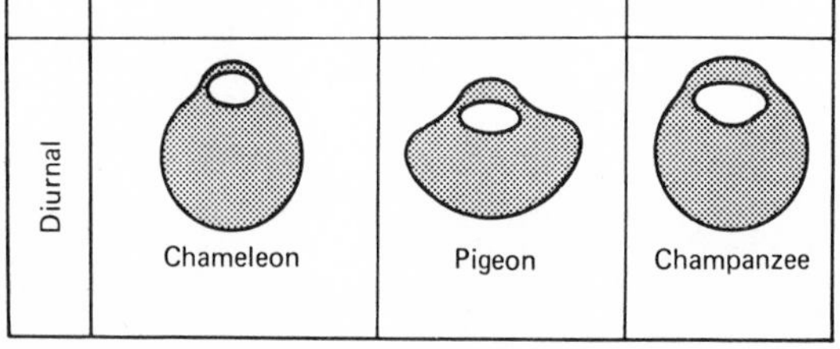

The Retina

Light passes through the lens to the retina at the back of the eyeball. The retina, which covers nearly 200° of the inside of the eyeball, is composed of a coating of interconnected nerve cells and photoreceptors that are responsive to light energy. Two morphologically distinct types of photoreceptors have been identified: *rods* and

Fig. 11.9 *Relative sizes of lenses in eyes of some nocturnal and diurnal animals. (Source: Marler and Hamilton, 1966, p. 319; after Duke-Elder, 1958, p. 605.)*

Group		
Lizards	Birds	Mammals
Nocturnal Gecko	Owl	Opossum
Diurnal Chameleon	Pigeon	Champanzee

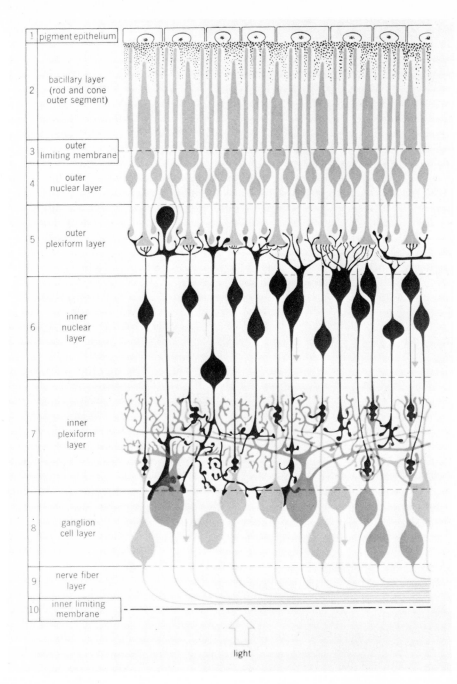

1	pigment epithelium
2	bacillary layer (rod and cone outer segment)
3	outer limiting membrane
4	outer nuclear layer
5	outer plexiform layer
6	inner nuclear layer
7	inner plexiform layer
8	ganglion cell layer
9	nerve fiber layer
10	inner limiting membrane

light

Fig. 11.10 *Schematic diagram of the neural structures and interconnections of the vertebrate retina. Notice that the photoreceptors do not face the light but point toward the choroid layer (not shown). (From Human Anatomy and Physiology, by J. Crouch & J. R. McClintic, Wiley, New York, 1971, p. 581. Reprinted by permission of the publisher.)*

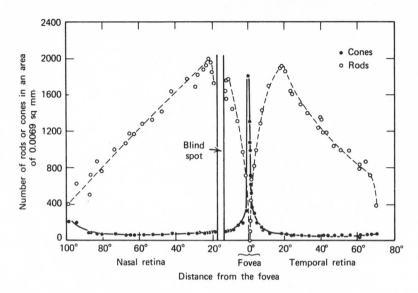

Fig. 11.11 *Distribution of rods and cones throughout the retina. The number of receptors per unit area from the fovea to the extreme periphery has been plotted. Cones are represented by solid, rods by open, circles. (Source: Chapanis, 1949, p. 7.)*

cones, named for their cylindrical and conic shapes respectively (see Figure 11.10). Rods, which in the primate retina number about 120 to 130 million, are heavily concentrated in the peripheral region of the retina. Cones, which number about 6 to 8 million, are primarily concentrated in a small pit or indentation about 0.3 mm across (subtending a visual angle of between 1° and 2°) called the *fovea.* The central region of the retina that includes the fovea is marked by a yellow pigment, the *macula lutea,* over an area 2 to 3 mm in diameter. The macula subtends a visual angle of about 6° to 8°. The cones vary in length from 0.020 to 0.090 mm and, aside from those at the fovea, vary in width between 0.002 and 0.008 mm. At the fovea they are as thin as 0.001 mm. The length of rods varies between 0.040 and 0.060 mm, and the average width is about 0.002 mm. The distribution of rods and cones over the retina is illustrated in Figure 11.11. The gap in the curve corresponds to that part of the retina where the optic nerve fibers leave the eye. There are no photo-

receptors in this area, and accordingly there is no vision when light strikes this region of the retina. It is appropriately termed the blind spot (sometimes called the *optic disc;* see Figure 11.12).

As illustrated in Figure 11.10, there is an apparently illogical relation between the location of the photoreceptors and incoming light in that the receptors do not face the light. In most

Fig. 11.12 *The blind spot. Close the left eye and fixate the right eye on the cross. Slowly move the page back and forth from the eye between 5 and 15 in (12.6 to 38 cm) until the position is reached at which the spot disappears. The spot is then falling on the region of the retina where the nerve fibers group together and leave the eye. There are no rods or cones at this region.*

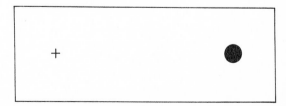

vertebrates, the photoreceptors are located in the back of the retina and nerve fibers connected to them are gathered together in front. This means that light must travel through the network of nerve fibers, blood vessels, and other supporting cells before it reaches the photoreceptors: The retina is thus functionally inside out. However, in operation this poses little problem, for the blood cells are quite small and the nerve fibers and related cells are more or less transparent. Furthermore, as Figure 11.13 points out, the nerve cells of the fovea are arranged in a spoke-like fashion so that they do not interfere with the incoming light rays.

Two major kinds of connections, as illustrated in Figure 11.10, exist between photoreceptors and the nerve fibers leading to the brain. Groups of rods (sometimes with cones) and cones (sometimes singly) connect with intermediate neurons, *bipolar cells* (not labeled in the figure but are in the *inner nuclear layer*), which in turn connect to *ganglion cells,* whose axons are the optic nerve fibers. The total number of bipolar and ganglion cells that is present in the periphery of the retina is much less than the number of rods. It follows that each bipolar and ganglion cell receives the input from a large number of rods. In the extreme peripheral regions of the retina, as many as several hundred rods may be connected to one bipolar cell. In contrast, in the cone-rich area of the retina, the fovea, the number of cones more or less matches the number of intermediate neurons. Thus, the most direct transmission between the retina and the brain is with cones at the fovea. However, it would be an oversimplification to assume that foveal cones are independently or directly linked to cortical cells. There are many lateral connections between foveal cones at the level of the ganglia. ". . . The activity in each ganglion cell is affected by the actions of a large number of different cones, and further, each cone influences the activity of a large number of ganglion cells" (Cornsweet, 1970, p. 139). The most reasonable assumption is that

Fig. 11.13 *Cross section of the central fovea of the human retina. The centermost region contains only cones, which are thin, long, and tightly grouped. Notice the spoke-like arrangement of the blood vessels and nerve fibers at the center region. This reduces the interference and distortion of the incoming light rays. (Source: Polyak, S., 1957, The Vertebrate Visual System, Chicago: University of Chicago Press, p. 276 Reprinted by permission of the publisher.)*

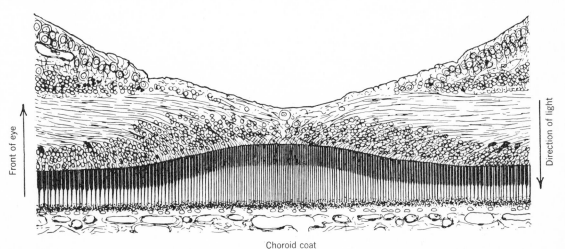

Front of eye

Direction of light

Choroid coat

cones have fewer intermediate connections than do rods.

There is some functional significance of the neural connections of rods and cones to the bipolar and ganglion cells. The fact that a number of rods share a common ganglion cell means that there is a convergence or pooling of receptor information from an appreciable part of the retina at a single ganglion cell. This summation of stimulation results in an increase in the likelihood of the common ganglion cell reaching the energy level necessary to fire (see Figure 11.14). This is an aid to *sensitivity,* to perceiving in low levels of illumination. Of course, the pooling of stimulus information from a number of rods at the ganglia detracts from the discrete information given by any single rod; hence, image resolution or *acuity* is correspondingly coarse. In contrast to the neural connections of rods, if only one or a very few receptors are connected to a single ganglion cell, which is the case for foveal cones, the photoreceptors are then capable of contributing more independent information, such as that required for resolving stimulus patterns. Accordingly, a foveal cone, owing to its neural connection, is capable of relaying more information about its source of stimulation than is a rod. In short, at the fovea there is a heavy concentration of cones, hence a greater number of independently stimulated nerve fibers and a greater capacity for differentiating an image. Indeed, when we look directly at a target we position our eyes so that the target image falls directly on the foveal cones. The result, of course, is increased acuity but at a sacrifice to sensitivity. Figure 11.14 points this out schematically.

Eyeball Mobility

Human eyes are set in orbits and are capable of rotating within the skull. The eyes are moved about by three pairs of oculomotor muscles, as illustrated in Figure 11.15. Eyeball mobility is a useful mechanism for it allows a person to track moving objects by moving the eyes smoothly without turning the head or body. Possession of

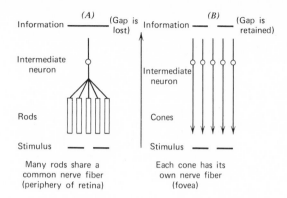

Fig. 11.14 *Highly simplified schematic diagram of neural connections of rods and cones to intermediate neurons. In (A) the stimulation from a number of rods converge on a single neuron. Thus sensitivity is high but acuity is low and information of the gap in the stimulus line is lost. In (B) there is no convergence of cone stimulation, and acuity is high. (From Psychology: Man in Perspective, by A. Buss, Wiley, New York, 1973, p. 191. Reprinted by permission of the publisher.)*

this capability enables a person to visually anchor on environmental stimuli even when undergoing postural changes. The eyes of many lower organisms are more rigidly attached to neighboring tissue. For example, the eyes of certain crustacea are rigid parts of the head, fixed and immobile. Ocular movements of these organisms must necessarily involve movement of the head or the entire body, thereby restricting the ability to track moving targets. Eye movement will be the topic of a separate section in the next chapter.

Placement of the Eyes and the Visual Field

Thus far we have discussed the functional anatomy of a single eye. However, vision typically involves two eyes. Vertebrates have either two laterally directed eyes at the sides of the head or two frontally directed eyes (see Figure 11.16). In the case of laterally directed eyes, this results in two separate fields of vision, a small degree of binocular overlap (the area seen by both eyes),

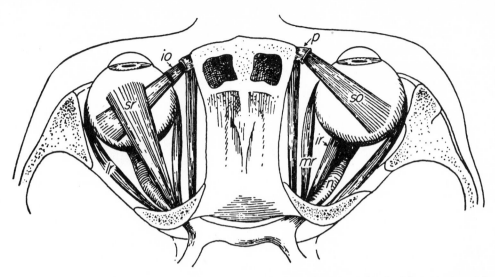

Fig. 11.15 *Oculomotor muscles of man, as seen from above in a dissected head. On the left, a portion of the superior oblique has been cut away to reveal the inferior oblique; on the right, the superior rectus has been removed to permit a view of the inferior rectus. io-inferior oblique; ir-inferior rectus; lr-lateral (external) rectus; mr-medial (internal) rectus; n-optic nerve; p-pulley through which tendon of superior oblique passes; so-tendinous portion of superior oblique; sr-superior rectus. (Source: Walls, 1963, p. 37.)*

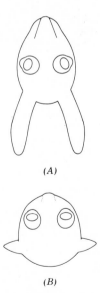

(A)

(B)

Fig. 11.16A *Laterally-directed eyes of the rabbit, typical of prey animals. Each eye looks in a different direction.*

Fig. 11.16B *Frontally-directed eyes of the cat, typical of predatory animals. Both eyes look in the same direction.*

and a relatively large total view. Laterally directed eyes are an obvious anatomical adaptation, especially for prey animals that must maintain continual vigilance against predators (see Figure 11.17). The panoramic vision of the rabbit, one of the most defenseless of mammals, is an example of this. In contrast, the frontal placement of the eyes, more typical of predators, creates a relatively narrow total visual field, but it also produces a greater degree of binocular overlap. Binocular overlap enhances the perception of depth and distance and provides for an accurate means of locating objects in space, two factors that are especially important to predatory animals and animals like primates, that require acute depth perception to perform manipulatory skills with their hands such as holding and grasping, and effecting leaping.

With frontally directed eyes there is a tendency toward conjugate (coupled) eye movements, carried out by the action of the eye muscles that control the rotation of the eyes in their orbits. The result is that movement of both eyes is

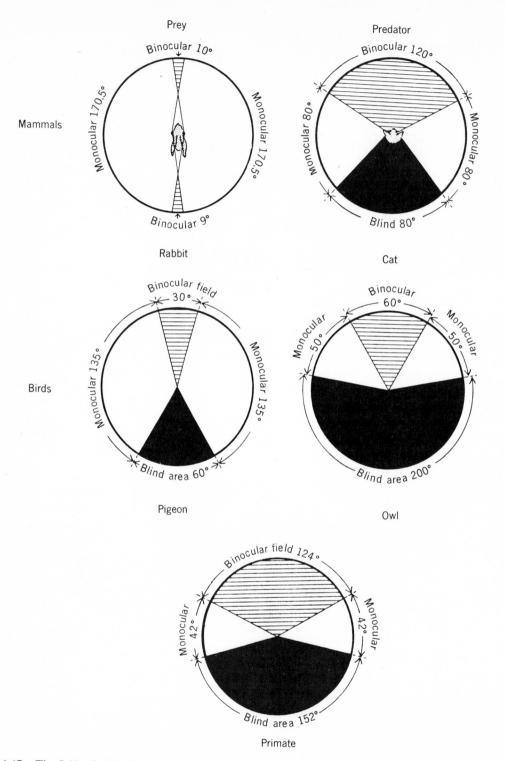

Fig. 11.17 *The fields of vision for some prey and predatory mammals and birds and for the primate. Binocular field refers to the area seen by both eyes. (Source: Duke-Elder, 1958, pp. 673, 682, 689.)*

equal—each eye cannot independently explore the visual field. This style of viewing is necessary if both foveae are to register the same pattern of environmental signals.

In sum, then, there is a tendency for prey animals to possess laterally directed eyes. This results in a larger total visual field and less binocular overlap than is the case for predatory animals or animals with a high degree of manipulative skills. The latter, in contrast, possess frontally directed eyes, a reduced overall visual field, and a greater degree of binocular overlap. Thus, there is a trade-off between frontal and lateral viewing, the style adopted depending on the survival needs of the species (Duke-Elder, 1958).

ACCOMMODATION

Two optical mechanisms of the anterior portion of the eye are of special importance to perception: accommodation and pupil mobility. As light enters the eyeball, it is initially refracted or bent by the cornea. It is further refracted by the lens in a dynamic process termed *accommodation*. Accommodation refers to the variable refractive capacity of the lens, that is, the change in the shape of the lens necessary to bring an image into sharp focus on the retina. When fixating on a near target, the lens refracts differently from when fixating on a far one. In the normal human, variations in lens shape permit a range of accommodation from 20 feet (6 m) to about 4 in (10.2 cm) (Brown, 1965).

The refractive power of the eye is expressed in units called *diopters* (*D*). A lens with a focal length of 1 meter is designated as having the refractive power of 1 diopter (1 *D*). (The *focal length* of a lens is the distance between the lens and a sharp image it forms of a very distant object; see Figure 11.18.) The refractive power of a lens is expressed as the reciprocal of its focal length (in meters). Thus, lenses whose focal lengths are 1/10 meter, 1/4 meter, or 5 meters have the refractive or dioptric power of 10 *D*, 4 *D* and 0.2 *D*, respectively. Notice that the higher the dioptric power of the lens, the greater the amplitude of accommodation and the closer an object can be to the eye and produce a clear image. The total refractive power of the normal adult eye is approximately 66 *D* with the cornea contributing about twice as much refractive power as the lens.

Accommodation is not found in all levels of vertebrates, and it may differ somewhat for different animals. In general, there are two different accommodative techniques used by vertebrates for

Fig. 11.18 *The focal length of a lens is the distance between the lens and the sharp image it forms of a distant object. In the figure, the lens has been moved back and forth until the image of the tree is in sharp focus on the wall. The distance between the lens and the wall is the focal length of the lens. (Source: Cornsweet, 1970, p. 38. Reprinted by permission of the author and publisher.)*

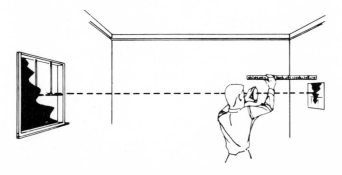

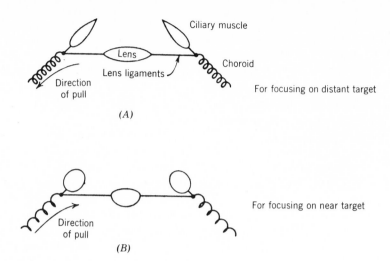

Fig. 11.19   *Changes occurring during accommodation. (A) Ciliary muscle is relaxed for focusing on distant target. Elastic pull of choroid places tension on lens ligaments, flattening lens. (B) Ciliary muscle contracted for focusing on close target. Tension removed from lens ligaments, choroid is stretched, and the lens rounds up of its own elasticity. (Source: Crouch & McClintic, 1971, p. 584.)*

achieving a focused image—moving the lens in relation to the retina, or changing the curvature of the lens. The former technique is similar to the focusing mechanisms employed in the camera. The camera lens moves forward for focusing on a nearby target and moves backwards for focusing on a distant target. This accommodative technique involving movement of the lens is used by fish. The second technique of accommodation, used by higher species, is to change the curvature of the lens—flattening the lens for focusing on distant targets and thickening it when focusing on nearby ones. This change in lens shape is related to relaxing or contracting the ciliary muscle, which is attached to the zonular ligaments that suspend the lens in place (see Figures 11.8 and 11.19).

An interesting accommodative-type adaptation to viewing through more than one medium (air and water) has evolved with some ducks. Because water reduces the refractive capacity of the cornea, targets appear out of focus when viewed in water. However, as Cornsweet (1970) notes,

some diving ducks have a compensatory mechanism for this: Their eyelids are transparent and serve as additional lenses. These ducks dive with closed lids, thus adding to the total refractive power of their eyes. Indeed, this combination of the refractive power of the lid, cornea, and lens is sufficient to form images in the retinal plane when viewing is done under water.

For man the accommodative ability develops in infancy. The newborn human infant, less than one month of age, can accommodate but only on targets at one distance, whose median value is 19 cm (Haynes, White, & Held, 1965). Images of targets nearer or farther away are proportionately blurred. However, during the second month of infancy the accommodative system begins to respond adaptatively to changes in target distance and approximates adult performance by the fourth month.

Accommodation has limits—as an object is brought toward the face, the ciliary muscle undergoes contraction and the curvature of the lens increases, but when it cannot contract further, the object goes out of focus. If we are forced to maintain continued focus on near objects, say six inches (15.2 cm) or less, the ciliary muscles soon fatigue and eye strain sets in. Generally, we must resort to optical devices to enable prolonged examination of objects that are located quite close to the eye.

As a target is gradually brought close to the eye, a distance is reached at which even the strongest contraction of the ciliary muscle will not produce a distinct image of the target. This is because the resultant light rays are so divergent that, even with full accommodation, the lens system cannot bring them to a focus on the retina. The nearest distance at which a target can be seen clearly, with full accommodation, is called the *near point.*

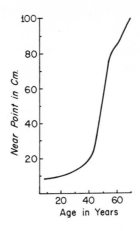

Fig. 11.20   *Increase in distance to near point of vision with age. Near point refers to nearest distance at which a target can be seen clearly. (From Ruch, T. C., et al: Neurophysiology, Philadelphia, W.-B. Saunders Company, 1965, p. 406. Reprinted by permission of the publisher.)*

Refractive Errors

Accommodation of the human eye deteriorates with age and a form of refractive error called *presbyopia* occurs. With increasing age the elasticity of the lens progressively diminishes so that it becomes more difficult for the ciliary muscle to change the lens' curvature to accommodate for near objects. One result of presbyopia is that the near point increases (see Figure 11.20) with the aging process. Hence, older persons with uncorrected lenses must often hold reading material abnormally far from their face in order to focus adequately.

As we noted above, when the ciliary muscle is relaxed an optically normal or *emmetropic* eye forms an image of a distant target on the retina (Figure 11.21a). As the distance between target and eye is reduced, the lens must accommodate or the focal plane of the image will be behind the retina, resulting in a blurred retinal image. In this instance, the lack of proper accommodation is called *hypermetropia,* or farsightedness (see Figure 11.21b). This occurs because the eyeball is too short for the accommodative capacity of the lens. Though the eye can focus on a distant target,

it cannot focus accurately on one nearby. To correct for hypermetropia a converging (convex) lens must be worn to increase the refraction of the lens. A second refractive error, shown in Figure 11.21c, is called *myopia* or nearsightedness. The image of a distant target is brought to a focus in front of the retina because the eyeball is too long for the accommodative capability of the lens. Thus, the myopic eye can focus on near targets well but cannot focus accurately on distant ones. To correct for myopia a diverging (concave) lens is required to diminish the refraction and focus the image on the retina. A note of interest concerns the recent research on the origin of myopia. Although generally recognized to be due primarily to heredity, Young (1970) has indicated that myopia may be partly due to a substantial amount of near viewing during childhood, requiring continuous accommodation (e.g., as in learning to read).

Other forms of refractive errors, though not related to accommodation, are called *lens aberrations.* As Figure 11.22a shows, light rays passing through the peripheral parts of a spherical lens are

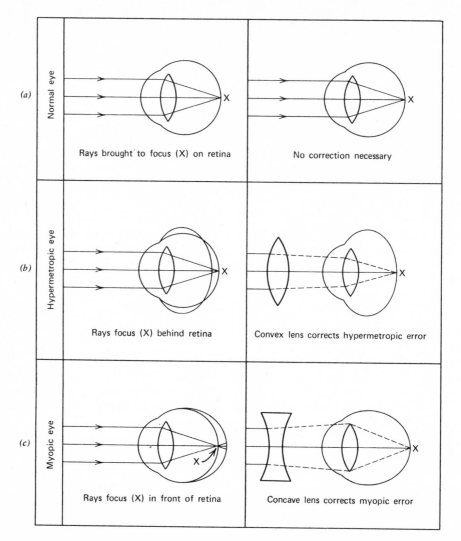

Fig. 11.21 *Diagram of the three refractive states of the eye. a: Emmetropic (normal); b: Hypermetropic (farsighted); c: Myopic (Nearsighted). The diagram indicates the kind of lens required to bring the light rays to a focus on the retina. (From Basic Anatomy and Physiology of the Human Body, by J. R. McClintic, Wiley, New York, 1975, p. 302. Reprinted by permission of the publisher.)*

refracted more strongly and brought to a focus at a closer plane than those rays passing through the central regions, a phenomenon called *spherical aberration*. That is, the rays from the marginal portion of the lens meet at a point nearer the lens than do the inner rays. Uncorrected, this can result in a blurred image. However, there are a number of corneal and lens mechanisms that serve in part to compensate for spherical aberration. Furthermore, under moderately good lighting conditions, the pupil contracts to limit the rays of light to the central part of the lens (Riggs, 1965). A second form of lens aberration, called *chromatic aberration,* shown in Figure 11.22*b,* is due to the fact that lenses made of a single material refract rays of short wavelengths more strongly than those of longer wavelengths. Thus blue, for example, is brought to a shorter focus than red. However, this is rarely a problem, since some of the very short wavelengths, where the chromatic error is greatest, are filtered out by the lens' yellow pigmentation acting as a color filter. About 8% of the visible spectrum is so absorbed by the lens. (Indeed, persons who have their lenses removed, as in cataract surgery, have excellent ultraviolet vision.) However, as Wald (1950) points out: "This boon is distributed over one's lifetime, for the lens becomes a deeper yellow and makes more of the ordinary violet and blue invisible as one grows older." (p. 36).

Astigmatism

Ideally the refractive surfaces of the cornea and the lens are spherical with the curvatures equalized along all meridians. When the corneal surface is not spherical, an error of refraction called *astigmatism* occurs. Basically the astigmatic surface produces meridians of differing curvatures. In most instances of astigmatism the corneal surface is flatter from side to side than it is vertically. This produces a meridian of least curvature at right angles to a meridian of greatest curvature. The effect is that light rays falling along the meridian of greatest curvature will tend to reach a focus before those rays falling along the meridian of least curvature, resulting in the blurring and distortion of parts of images. The correction for astigmatism is to employ a lens that af-

Fig. 11.22*a* *Schematic of spherical aberration. The light rays that pass through the edge of a spherical lens are brought to a shorter focus than those that pass through the center. The result is that the image formed of a point is a blur circle.*

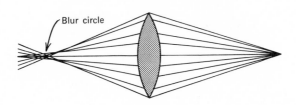

Fig. 11.22*b* *Schematic of chromatic aberration. When light of various wavelengths is refracted by a lens made of a single material the light of shorter wavelengths is refracted more than that of longer wavelengths, for example, blue (B) is brought to a shorter focus than red (R). The result is that the image formed of a white point is a chromatic blur circle.*

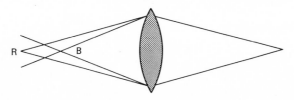

fects one set of rays more than the other, that is, to equalize the refraction in the meridians of least and greatest curvature.

PUPIL MOBILITY

The variable pupil, controlled by the iris, is ordinarily recognized as having two reflexive functions. It maintains an optimal intensity of light entering the eye. Too little light will not sufficiently excite the photoreceptors in the retina, and too much light will render them inefficient or perhaps injure them. When there is little available light, the pupil opens wide—dilates. When there is much light, the pupil closes down or constricts. A second function of the pupil's mobility is to restrict the incoming light mainly to the central and optically best part of the lens, the part that provides the best focus. As we noted with spherical aberration, the constriction of the pupil tends to keep out light that strikes the periphery of the lens, such light as would be focused at a different plane from that coming through the center of the lens. A small pupil also enhances acuity by keeping out extraneous light. We perform this function when squinting in the presence of glare, thereby cutting down the light that enters the eye. The same effect may be achieved by viewing through a long tube, a procedure that yields somewhat sharper images than can be obtained with the naked eye. Of course, the restriction of peripheral light cannot occur when lighting is poor and a full aperture opening is required. Thus, acuity or image resolution is greatest when the available light is bright and the pupil is appropriately constricted.

The amount of available light is not the only determiner of pupillary variation. Heinrich in 1896 (see Bakan, 1967) and more recently Hess (e.g., 1965) have noted that the size of the pupil varies in response to strong emotional states, certain forms of ongoing mental activity and, in general, serves as a measure of arousal. Hess

(1965; Hess & Polt, 1960, 1966) demonstrated that while a subject is viewing visual stimuli his pupil size may serve as an indication of the interest value of the content of the stimuli. For example, the pupils of males dilated in reaction to viewing pictures of sharks and female pinups, and they constricted slightly to male pinups. In contrast, the pupils of female subjects constricted to the pictures of sharks and the female pinups but dilated to the male pinups. Differential pupillary changes to the same stimuli have also been reported by sexual orientation of the viewer. Thus the pupils of heterosexual males dilated more to the viewing of pictures of nude women than of nude men, whereas homosexual males showed the opposite response, dilating their pupils more to pictures of nude men than to nude women (Hess, Seltzer, & Schlien, 1965). Correlated attitude and pupillary reactions have also been observed for such diverse stimuli as foods (Hess & Polt, 1966) and political figures (Barlow, J. D., 1969).

Mental activity also produces changes in pupil size. Hess and Polt (1964) had subjects solve a graded series of verbally presented multiplication problems. Typically, the size of the pupils of each subject showed a gradual increase beginning with the presentation of the problem and reaching maximum diameter immediately before the subjects' verbal answer was given. This is shown in Table 11.2, which presents the percentage of increase in pupil size by problem. In addition the table indicates that pupil size increases with problem difficulty. The notion that pupil size reflects mental effort has generally been supported (e.g., Kahneman & Beatty, 1966; Kahneman, Onuska, & Wolman, 1969; see also Goldwater, 1972, p. 345).

It is clear from our discussion that attentional and emotional factors are reflected in pupil mobility. However, an exact formulation of the cause-and-effect relationship of attitudes and mental activity to pupillary reactions has yet to be worked out (see Goldwater, 1972).

Table 11.2
THE PERCENTAGE OF INCREASE IN
PUPIL DIAMETER[a]

Subject	Problem			
	7 × 8	8 × 13	13 × 14	16 × 23
H.H.	15.2	15.8	20.2	22.9
E.K.	9.8	14.1	24.9	21.2
T.H.	10.0	8.9	13.5	23.1
G.B.	4.0	8.8	7.8	11.6
P.M.	16.2	9.1	25.1	29.5
Mean	10.8	11.3	18.3	21.6

[a] At the point of a solution of a problem as compared with the diameter of the pupil before the problem was posed. Source: Hess & Polt, *Science*, *140*, 1964, 1191, December 1970. Copyright © 1970 by the American Association for the Advancement of Science.

EYE AND BRAIN

There is a series of complex connections in the pathway between the retina and the visual projection area of the brain's occipital lobe. A schematic diagram of the human visual system is shown in Figure 11.23. The axons of the ganglion cells group and leave the eye via the blind spot and converge at the *optic chiasma*. At the chiasma, in man, fibers from the inner or *nasal* halves of each retina decussate (cross) whereas those from the outside or *temporal* halves of each retina do not. After this partial decussation the nerve fibers, called *tracts*, make connections at several relay stations. The most important is the *lateral geniculate nucleus*, the relay center for vision in the thalamus. Visual radiations from the lateral geniculate nucleus extend to the visual area (occipital lobe) of the cerebral cortex; some fibers also connect to vision areas in the midbrain that are involved with ocular reflexes.

As shown in Figure 11.24, light from the right visual field stimulates the left halves of each retina (i.e., the temporal and nasal halves of the left and right eyes, respectively) and light from the left visual field stimulates the right halves of each retina (the nasal and temporal halves of the left and right eyes, respectively). It follows that stimulation of the left halves of each retina activates the left occipital lobe. Similarly, stimulation of the right halves of each retina activates the right visual cortical area. This means the right

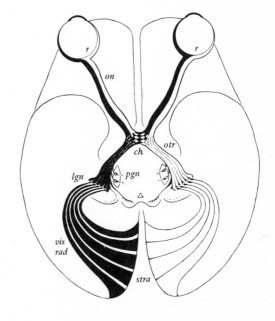

Fig. 11.23 *Diagram of the human visual system drawn into an outline of the brain. Shown are the eyes, including the retinae (r), optic nerves (on), optic chiasma (ch), optic tracts (otr), terminating in subcortical visual centers, the principal one of which is the lateral geniculate nucleus (lgn); visual radiations (vis rad), originating in the lateral geniculate nucleus terminate in the striate area (stra) of the occipital lobes. Some optic tracts terminate in the pregeniculate nucleus (pgn). Observe that fibers originating in the inner or nasal halves of the retinae intercross at the chiasma, whereas fibers originating in the outer or temporal halves of the retinae do not cross. (Source: Polyak, S., 1957, The Vertebrate Visual System, Chicago: University of Chicago Press, p. 289. Reprinted by permission of publisher.)*

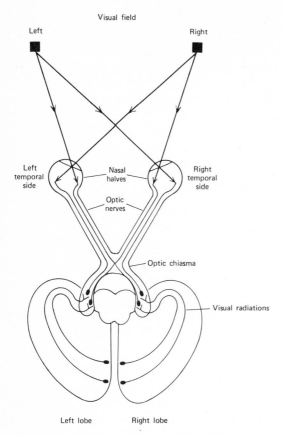

Visual field

Left   Right

Left
temporal   Nasal   Right
side   halves   temporal
                                     side
                  Optic
                  nerves

Optic chiasma

Visual radiations

Left lobe   Right lobe

Fig. 11.24 *Highly simplified schematic diagram of the human visual system showing the projection of the visual fields through the system. Observe that the right half of the visual field projects on the left half of each retina (and to the left of the brain). Similarly, the left half of the visual field projects on the right half of each retina. (From Basic Anatomy and Physiology of the Human Body, by J. R. McClintic, Wiley, New York, 1975, p. 305. Reprinted by permission of the publisher.)*

visual field is represented on the left side of the brain, and the left visual field on the right side of the brain. Thus, only half of the total visual field is projected on each occipital lobe.

The relation of the visual field to the visual pathway is indicated when plotting the results of lesions in various parts of visual projection

pathways. In Figure 11.25*A*, the optic nerve has been cut on the right side, which produces complete blindness in that eye. In Figure 11.25*B*, the cut has been made through the optic chiasma, which severs the crossed fibers from the nasal halves of the two retinae. This produces blindness for the temporal parts of the visual field. In Figure 11.25*C*, the right optic tract is cut and the subject is blind for the left side of the visual field, that is, visual function is lost in the right halves of both the retinae. This is a condition known as *homonymous hemianopia* and it may occur for either the left or right visual field, depending on which tract has been cut.

Our discussion of the partial crossing of optic fibers at the chiasma holds only for mammals. According to Walls (1963), for most vertebrates below mammals (e.g., fish and birds) all the optic nerve fibers from each eye cross over at the chiasma in a total decussation to form optic tracts on the opposite side. Thus, each eye is connected only with the opposite half of the brain. For mammals the relative amount of uncrossed fibers is closely proportional to the degree of frontal direction to the eyes. Walls (1963) writes that about 12 to 16% of the fibers remain uncrossed in the horse, 20% in the rat and opossum, 25% in the dog, one-third in the cat, and it reaches a maximum of one-half in higher primates.

Receptive Fields

As we have noted, there are numerous complex interconnections between the photoreceptors of the retina and the cortical cells of the visual area of the brain. However, the incoming pattern of light projected on the retina provides the sort of information that the nervous system is adapted to receive and this information does reach the brain in a more or less intact form. A direct means of studying the relationship between the retina and various loci of the visual system is by recording the electrical responses of single nerve cells to light patterns. Basically a microelectrode is implanted, ideally, in a single cell of the ganglia,

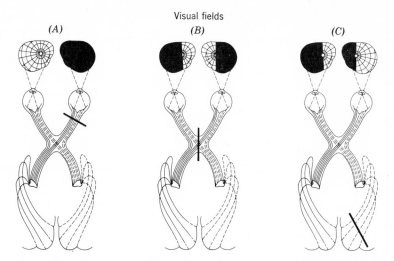

Fig. 11.25 *Visual field defects resulting from lesions at three locations of the visual pathway. Affected areas of the visual field are darkened.*

some relay station, or in the visual area of the cortex of an experimental animal. The animal is then shown an assortment of stimuli varying in size, orientation, and pattern, each projecting over a different region of the retina, until one of the stimuli produces some electrical activity in the cell or neuron (see Figure 11.26). The result is that an area of the visual field called a *receptive*

field is mapped out on which the presentation of a stimulus of sufficient intensity or quality will produce the firing of a sensory cell (Henry & Bishop, 1971). In short, the receptive field for a given receptor cell is that part of the visual field that excites or inhibits the cell. Employing such a technique it has been possible to map the receptive field for various loci of the visual system.

Fig. 11.26 *Experimental arrangement for mapping receptive fields. An electrode is inserted into a cell at some point in the visual system of the experimental animal. Various light stimuli are projected on a screen in front of the animal's eyes. The impulse activity of individual cells in response to the stimuli indicates the characteristics of the receptive field. (Reprinted by permission of the publisher from Mussen, P., & Rosenzweig, M. R., Psychology: An Introduction, 1973, Lexington, Mass.: D. C. Heath and Company, p. 672.)*

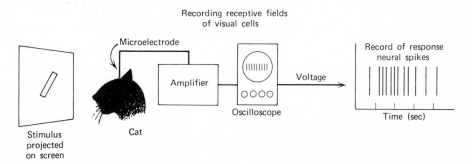

Consider the receptive fields for ganglion cells. Typically ganglion cells fire at fairly steady rates in the absence of any light stimulation (20 to 30 times per second). In one investigation a microelectrode was inserted in a ganglion cell of a cat (Kuffler, 1953). When a tiny spot of light was then projected into the cat's eye and was moved over various regions of the retina, the steady state was observed to vary. That the ganglion cell's rate of discharge was maximally altered by shining a small spot of light on a small circular retinal area indicates that the cell's receptive field is small and approximately circular. However, as Figure 11.27 illustrates, the light stimulus alters the ganglion cell's discharge rate in different ways, depending on the part of the receptive field that is stimulated. In one type of ganglion cell, the receptive field consists of a small circular "on" area, in which the impulse rate of the cell increases at the onset of the light. Light stimulation to a surrounding peripheral "off" zone inhibits the ganglion cell's neural activity, and the cell shows a burst of impulses when the light stimulus is removed. Another type of ganglion cell has a reversed form of receptive field, consisting of an inhibitory "off" center and an excitatory "on" periphery. Light striking only an "on" region produces a strong excitatory response. The more "on" area thus stimulated, the more vigorous the response. However, "on" and "off" regions are mutually antagonistic: If one spot of light is shone on an "on" area and a second spot on its adjacent "off" area, the two effects tend to neutralize each other, resulting in very weak "on" or "off" responses. Thus, diffusely lighting up the whole retina, thereby simultaneously affecting receptors throughout the retina, does not affect a single ganglion cell as much as does a small spot of light precisely covering its receptive field center.

As receptive fields are plotted for cells lying closer to the brain, the optic array necessary for excitation becomes finer and more precise. Many of the significant findings on the functioning of the visual cortex come from the work of Hubel and Wiesel with cats (e.g., 1959, 1962; Hubel, 1963). They have reported that instead of having circular receptive fields with concentric "on" and "off" regions, as in the case of retinal ganglion cells, the neurons of the visual cortex of the cat's brain (and presumably most mammals) possess receptive fields of a very different character. Some cortical neurons possess very small receptive fields (e.g., subtending less than a degree of arc) and some possess relatively large receptive fields, especially in the peripheral parts of the retina (e.g., 32° of arc) (Hubel and Wiesel, 1962). Some cells have comparatively simple receptive fields (see Figure 11.28) in that an optimum cortical response will occur only from a narrow slit or bar of light (e.g., a dark bar of light against a light

Fig. 11.27 *An oscilloscope record shows strong firing by an "on" center type of cell when a circular spot of light strikes the field center. If the spot hits an "off" (or peripheral) area, the firing is suppressed until the light goes off. (Reprinted by permission of the publisher from Mussen, P., & Rosenzweig, M. R., Psychology: An Introduction 1973, Lexington, Mass.: D. C. Heath and Company, p. 627.)*

Examples of receptive fields

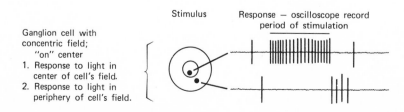

Ganglion cell with
concentric field;
    "on" center
1. Response to light in
   center of cell's field.
2. Response to light in
   periphery of cell's field.

Stimulus

Response — oscilloscope record
period of stimulation

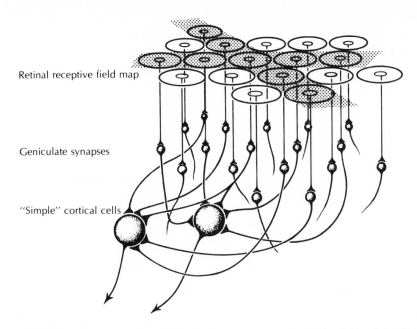

Retinal receptive field map

Geniculate synapses

"Simple" cortical cells

Fig. 11.28 *Semischematic diagram of a set of neural connections for the receptive fields of simple cortical cells in the brain of the cat (as suggested by Hubel and Wiesel). Two simple cells are shown, each of which collects inputs from cells in the geniculate whose receptive fields are all in a row. The simple cells fire if any one or more of their input neurons are firing. (Source: Cornsweet, 1970, p. 432. Reprinted by permission of the author and publisher.)*

background or the reverse). Some cortical cells have receptive fields that require that the bar of light be of a particular length or be placed in a certain orientation or position (see Figure 11.29). Still more complex cells have receptive fields that will produce cortical activity only if the light stimulus is of a limited length, is properly orientated, *and* moves in a certain direction across the retina (See Figure 11.30). Deviations from these requirements may yield weak responses or none at all. In addition, cortical cells have been identified that are differentially sensitive to the size, shape, direction of movement, orientation, and color dimensions of the receptive field (Gross, Bender, & Rocha-Miranda, 1969; Gross, Rocha-Miranda, & Bender, 1972).

In addition, there are cortical cells that react to precise and distinct stimulus configurations that fall within a relatively large region of the visual field, regardless of orientation and location.

This suggests that these cells are generalizing or abstracting a common feature from a number of cortical cells and their respective fields. Perhaps these complex cells are in turn fired by the initial activation of a number of more specific cortical cells, suggesting a hierarchical organization of the visual cortex. These findings indicate that visual patterns are represented neurophysiologically by complex combinations of cortical cell activity and furthermore that there are analyzing mechanisms in the brain that select out certain features of the visual stimulus.

There is much evidence that the complex cortical organization described for the cat's visual system applies to many other species, especially phylogenetically higher species, for example, primates (Hubel & Wiesel, 1968; Bridgeman, 1972), including man (Thomas, 1970). However, it is not typical of the visual systems of lower species. In contrast, animals possessing a com-

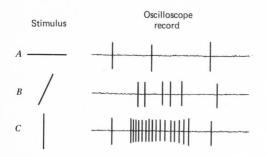

Fig. 11.29 *Oscilloscope record of a cortical cell whose maximal response is to a vertically oriented stimulus. Horizontal stimulus at (A) produces no response; slight tilt at (B) produces a weak response; vertical stimulus (at C) produces a strong response. (Reprinted by permission of the publisher from Mussen, P., & Rosenzweig, M. R., Psychology: An Introduction, 1973, Lexington, Mass.: D. C. Heath and Company, p. 627.)*

paratively primitive visual cortex (e.g., the rabbit and ground squirrel) or lacking it completely (e.g., the pigeon and frog) usually have more highly developed integrative mechanisms in the retina (Michael, 1969).

Lettvin and his colleagues (see Lettvin, Maturana, McCullough, & Pitts, 1959) have published an important neurophysiological analysis of the frog's vision that identifies several distinct kinds of pattern or form detectors in the retina of the frog. By recording the neural activity of single fibers in the frog's optic nerve in response to different visual stimuli, several distinct types of fibers have been identified, each type concerned with a different sort of pattern or visual event. There were fibers that reacted to sharp edges and borders, movement of edges, general dimming of illumination, or rapid general darkening. Most interesting were the "bug perceivers," so called by the authors because these were nerve fibers that responded best to small dark objects intermittently moving across the visual field. In the authors' words:

> Such a fiber responds best when a dark
> object, smaller than a receptive field, enters

that field, stops, and moves about intermittently thereafter. The response is not affected if the lighting changes or if the background (say a picture of grass and flowers) is moving, and is not there if only the background, moving or still, is in the field. Could one better describe a system for detecting an accessible bug? (P. 1951)

The functional value of bug perceivers to the frog, primarily an insect eater, is obvious. Thus the frog, possessing a primitive brain, has a highly complex retina that enables much of the processing, organizing, and interpretation of visual stimuli to occur peripherally. It appears that whether visual information is processed at the retina or in the brain depends on the evolutionary development of the species.

This chapter served as the introduction to the nature of the visual stimulus, light or radiant electromagnetic energy. Color or hue is the psychological correlate to the wavelength of light, and brightness is the psychological correlate to

Fig. 11.30 *Cortical cell sensitive to the direction of motion. This cell responds strongly only when the stimulus is moved down. It responds weakly to upward motion, and does not respond at all to sideways motion. (Reprinted by permission of the publisher from Mussen, P., & Rosenzweig, M. R., Psychology: An Introduction, 1973, Lexington, Mass.: D. C. Heath and Company, p. 627.)*

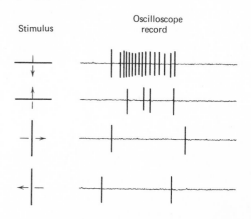

the physical intensity or the amount of radiant energy. The specification and measurement of the intensity dimension of light was examined in terms of the radiant energy falling on a surface—incident light or illuminance, and the intensity of a light reaching the eye from a surface—reflected light or luminance.

The basic anatomical structures of the eye were outlined and the functioning of certain parts were elaborated. The major parts given were the cornea, the iris and pupil, the lens, and their supporting structures. The retina and its neural connections and photoreceptors, the rods and cones, were identified and described. The functional significance of the neural connections of rods and cones for effecting sensitivity and acuity, respectively, was examined.

Some evolutionary trends in the placement of the eyes and binocular overlap were given. It was noted that there is a tendency for prey animals to possess laterally directed eyes resulting in a larger total visual field and less binocular overlap than is found in predatory animals or animals with a high degree of manipulative skill, such as primates.

The dynamic processes of pupil mobility and accommodation were described. Some errors of lens refraction were specified: presbyopia, hypermetropia, myopia, spherical and chromatic aberration, and astigmatism.

Finally, the complex connections in the neural pathways between the retina and the visual projection area of the brain were examined and the notion of receptive fields for various loci of the visual system, including the occipital lobe, was discussed.

The emphasis in the previous chapter was on structures and related mechanisms of the visual system. In this chapter we will discuss the functioning of these structures and some resultant basic visual phenomena.

SCOTOPIC AND PHOTOPIC VISION

The distinctions between rods and cones with respect to anatomy, relative distribution, and neural connections were described in the preceding chapter. These distinctions are also reflected in their functional properties. Vision accomplished with cones has been termed *photopic* vision and that with rods *scotopic* vision. A summary of the anatomical and functional properties of photopic and scotopic vision is given in Table 12.1. The relative number of rods and cones found in many species shows certain ecological trends. Nocturnal animals have primarily rod retinae. Accordingly, nocturnal animals possess retinae that are best suited for night vision—a high degree of light sensitivity rather than acuity. In contrast, diurnal or day-active animals have either relatively rod-free retinae (e.g., birds) or as

in the case of some species such as primates, possess retinae with both rods and cones.

ADAPTATION

One of the functional differences between rods and cones occurs in response to the general conditions of lighting.

When moving abruptly from a well-lighted to a poorly lit or dark environment, we initially experience a condition of temporary blindness. However, gradually some of the visual features in the dim surroundings become perceptible and we are able to resolve details. The process of adjustment to a dimly illuminated environment is called *dark adaptation*. One means of measuring the course of dark adaptation is as follows: The subject is first exposed to a brightly illuminated surface for a short period of time. This reduces the subject's sensitivity and also provides a well-defined starting level from which the temporal course of dark adaptation can be traced. The subject is then exposed to a dark environment, and at various intervals over the course of time, measurements are made of the absolute threshold for a light stimulus. The stimulus is of a specific wave-

Table 12.1
PROPERTIES OF PHOTOPIC AND SCOTOPIC VISION OF THE HUMAN EYE[a]

	Photopic (cone)	Scotopic (rod)
Receptor	Cones (ca. 7 million)	Rods (ca. 120 million)
Retinal location	Concentrated at center, fewer in periphery	General in periphery, none in fovea
Neural processing	Discriminative	Summative
Peak wavelength	555 nm	505 nm
Luminance level	Daylight (1 to 10^7 mL)	Night (10^{-6} to 1 mL)
Color vision	Normally trichromatic	Achromatic
Dark adaptation	Rapid (ca. 7 min)	Slow (ca. 40 min)
Spatial resolution	High acuity	Low acuity
Temporal resolution	Fast reacting	Slower reacting

[a] Source: L. A. Riggs, in *Experimental Psychology* (3rd ed.), edited by J. W. Kling and L. A. Riggs, Holt, Rinehart & Winston, 1971, p. 283.

length, duration, and energy level and strikes a precise area on the retina. The result is a curve relating the minimum energy required to reach threshold as a function of time in the dark. Figure 12.1 presents a typical dark adaptation curve. The figure shows the decrease in the threshold (or increase in sensitivity, plotted on the ordinate) with continued exposure to the darkened environment (shown on the abscissa).

The dark adaptation curve of Figure 12.1 is composed of two segments, reflecting the two different rates of adaptive change taking place. The upper branch is for cones and the lower one for rods. During the early stages of adaptation there is an initial rapid fall in threshold which quickly reaches a stable plateau; this reflects the increase in sensitivity for cones. The total gain in the sensitivity of cones is much less extensive than that of the rods and it occurs in about 5 min of dark exposure. The lower segment of the curve of Figure 12.1 represents the dark adaptation of rods. The increase in sensitivity over time for rods requires from 20 to 30 min of continual exposure to the dark. Thus, after about a half-hour of dark adaptation the sensitivity of the eye is many times greater than what it was at the onset of the dark adaptation process. A speculation on the temporal course of dark adaptation is offered by Buss (1973):

At first glance the half hour required to adapt fully to the dark of night would appear to be maladaptive. A visually deficient animal would surely fall prey to other animals under these conditions, but . . . rapid changes from light to dark occur mainly in man's technologically advanced civilization. In nature a rapid change from light to dark would occur only when an animal entered a cave, and most animals tend to avoid caves. The natural transition from light to dark requires approximately 20

Fig. 12.1 *Change in the visual threshold during the course of dark adaptation. The top branch of the curve is for cones, the bottom one for the rods. (After Hecht & Shlaer, 1938.)*

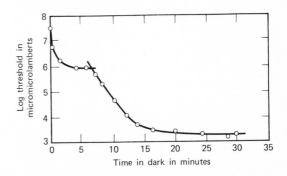

minutes—the period of twilight between the sun's setting and darkness of night—and this period matches the time it takes for dark adaptation to be completed. (Pp. 196–197)

Of interest is the finding cited by Blough (1955, 1961) that when tested under conditions suitable for assessing the visual thresholds of infrahumans, the pigeon manifests a course of dark adaptation very similar in general form to that of the human. The primary difference between the dark adaptation of the human and the pigeon is owing to the fact that the pigeon, unlike man, is quite inactive in conditions of dim lighting and has comparatively fewer rods than cones. Consequently, the rod segment of the dark adaptation curve (Figure 12.1) is more shallow for the pigeon than for the human.

In general, photopic vision is poor in a dimly lit environment and scotopic vision dominates. Thus, when looking at a faint star in the dim light of the moon, we are more successful when we do not fixate directly on the star. By doing this we ensure that the image falls on the sensitive rods in the peripheral regions of the retina rather than the cone-concentrated fovea.

The Photochemical Basis of Dark Adaptation

Adaptation to the dark involves a complex chemical change within the rods. The rods of most vertebrates contain a light-absorbing pigment called *rhodopsin* or *visual purple* because of its color in isolation. It is an unstable chemical readily altered by light energy; it is bleached by exposure to light and regenerates in darkness. Although there are important neural changes relevant to dark adaptation, it is recognized that rhodopsin regeneration is the basic *photochemical* process underlying dark adaptation. The multistate cycle of bleaching and the synthesis of rhodopsin as a function of the light environment of the eye is diagramed in Figure 12.2. Rhodopsin is bleached by light to form retinene (or retinal), a yellow carotenoid (one of a class of plant pig-

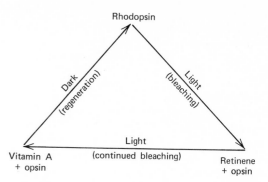

Fig. 12.2 *Photochemical basis underlying dark adaptation.*

ments) and *opsin,* a colorless protein. With continued bleaching retinene is converted to a form of vitamin A (also called retinol or 11-cis retinaldehyde) (Hsia & Graham, 1965; see also Alpern, Lawrence, & Wolsk, 1967, p. 30). In the anabolic (regenerative) portion of the cycle, when the eye is kept in the dark, vitamin A joins with opsin to reconstitute rhodopsin. Thus, an equilibrium is established between the composition of rhodopsin and its subsequent synthesis from its constituent elements (see Rubin & Walls, 1969). It should be noted that during the bleaching process a fraction of the rhodopsin is released into the blood and becomes unavailable for subsequent rhodopsin regeneration (Noell, Delmelle, & Albrecht, 1971).

This photodynamic process is consistent with the fact that a critical deficiency of vitamin A can produce a condition of pathological insensitivity to dim lighting called *nyctalopia* (sometimes *hemeralopia* or merely "night blindness"). There is evidence of extensive retinal damage due to continued vitamin A deficiency. Dowling and Wald (1960) deprived rats (who have only rod retinae) of vitamin A and found that after 8 weeks of deprivation the rats' sensitivity decreased radically, requiring up to 1000 times more light to produce a retinal neural response. With continued vitamin A depletion the poor cell nutrition became irrevocable, the rods degenerated, and the rats became permanently blind (see also Dowling, 1966).

As exposure to the dark increases the sensitivity of the retina, exposure to the light decreases it in a process called *light adaptation*. The exposure of the dark-adapted eye to light results in an initial rapid elevation of the threshold that continues to rise briefly but at a slower rate and then levels off to completion in several minutes. When the dark adapted retina is suddenly confronted with intense light, as when entering bright daylight from the interior of a dark auditorium, the experience of light adaptation is disagreeable and may even be painful.

It must be pointed out that factors other than changes in the concentration of rhodopsin are involved in adaptation. There is evidence from the frog's retina that visual sensitivity may vary significantly without correspondingly large changes in the concentration of rhodopsin (Granit, Holmberg, & Zewi, 1938). Moreover, the cycle of rhodopsin bleaching and regeneration occurs more slowly than does an actual change in threshold or sensitivity (Baker, 1953). A number of *neural* mechanisms as opposed to photochemical ones have been suggested. Rushton (1963) has proposed that the total activity of a number of neurally related receptors regulates the adaptive state of the eye. One important finding that argues for Rushton's "pooling of adaptation signals" is that light falling on one set of receptors produces a state of light adaptation that affects the response of receptors outside the region directly stimulated by the adapting light; that is, the sensitivity of receptors that share the same neural pool but are not directly stimulated is reduced nearly as much as that of receptors in areas that are strongly bleached (Rushton & Westheimer; 1962). Dowling (1967) has suggested that some of the neural events responsible for adaptation transpire in the bipolar cell layer of the vertebrate retina. Others have found that some adaptation occurs at the receptors themselves (Grabowski, Pinto, & Pak, 1972). Although a precise neural mechanism is not available, it is clear that there are some nonphotochemical mechanisms involved in adaptation.

Purkinje Shift

A fundamental distinction between photopic and scotopic vision is that rods and cones are not uniformly sensitive to the entire visible spectrum. Different wavelengths of light differ markedly in the extent to which they stimulate the eye. In Figure 12.3 the threshold values are plotted against wavelengths to obtain *spectral threshold curves*. This is a complex functional relationship because threshold level is dependent on the adaptive state of the eye and the kinds of receptors under stimulation. The threshold function for photopic vision, shown in the upper curve, results when the eye is light-adapted to moderately high intensities. It is quite elevated relative to the function for scotopic vision of the dark-adapted eye, shown in the bottom curve. Reading from the figure, the wavelength of maximal sensitivity (lowest threshold) for photopic vision is in the region of 550 nm (appearing as a yellow-green color) whereas the threshold curve for scotopic vision indicates that maximum sensitivity lies within the region of 500 nm (green). In other words, the rods are more sensitive to short wavelengths than are cones, and in general, the relative brightness of different wavelengths is related to the overall level of illumination.

It should be noted that it is only when light levels are sufficient to activate photopic vision that the perception of colors or hues occurs. When visual stimulation reaches only scotopic levels of radiant energy, stimulating only rods, weak lights are visible but not as colors; that is, all wavelengths are seen as a series of grays. The colorless interval in radiant energy for a given wavelength—the interval between seeing only a light and seeing a color—is given as the vertical difference between the scotopic and photopic threshold curves in Figure 12.3, and it is called the *photochromatic interval*. The photochromatic

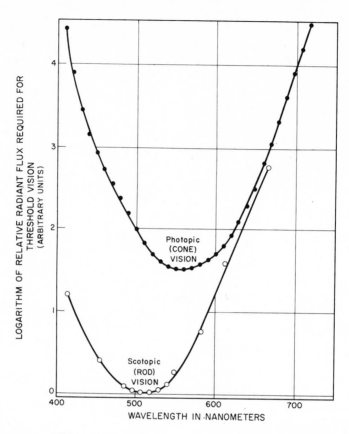

Fig. 12.3 *Relative amounts of light energy required to reach threshold as a function of wavelength. The top spectral threshold curve is for photopic vision, the bottom one for scotopic vision. Observe that the rods require less radiant energy than the cones for threshold visibility at all wavelengths except for the very long ones where the photopic and scotopic thresholds are about the same. Also, the photopic curve is shifted about 50 nm to the right with respect to the scotopic curve, indicating that the rods are maximally sensitive to wavelengths of 500 nm, the cones to wavelengths of about 550 nm. The vertical distance between the two curves represents the photochromatic interval. (Source: Chapanis, 1949, p. 12.)*

interval is largest at the short wavelength end and is smallest at the long wavelength end of the spectrum, where rods and cones are about equally sensitive to radiant energy. This latter point means that a light whose wavelength is 650 nm or above, if it is of sufficient radiant energy to be seen at all, is also chromatically seen (as red). In fact beyond 650 nm, the cone threshold may be a little lower than the rod threshold (Cornsweet, 1970).

These facts help to explain the phenomenon that when light energy is decreased so that visual function changes from photopic to scotopic levels, bright colors usually appear darker. For example, two equally bright surfaces matched in daylight, one red and one green, appear to differ in brightness when viewed in dim lighting; the bright red surface appears to be darker than the green. This is called the *Purkinje shift* after J. E. Purkinje, the physiologist who described it in 1825. Of course, what is occurring is a change in the apparent brightness of various wavelengths coincident with the shift from photopic to scotopic vision. We noted that the part of the spectrum to which the eye is most sensitive in bright illumination is different from that to which the eye is most sensitive in reduced illumination. It follows that under conditions of reduced illumination utilizing scotopic vision, the light composed of shorter wavelengths appears to be relatively brighter than when it is observed in bright illumination. Thus, during the approach of twilight, reds initially appear relatively bright compared to greens, but as twilight progresses the reddish colors appear darker. Since scotopic vision is colorless, within a certain illumination interval daylight greens change to moonlight grays and daylight reds change to moonlight blacks.

An aspect of dark adaptation that warrants comment owing to its practical consequence is the wavelength of the preadapting light. If the lighting just prior to adaptation consists of only a single long wavelength of light (monochromatic red), dark adaptation proceeds much more rapidly after the preadapting light is turned off than if other wavelengths, including white light, are used (Chapanis, 1949; Bartley, 1951). This is because the rods are relatively insensitive to the long wavelength end of the spectrum; hence, they suffer little light adaptation effects. There is an interesting practical application to this. If one must rapidly go from a well-lighted to a dimly lit environment, the process of dark adaptation may be begun in the light by wearing red goggles prior to entering the darkened environment. That is, if restricted only to long wavelengths, the eyes become fairly dark-adapted while exposed to ordinary levels of illumination. Indeed, it is held that preadaptation with monochromatic red light is nearly as effective preparation for night vision as being in complete darkness. The red goggles serve several related functions: As with any light filter they reduce the overall amount of light reaching the eyes so that the eyes are light-adapted to a lower energy level. More important,

however, red goggles allow in only red light, to which the rods are relatively insensitive. Thus, it is mostly the cones that must subsequently undergo dark adaptation when the goggles are removed in the dark, and, as indicated in the top branch of Figure 12.1, dark adaptation proceeds most rapidly for photopic vision.

THRESHOLDS FOR VISION

Under optimal conditions of testing, the least amount of radiant energy necessary to produce a visual sensation—the absolute threshold—is a strikingly small amount. The definitive and somewhat dramatic experiment on threshold determination was performed by Hecht, Shlaer, and Pirenne (1941, 1942). Owing to its significance, the experiment merits a brief discussion. Subjects were first dark-adapted, then were tested with a patch of light 10 minutes of arc in diameter (an area in angular measure of 10 minutes on the retina consists of from 300 to 500 rods). The light was applied to the most sensitive part of the retina, an area situated 20° from the fovea. The wavelength of the test patch of light, 510 nm, was optimal for scotopic vision, and the test exposures were flashes of 1 msec duration. A series of intensities of the test patch was presented many times, and the frequency of seeing the flash was determined for each intensity. From the subject's point of view, the experiment involved the report of whether or not he saw a flash of light. The experimenter chose as the threshold value the amount of light that could be seen 60% of the time. When translated into basic energy terms— the number of quanta striking the eye—threshold values were found to range from 54 to 148 quanta. However, the authors argue that although this amount of energy is required at the cornea, it does not represent the actual energy necessary for threshold vision. About 4% of the incident light is reflected by the cornea and about another 50% is absorbed by the lens and other ocular media. Thus, about 46% of the light energy incident on the eye actually reaches the rods. Furthermore, from independent studies it was estimated that about 80% of this remaining energy passes through the retina without being absorbed by rhodopsin. With a few simple calculations the threshold range of 54 to 148 quanta incident on the eye is corrected to an effective range of 5 to 14 quanta absorbed by the rods (in luminance terms the absolute threshold for this condition is of the order of 0.000001 mL). Since such a small number of quanta are distributed over an area containing a comparatively large number of rods, it is very unlikely that two quanta will be absorbed by the same rod. Thus, a single quantum of radiant energy must be sufficient to activate a single rod, and in order to initiate a visual sensation (at threshold level) it is necessary for only 1 quantum of light to be absorbed by each of five to 14 rods.

The limiting capacity of threshold vision appears to be linked to the physical nature of light in that if the eye were any more sensitive, the discreteness of photon emission would be perceptible and light would not be perceived as continuous or steady.

> *The fact that for the absolute visual threshold the number of quanta is small makes one realize the limitation set on vision by the quantum structure of light. Obviously the amount of energy required to stimulate any eye must be large enough to supply at least one quantum to the photosensitive material. No eye need be so sensitive as this. But it is a tribute to the excellence of natural selection that our own eye comes so remarkably close to the lowest limit. (Hecht, Shlaer, & Pirenne, 1942, P. 837)*

ABSOLUTE THRESHOLD OF BRIGHTNESS

The threshold determination discussed above was made under optimal conditions of testing.

However, there are a number of variables that affect threshold levels such as the area and duration of the light stimulus and the region of the retina on which the stimulus is presented.

Area of Retina Stimulated

For relatively small visual areas, covering visual angles of 10 min of arc or less, a constant threshold response can be maintained by the reciprocal interaction between area (for both fovea and periphery) and stimulus intensity. The relationship, known as *Ricco's Law*, is as follows: $A \times I = C$, where the product of area (A) and intensity (I) produces a constant threshold value (C). In general the law states that a constant threshold value is maintained by increasing the area stimulated while decreasing stimulus intensity, or the reverse. For larger retinal areas, *Piper's Law*, $\sqrt{A} \times I = C$, holds. For still larger areas of the retina, covering substantial regions, the threshold depends on intensity alone. That is, $I = C$ (Bartlett, 1965). No one law appears to extend over the full range of retinal area. The areal or spatial summation indicated by these relations holds best in the peripheral retina, and it is likely a result of neural interactions in the retina.

Duration of the Stimulus

Within limits, a form of temporal summation also occurs. For durations of about 100 msec or less, stimulus intensity and time bear a reciprocal relationship for a constant threshold value. Thus, a less intense light acting for a relatively long time and a more intense light acting for a relatively short time produce a constant effect. This is known as the *Bunson-Roscoe* (or *Bloch's*) *Law*. Thus, with I and C as above, and T as the stimulus duration, $T \times I = C$. This relationship holds for both foveal and peripheral retinal regions. The effective temporal range over which the law holds may be as long as 100 msec. Obviously, the law cannot hold over an indefinite

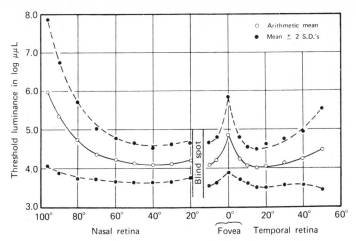

Fig. 12.4 *Luminance of the just perceptible light at various retinal locations. The solid line is the average curve for 101 subjects; the dotted lines enclose the measurements of 95% of the subjects. The measurements were made with a 1°, white test light. A comparison with Figure 11.11 indicates that, in general, the sensitivity of the eye is greatest where the density of rods is maximal. (Source: Chapanis, 1949, p. 9.)*

range for that would imply that we could detect a light stimulus of almost infinitesimal intensity provided it was exposed for a sufficient duration.

Retinal Locus

As we noted earlier with the spectral threshold curves (Figure 12.3), the absolute threshold is dependent on the part of the retina stimulated. As Figure 12.4 shows, areas primarily containing cones have a much higher threshold than do areas containing rods. In general, the sensitivity of the eye is greatest where the density of rods is maximal (compare Figure 12.4 with Figure 11.11 in the preceding chapter).

Two additional points noted earlier must be reiterated: The absolute threshold is not equally sensitive to radiant energy from all portions of the spectrum, but (see Figure 12.3) it is very much dependent on the wavelength of the light. Furthermore, the absolute threshold also depends on the adaptive state of the eye immediately preceding threshold determination. Of course, light adaptation produces an elevated threshold, whereas adaptation to the dark produces the opposite effect.

DIFFERENTIAL THRESHOLD OF BRIGHTNESS

The differential threshold for brightness discrimination refers to the smallest change in radiant energy that can be detected. As with the absolute threshold, the differential threshold varies with the degree of stimulus intensity. Basically, determination of the differential threshold involves computing the smallest increment of intensity (ΔI) necessary to detect a brightness change in a test stimulus. Differential thresholds have been found by using a bipartite or a divided light field in which there are two adjacent parts, each of which can be independently varied in intensity. Each half begins at the same energy level (and brightness), I; then the experimenter changes the energy level of one side. The smallest incremental change in intensity (ΔI) by which the viewer just perceives the two fields as different in brightness specifies the differential threshold; this is a distance on the intensity scale corresponding to a *jnd* (just noticeable difference). Thus, the intensity level of one half of the bipartite visual field may be designated as I and the intensity of the just discriminable one as $I + \Delta I$.

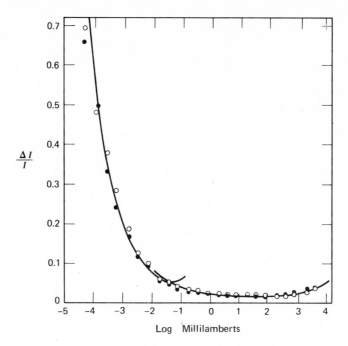

Fig. 12.5 *Weber fractions as a function of intensity (log I). At any given intensity level, the differential threshold is expressed relative to the intensity level at which the determination is made. (From Geldard, 1972, p. 42)*

One means of examining the differential threshold is to compute the Weber fractions, $\Delta I/I$, for various energy levels. Figure 12.5 presents a plot of Weber fractions as a function of energy level for white light. Quite obvious in the figure is that the Weber fractions are not a constant function of intensity. In general as the light intensity, (I), increases, so does discriminative capacity; that is, the $\Delta I/I$ fraction decreases. The disjunction in the lower portion of the curve of Figure 12.5 reflects the duplex character of the retina. The upper branch, at low intensities, relates to scotopic vision, whereas the lower one, where the Weber fraction is lower and discrimination is much finer, represents photopic vision. In addition to the initial level of radiant energy, the differential threshold also depends on several variables such as the area, wavelength, amount of area, duration of the test stimulus, and, of course, the locus of the retina stimulated.

Relevant to threshold determination and brightness discrimination is the psychophysical relation of the physical intensity to the perception of brightness. When measured by direct magnitude estimates of the subjective brightness associated with different values of intensity (see Chapter 2), the relationship of brightness to intensity approaches a power function with an exponent of 0.33, for the dark-adapted eye (Stevens, 1960; Marks & Stevens, 1966). This means that subjective brightness increases much more slowly than does stimulus intensity.

PERCEIVING CONTINUITY FROM INTERMITTENT LIGHT: THE CFF

As indicated earlier, the intensity and duration of a stimulus interact, and with certain specifications may be interchanged in order to reach a threshold response. This interaction extends beyond unitary stimuli. Under certain conditions of intensity and duration, an intermittent or flashing light stimulus may be perceived as continuously lit. This is owing to the fact that once initiated a visual image persists for a brief period after the physical stimulus is terminated. This effect can be easily demonstrated by interrupting a steady beam of light with an *episcotister,* a rotating disk that has sectors cut out so that light passes through during part of the disc's revolution (Figure 12.6). The number of flashes per second can be controlled by the speed of rotation (generally stated in cycles per second or Hz); the amount of reflected light is primarily determined by the size of the sector. Whether the light stimulus appears continuous or flickering depends primarily on the frequency of the rotation. When the frequency of rotation is relatively slow, the image of each light flash fades before the next one appears, and a viewer perceives the interrupted light source as flashing, that is, as an alternation of light and dark phases. However, when the frequency of rotation of the disk is sufficiently high, the image of a given light is added to a following one prior to its fading, and the physically interrupted light apparently fuses and appears continuous. Under the latter conditions the following generalization, called *Talbot's Law,*

holds: A flashing light, shown at a rate sufficient to produce fusion, that is "on" p % of the time, has the same apparent brightness as the light if continuously lit but only p % as intense. In other words, the brightness of the physically intermittent but apparently continuous light is the same as if the total amount of light had been uniformly distributed over a whole revolution of the disk. For example, the light flashing on and off equal times (allowing 50% of the light to pass through by having equal open and closed sectors of the episcotister) appears to have the brightness of a continuous light that is only half as intense; that is, the apparently continuous light appears to be half as bright as the illuminated sector of the disk. Talbot's Law holds equally well for other relative durations of the on and off phases in a revolution, indicating that in some manner the visual system is averaging the amount of total illumination received during the light and dark phases.

There is a certain minimum frequency of intermittent light necessary for it to be perceived as continuous. The rate at which flicker disappears and the interrupted light appears steady is known as the *critical fusion frequency* (CFF). Aside from the obvious variable of frequency of revolution, values of CFF depend on a number of factors, chief among them being the intensity of the flash. Some typical values of CFF as a function of intensity are given in Figure 12.7a.

Over a considerable range and for a number of spectral regions, the relationship between the logarithm of intensity and fusion frequency is nearly linear: CFF is proportional to Log I. The lower and upper branches in the curve refer to rod and cone segments, respectively. Weak flashes show greater persistency and fuse at comparatively slow rates. The rods, which maximally function at low levels of illumination, thus have a lower CFF than cones. Generally, the more intense the stimulus, the greater the frequency required for the threshold of fusion to be reached. Beyond 60 Hz fusion occurs regardless of intensity. In addition to intensity, CFF varies with light deprivation (Zubeck & Bross, 1972), the retinal locus of stimulation, stimulus size and

Fig. 12.6 *Stationary episcotister disk. The size and the number of sectors of a rotating episcotister determine the amount of reflected light.*

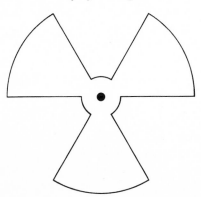

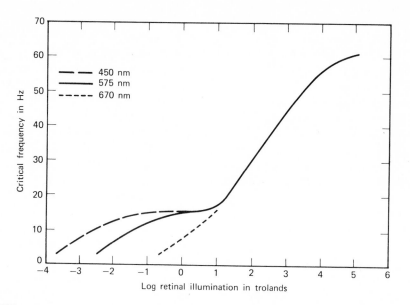

Fig. 12.7a *CFF as a function of intensity for several wavelengths. The lower branches of the curve are the responses of the rods; the upper branch is for cones. Notice that as illumination increases the CFF is independent of the wavelength of the light. (Source: modified from Hecht & Shlaer, 1936, by the Rockefeller University Press.)*

Fig. 12.7b *When this figure is rotated at gradually increasing speed, the thin ring continues to flicker after the rest of the black and white field has fused to yield a uniform gray. Through contrast the difference between the white and black of the ring has been heightened by their respective backgrounds. Hence they are slower to fuse. (Source: Krech & Crutchfield, 1958, p. 75. Reprinted by permission of the authors.)*

contrast (see Figure 12.7b), the adaptive state of the eye, body temperature, age, and with numerous other complex variables (see Geldard, 1972, pp. 134–142).

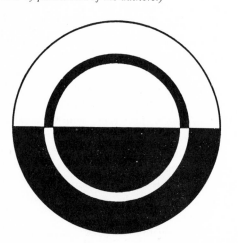

THRESHOLD FOR COLOR

Although we reserve a detailed discussion of color perception for the next chapter, there are some threshold-relevant facts regarding color that are best described in the present context. The perception of color or hue is a psychological experience that is primarily related to the spectral stimuli. The threshold for the discrimination of colors—the least perceptible difference in wavelength that the eye can detect—is determined by using a bipartite field whose halves are of equal intensity. The procedure is to gradually and incrementally change the wavelength of one side

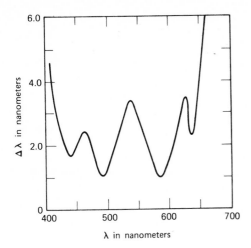

Fig. 12.8 *Wavelength discrimination by the human eye. The change in wavelength which can be just detected (Δ λ) is plotted as a function of wavelength. (From The Human Senses, by F. A. Geldard, Wiley, New York, 1973, p. 63. Reprinted by permission of the publisher.)*

until it is perceived as different in color from the other (Δλ is the term for an increment of wavelength). When this is done, Δλ, the increment of wavelength, defines the *jnd*. Beginning with a red light of 700 nm on both sides of the bipartite field and shifting the wavelength on one side of the field downward until a discrimination between the two fields can be just detected produces the first *jnd* (Δλ = 22 nm) and sets the level for the next determination (700 nm − 22 nm = 678 nm). Proceeding in this way through the visible spectrum yields 128 *jnd*'s, some Δλ's only 1 nm, most below 4 nm and some, at the extreme red end of the spectrum, greater than 6 nm. The magnitude of Δλ for various spectral regions is shown in Figure 12.8. In general, discriminability is best at about 480 to 490 nm (blue-green) and 580 to 590 nm (yellow), whereas poor discriminability appears at the spectral extremes of visibility and at a region near 540 nm (green-yellow).

Fig. 12.9 *Equal color contours. All combinations of intensity and wavelength lying on a given contour appear as the same color. The three spectral points, Y (yellow), G (green) and B (blue), yield a constant color regardless of the level of intensity. All other colors vary in accordance with the Bezold-Brücke shift. (Source: Purdy, 1937, American Journal of Psychology, 49, 313–315.)*

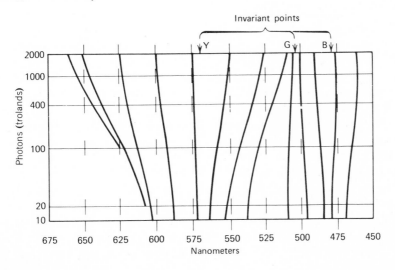

Bezold-Brücke Shift

Although spectral wavelength is the most important single contributor to the perception of color, the intensity of the wavelength is also an important factor. An effect that occurs when spectral wavelengths are intensified is that, except for the colors of three wavelengths, all colors shift slightly toward either yellow or blue. This change in hue as a function of intensity is called the *Bezold-Brücke shift*. One means of demonstrating the apparent change in color is to have subjects match the colors of two patches of identical wavelengths that differ in intensity. The wavelength of a standard patch is kept fixed, and the subject matches its apparent color by varying the wavelength of the second comparison patch. Figure 12.9 shows the results of this procedure for various regions of the spectrum and for various intensity levels with a plot of equal color contours. All combinations of intensity and wavelength lying on a given curve are perceived as the same color. With greater intensity, yellow-reds and yellow-greens shift toward yellow, and blue-greens and violets appear bluer (see Judd, 1951).

THRESHOLD FOR SATURATION

The visible spectrum contains many wavelengths, each of which is seen as a particular color. Light that is composed of a single wavelength (monochromatic light) is called spectrally *pure*. In contrast, white light, composed of radiant energy distributed among all wavelengths, lacks purity. The narrower the band of wavelengths comprising a light, the greater is its purity. When the purity of a light stimulus is varied, the light changes in its apparent grayness: The less pure the light, the more gray it appears. The degree to which a chromatic stimulus differs from an achromatic or gray stimulus of the same intensity specifies the subjective or psychological

attribute called *saturation*. Saturation, as a dimension of color experience, may be thought of as the relative absence of grayness in a color. In short, the perceived saturation of a color is directly related to its spectral purity. As an example, a monochromatic green light of 510 nm, composed of a single wavelength, is spectrally pure and appears as a highly saturated color. However, if its intensity is held fixed as other wavelengths are systematically added to it, its saturation will decrease and the green color will begin to appear grayish. Notice that as long as the 510 nm green light remains the dominant wavelength, the light will continue to appear green.

The absolute threshold for saturation is the least amount of a pure spectral wavelength that must be mixed with white light in order to produce a perceptible color. The greater the amount of pure spectral light required in mixture with white light to just produce a color, the lower is the spectral light's saturation. In general, the yellow region of the spectrum is less saturated than the red or violet region. As shown in Figure 12.10, approximately 0.05% yellow (about 570 nm) must be added to white light to just produce a color that is perceived as yellow, whereas only about 0.001% violet and blue light (400 to 450 nm) and 0.005% red light (650 nm) are needed to just produce their respective colors. Put in another way, 0.05% yellow, 0.005% red, and 0.001% violet or blue light will perceptibly "color" white light. Thus, the spectrum is maximally saturated at the extremes (violet and red) and minimally at yellow.

The degree of saturation also is affected by the intensity of the light. As indicated earlier, at low intensity levels (see the photochromatic interval, Figure 12.3) all but the very long wavelengths (reds) produce a visual response before they appear chromatic; that is, except for the extreme reds, a visual stimulus is seen as a light before it is seen as a color. Wavelengths at such low intensity levels produce lights that are quite

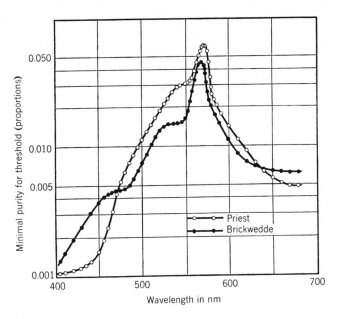

Fig. 12.10 *Saturation thresholds. Minimum proportion of pure spectral light that must be added to white light in order to yield a just perceptible color. The curves are based on the data of two researchers. (Source: Osgood, 1953, 145; after Murchison, Handbook of Experimental Psychology, Clark University Press, Worcester, Mass., 1934, p. 801.)*

desaturated. As intensity increases, saturation also increases and the stimulus is chromatically perceived, until a maximum in saturation is reached in the middle ranges of intensities. Notice, however, that for each wavelength there is a different intensity that produces a maximum saturation. With still further increases in intensity saturation begins to decline.

ACUITY

We discussed briefly some of the anatomical bases of visual acuity in the previous chapter; we deal here with its measurement. Visual acuity, in a broad sense, refers to the ability to resolve fine details and to distinguish different parts of the visual field from each other (Figure 12.11).

Actually there are a number of acuities, each involving a different task—detection, localization, resolution, and recognition. *Detection* acuity refers to the task of detecting the presence of a target stimulus in the visual field. Often a small object of a specified size must be detected against a darker background. *Localization* or *vernier* acuity concerns the ability to detect whether two lines, laid end to end, are continuous or whether one line is offset relative to the other. The amount of displacement can be varied, and the level at which the viewer cannot perceive the misalignment of the two lines sets the level of acuity (see Figure 12.12). *Resolution* acuity refers to the ability to perceive a separation between discrete elements of a pattern (see Figure 12.13). Thus, one might determine whether a pattern of line gratings can be seen as distinct and lying in a certain orientation (Figure 12.13c). As the lines

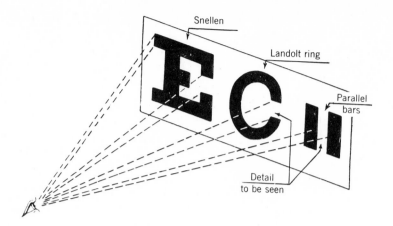

Fig. 12.11 *Details of targets used in the measurement of visual acuity. The Snellen letters measure recognition acuity; the other two targets assess resolution acuity. The viewer must report the position of the break in the Landolt ring and the orientation of the parallel bars. (Source: Chapanis, 1949, p. 26.)*

become thinner or closer together, the grating pattern appears to lack any discrete lines or orientation; that is, the pattern cannot be resolved. The *Landolt rings,* shown in Figure 12.14, are also used to assess resolution acuity. *Recognition* acuity is perhaps the most familiar of the acuities. The usual task of recognition acuity requires the viewer to name the target stimuli. The *Snellen* letters (Figure 12.15) of the familiar eye chart are examples of test stimuli used to measure recognition acuity.

Visual Angle

The degree of acuity differs for the different types. However, before discussing them further we must

introduce a measure for specifying acuity that applies to all types. The size of the just discriminable critical detail of the test targets is specified in terms of the *visual angle* its image subtends on the retina. The visual angle refers to the angle formed by the target on the retina. Visual angle, given in degrees, minutes, and seconds of arc, is a useful measure in that it gives the acuity value as a joint function of the target size and distance from the

Fig. 12.12 *Vernier acuity measurement with a movable line. (Source: Rubin & Walls, 1969, p. 147. Reprinted by permission of the authors and publisher.)*

Fig. 12.13 *Targets for resolution acuity (a) Parallel bars, (b) Double dot target, (c) Acuity grating, (d) Checkerboard. Most commonly used is a grating pattern (c) in which the widths of the dark and bright lines are made equal. A series of gratings from coarse to fine is presented and visual acuity is specified in terms of the angular width of the line of the finest grating that can be resolved. (From L. A. Riggs, in Vision and Visual Perception, edited by C. H. Graham, Wiley, New York, 1965, p. 325. Reprinted by permission of the publisher.)*

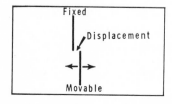

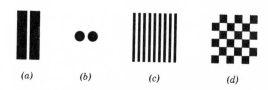

(a)   (b)   (c)   (d)

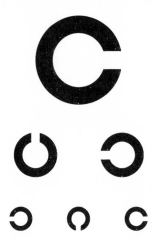

Fig. 12.14 *Landolt rings used for assessing resolution acuity. The rings consist of a line whose thickness is one-fifth the outer diameter. The gap width is also one-fifth the outer diameter. (From L. A. Riggs, in Vision and Visual Perception, edited by C. H. Graham, Wiley, New York, 1965, p. 324. Reprinted by permission of the publisher.)*

subject's eye. This precludes specifying both target size and target distance and enables direct comparisons to be made of different size stimuli located at different distances from the viewer. Notice, however, that even when expressed in terms of visual angle, the actual distance at which a target is located from the viewer is an important consideration. Because of lens accommodation differences between persons, acuity measurements are generally taken at a near distance, say 13 or 16 in (33 or 40.6 cm), and at a far distance, 20 ft (6.1 meters). For objects located at distances beyond about 20 ft (6.1 meters) accommodation remains fairly constant.

In order to specify the value of the visual angle (β) subtended by a target (see Figure 12.16) the following equation is used.

$$\tan \frac{\beta}{2} = \frac{y}{2x}$$

Where tan $\beta/2$ represents the trigonometric function for half of the visual angle, y represents the

size of the target, and x represents the distance of the target from the retina along the line of regard. Using the values of Figure 12.16, the target distance is 25 in, and target size is 2 in, hence tangent $\beta/2$ is $\frac{1}{25}$ or 0.04; that is, $\frac{1}{2}$ of the target length divided by the distance of the target from the eye or 1 in divided by 25 in. The angle whose tangent is 0.04 is 2° 18′. But this is only one-half of the target angle β, hence the full visual angle subtended by the target image at the retina is twice this value or 4° 36′. Often visual acuity is given as the reciprocal of the required visual angle in order to indicate that high numerical values reflect high levels of acuity.

In terms of visual angle the four types of acuity have approximately the following optimal acuity values for human vision: detection acuity—$\frac{1}{2}$ sec of arc; localization acuity—2 sec of arc; and for both resolution and recognition—30 sec of arc (Haber & Hershenson, 1973, p. 113). We noted in

Fig. 12.15 *Snellen letters used for measuring recognition acuity. The Snellen letters are composed of lines and serifs having a thickness that is one-fifth the height or width of the whole letter. The Snellen eye chart was devised by the Dutch ophthalmologist, Herman Snellen, in 1862. (From L. A. Riggs, in Vision and Visual Perception, edited by C. H. Graham, Wiley, New York, 1961, p. 324. Reprinted by permission of the publisher.)*

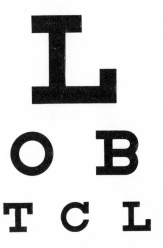

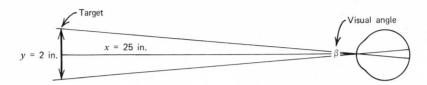

Fig. 12.16   *The angle, β, in radian measure, is the visual angle subtended by the target, y, that lies at a distance, x, from the retina.*

the previous chapter that many nocturnal animals have greater sensitivity in dim lighting than man. Accordingly, it has been estimated that the resolution acuity of some diurnal animals such as the eagle may reach 3.6 times human visual acuity (Shlaer, 1972).

Because of its widespread use we have a bit more to say about recognition acuity. The most common form of acuity measurement in clinical practice is recognition, and it is usually measured by means of the familiar eye chart. Typically, the chart contains lines of Snellen letters that vary in size. The viewer reads the line with the smallest letters that he can possibly read with accuracy. When this type of acuity is assessed, the resultant value is expressed as a ratio of the distance at which a line of letters can just be correctly seen to the distance at which the hypothetical average person with normal vision can read the same line. Accordingly, a ratio of 20/20 indicates that the viewer correctly sees at 20 feet letters that the average person can just read at 20 feet (20/20 = 1 min of arc). A ratio of 20/15 means that the viewer sees at 20 feet what the average person can just see at 15 feet—obviously better than average acuity. On the other hand, a ratio of 20/30 means that the viewer can just read at 20 feet what the average person can read at 30 feet—poorer than average acuity.

Acuity and Intensity

The dependence of visual acuity on the intensity of the illumination is shown by the curve of Figure 12.17. Acuity, plotted as the reciprocal of

visual angle, increases rather slowly at low intensity levels, then in the middle ranges (−2 to +2 log units, or 0.01 to 100 mL) visual acuity increases quite rapidly as intensity increases. Thereafter, increases in intensity produce very little increase in acuity. Observe, however, that because of the means of plotting the ordinate of the figure it does not give a true indication of the smallest detail that can be seen as a function of the luminance level. The left ordinate of the figure is the reciprocal of the visual angle in minutes. When the ordinate is plotted directly in terms of the smallest detail that can be seen—in units of visual angle—as shown at the right ordinate of the figure, it becomes clear that there is relatively little to be gained by increasing intensity in the range of, say 0 to 3 log units of intensity (1 to 1000 mL). Whereas when the same change in luminance is plotted in acuity values, the curve shows large increases in acuity.

Acuity and Retinal Locus

Visual acuity is best when the image falls on the fovea, where the cones are most densely packed, and acuity becomes increasingly poor as areas peripheral to the fovea are stimulated. The variation in visual acuity for different regions of the human retina is indicated by the 1894 classic figure by Wertheim, shown here in Figure 12.18. It is obvious that acuity is dependent on the distribution of cones when comparing this figure with a plot of the distribution of rods and cones in the retina, shown in the previous chapter, Figure 11.11. Though Figure 12.18 represents the general trend for acuity and retinal locus, it is likely that the periphery is not as poor as indicated. Recently several investigations have reported that the peripheral regions of the retina are two to four times higher in resolution acuity than Figure 12.18 indicates (Kerr, 1971). Furthermore, some degree of recognition acuity has been shown for the periphery, 80° from the fovea (Menzer & Thurmond, 1970).

Notice that although acuity depends on the stimulation of cones, it is not clear how cones effect such high levels of acuity. As we indicated earlier, targets subtending 0.5 sec of visual angle are sufficiently large for detection acuity yet according to Polyak's (1941) measures, this width is far smaller than the width of a single primate cone (12 to 18 sec of visual angle). Perhaps series of adjacent cones contribute to some sort of integrative process for detection acuity.

Stiles-Crawford Effect

Another anatomical determinant of acuity is the *Stiles-Crawford* effect, which refers to the fact that acuity depends on the part of the pupil through which the light enters. Light entering near the edge of the pupil must be much more intense than light rays entering at the center in order to evoke the same degree of perceived brightness. Indeed, light entering at the border of a fully dilated pupil has about one-fifth the stimulation effectiveness of a light coming straight through the center. However, the Stiles-Crawford effect is not a result of the pupil per se, but due rather to the fact that the effectiveness of a cone depends on the angle at which the light strikes it. In short, cones have directional sensitivity. Thus, light rays entering the eye nearer the center of the pupil stimulate the cones directly and yield the greatest visual acuity. On the other hand, rods show no directional sensitivity, and there is no Stiles-Crawford effect for scotopic vision.

A number of other factors influence acuity. Clearly, the brightness relation between the target and its background is an important consideration, as is the amount of time spent viewing the target; generally the more time spent looking at a target the more visible it is. Furthermore, the viewer's eye movements, the size of the pupil, the wavelength of the target stimuli and background, the

Fig. 12.17 *Visual acuity as a function of background luminance for resolution acuity. (Source: Chapanis, 1949, p. 28.)*

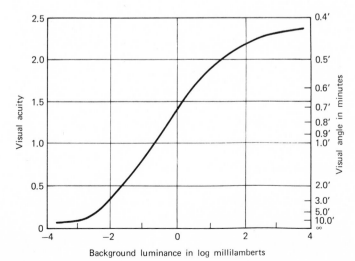

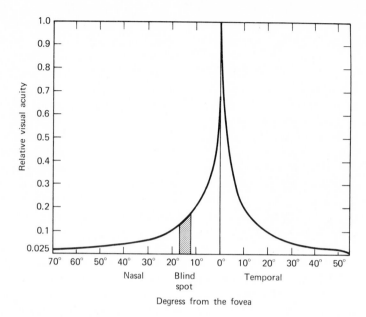

Fig. 12.18 *Visual acuity at different retinal positions. These results were obtained with a grating target. All values are expressed as proportions of foveal acuity. (Source: Chapanis, 1949, p. 27; after Wertheim, 1894.)*

age and experience of the viewer, and other psychological factors may have an important effect on the level of acuity (see Rubin & Walls, 1969; Riggs, 1965, Chap. 11). One of these factors, eye movements, is of sufficient importance not only to acuity but for a general understanding of the visual system to warrant some discussion.

EYE MOVEMENTS

As we noted in Chapter 11, the eyes are moved about by the action of the oculomotor muscles. This enables an observer to position his eyes so that they can fixate or focus on a target. In other words, the eyes move to a position so that the image of a target falls directly on the small central region of clearest, most acute vision, the fovea. Employment of sophisticated measuring devices and techniques have revealed several dif-

ferent types of eye movements (see Llwellyn Thomas, 1968; Alpern, 1971, pp. 371–375).

Saccades

The most common form of eye movement is called the *saccade,* which is a rapid and abrupt jump made by the eye as it moves from one fixation to another. Saccades may be small (less than 10 min of visual angle) and large (20° of angle). They are primarily used to search and explore in the visual field and occur in such tasks as reading and the examination of relatively stationary scenes (Figure 12.19*a*). As Figure 12.19*b* shows, the pattern of eye movement may be partially determined by the kind of information to be extracted from a scene (see also Mackworth & Morandi, 1967). There is also some evidence that the lateral direction of saccades may reflect some personality factors (see Day, 1967; Bakan, 1971). In addition, saccadic movements are initiated to stabilize eye position when there is movement of the head or body in

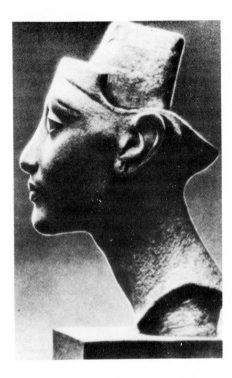

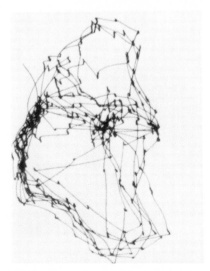

Fig. 12.19a *The bottom photograph is a record of eye movements made during free examination of the top photograph with both eyes for 3 min. (Source: Yarbus, 1967, p. 180. Reprinted with permission of Plenum Press.)*

space. In this case bodily movement is compensated for by eye movements.

Because vision is impaired during eye movements, it is not surprising that they are extremely rapid. Indeed, the muscles responsible for saccadic eye movements are among the fastest in the body. According to Robinson (1968), a 10° human saccade lasts 45 msec and the angular velocity may reach 400° per second. Typically, there are one to three saccades per second, but they occur so rapidly that they occupy only about 10% of the total viewing time (Noton & Stark, 1971b). Saccades are generally voluntary for they can be made with the eyes closed or in total darkness, and they can be suppressed (Steinman, et al., 1967). However, they also show a reflexive nature. A suddenly appearing, flickering, or moving stimulus seen out of the corner of the eye can result in a saccade that moves the gaze directly on the stimulus. This is of adaptive significance, "... for in the primitive world, a slight movement glimpsed from the corner of the eye ... might be the first warning of an attack" (Llewellyn Thomas, 1969, p. 406).

Pursuit Movements

Pursuit movements are almost completely automatic and require a physically moving stimulus. In contrast to saccades, pursuit movements are smoothly executed and are comparatively slow. Generally, they are used to track an object moving in a stationary environment, hence target velocity rather than target location is the appropriate stimulus. In this instance, the velocity of the pursuit movement of the eye matches the velocity of the moving stimulus. This serves to more or less cast and preserve the image of a stationary target on the retina. Moving the eye in accordance with the movement of a stimulus enhances the perception of the form of a stimulus. This reasonably follows because it is easier for the visual system to perceive the form of an image if it is relatively stationary on the retina rather than moving.

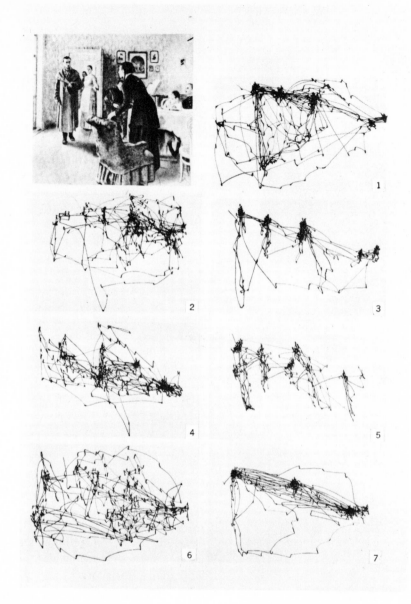

Fig. 12.19b *Seven records of eye movements by the same subject made to the same picture but viewed under different instructions. Each line represents a saccade. Each record lasted 3 min. The subject examined the reproduction with both eyes. (1) Free examination of the picture. Before the subsequent recording sessions, the subject was asked to: (2) estimate the material circumstances of the family in the picture; (3) give the ages of the people; (4) surmise what the family had been doing before the arrival of the "unexpected visitor"; (5) remember the clothes worn by the people; (6) remember the position of the people and objects in the room; (7) estimate how long the "unexpected visitor" had been away from the family. (Source: Yarbus, 1967, p. 174. Reprinted with permission of Plenum Press.)*

Vergence Movements

The eyes may either converge toward or diverge from each other in order to fuse the images of near and far fixated targets, respectively. Vergence movements move the eyes in opposite directions in the horizontal plane from each other so that both eyes can focus on the same target. A lack of proper vergence movements results in *diplopia* or "double vision." Vergence movements, of course, are important only to animals, including man, with frontally pointing eyes.

Miniature Eye Movements

There are also a number of so-called miniature eye movements that may be identified and measured during maintained fixation. When a person maintains deliberate fixation on a target, a pattern of extremely small but continual eye movements is observable with proper recording techniques. Although in continual movement during fixation, the eye does not wander very far from its average focal position. Three miniature eye movements have been identified: *microsaccades, drifts* with which the eye slowly drifts back and forth in the interval between the microsaccades, and in addition, the saccades and drift movements are superimposed on a high frequency tremor of an oscillatory nature called *physiological nystagmus*. It is recognized (as we will see in a later chapter) that if miniature eye movements were entirely eliminated, thus producing a condition on the retina identical to what would exist if the eye itself were motionless, then the image would fade and disappear. However, further attempts to implicate miniature eye movements as necessary for the attainment of such perceptual capacities as acuity and form perception have been seriously questioned (Steinman et al., 1973).

Eye Movements and Scanpaths

Eye movements may be more than simply motor actions that move the image of a pattern over the retina. The pattern of eye movements shown in Figure 12.19*b* suggests that the eyes follow regular pathways. The lines representing the saccades do not crisscross the picture at random but in paths from region to region. Noton and Stark (1971*a,b,c*) have reported a series of interesting studies showing that in scanning a pattern, certain sequences of saccadic eye movements are recurrent (see also Locher & Nodine, 1974).

In each of two experimental phases, the subjects were instructed that their visual processes would be studied while they viewed some pictures that they were to "simply observe." In the initial or "learning" phase, a subject viewed five different patterns each for 20 sec. In the second or "recognition" phase these five patterns were shown again along with five new patterns. The sequence of eye movements was recorded in both phases. Analysis of the eye movements made in the learning phase showed that when a subject was freely viewing a pattern, his eyes usually followed a course of repeated movements with discontinuities, revealing a path characteristic of that subject viewing that pattern. The fixed path characteristic of the sequence of eye movements of a subject for a given pattern is termed a *scanpath*. When the same pattern was presented to the subject during the recognition phase, eye movements usually followed the same path established during the learning phase. According to Noton and Stark, this suggests that the memory of the features of the patterns are linked together in sequence by the memory of the eye movements required to look from one feature to the next. Figure 12.20*a* shows a typical pattern viewed in the experiment. Figure 12.20*b*, presents two extracts from a subject's eye movements record during the 20 sec learning phase. The occurrence of fixed paths is obvious. In Figure 12.20*c*, are extracts of the initial eye movements executed by the same subject during the recognition phase viewings. Finally, in Figure 12.20*d*, is an idealized rendering of the scanpath for that pattern by that subject.

It should be noted that the same subject had

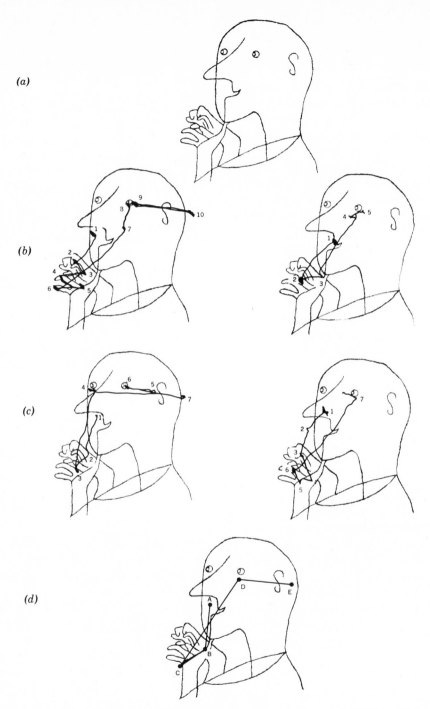

Fig. 12.20a   *Typical pattern viewed by a subject in experiment.*

Fig. 12.20b   *Extracts of subject's eye movements during 20-sec. learning phase.*

Fig. 12.20c   *Extracts of initial eye movements during recognition phase.*

Fig. 12.20d   *Idealized drawing of fixed path—or scanpath—of the subject for the pattern. (Reprinted with permission from Norton, D. & Stark, L., and Vision Research, 1971, 11, 932, Pergamon Press.)*

quite different scanpaths for different patterns, suggesting that scanpaths are not the result of some fixed habit of eye movements. Furthermore, scanpaths differed markedly between subjects for a given pattern, indicating that scanpaths do not result from some general physiological mechanisms (which would be expected to operate about the same way in all subjects) (see Figure 12.21).

In conclusion, in scanning a pattern a subject's eyes tend to follow a fixed path from feature to feature, resulting in a characteristic scanpath. This suggests that eye movements are more than mere motor components of the visual system. Indeed, the view that the neural activity responsible for eye movements plays a role in acuity and in the perception of shape and distance has a good deal of empirical support (e.g., Crovitz & Daves, 1962; Festinger, Burnham, Ono, & Bamber, 1967).

This chapter has focused on the phenomena and functioning of the visual system. The functional distinction between rods and cones introduced in the preceding chapter has been stressed throughout. Vision accomplished with only rods or only cones is termed scotopic or photopic vision, respectively.

One of the important functional differences between photopic and scotopic vision is in response to the general conditions of illumination. Adjustment to a dimly illuminated environment is termed dark adaptation; it has both a photochemical and neural basis. Related phenomena such as the Purkinje shift and spectral sensitivity were discussed.

Absolute threshold determinations for brightness were examined and the following relationships for the absolute threshold were described: Intensity and the amount of area of the retina stimulated (Ricco's and Piper's Law), intensity and the duration of the stimulus (Bunson-Roscoe or Bloch's Law), and intensity and retinal locus. It was noted that differential thresholds for brightness vary for photopic and

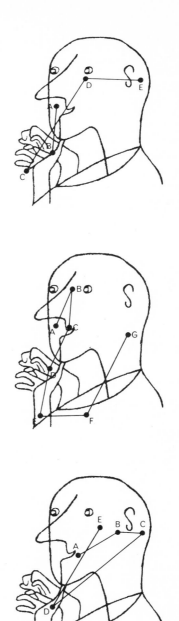

Fig. 12.21 *The figures show different scanpaths for three subjects viewing the same pattern. (Reprinted with permission from Norton, D. & Stark, L., and Vision Research, 1971, 11, 933, Pergamon Press.)*

scotopic vision; in general, differential thresholds decrease with an increase in light intensity. Thresholds for wavelength and saturation were also examined, and related phenomena such as the Bezold-Brücke effect were described.

The perception of continuous stimulation from intermittent light (CFF) was discussed, and the quantitative relationship specified by Talbot's Law was examined.

The notion of visual acuity was introduced and four types were identified: detection, localiza-tion or vernier, resolution, and recognition acuity. The measurement of visual acuity in terms of units of visual angle was presented as well as variables that affect acuity.

The last part of the chapter dealt with eye movements, and several were identified and dis-cussed: saccadic, pursuit, vergence, and miniature eye movements. The notion of scanpaths or the fixed-path characteristic of the sequence of eye movements of a viewer for a given pattern was outlined.

13

The Perception of Color

By color perception or color vision we refer to the capacity to perceive and discriminate between lights on the basis of their wavelength composition. Although we have had occasion to comment on several issues that concern color, we have not dealt with color perception as a separate topic. This is the purpose of the present chapter.

Few issues in perception have had as persistent, controversial, and inconclusive a history as has color perception. Artists, philosophers, poets, physicists, as well as physiologists and psychologists have contributed in one way or another to the present state of our knowledge. It is not difficult to see why so much interest has been generated by the problems of the nature of color perception. Color is a pervasive characteristic of the environment that not only specifies a certain fundamental attribute or quality of surfaces and objects, but in the case of man it has profound aesthetic and emotional effects. That is to say, it provides a highly personal experience affected by associations and preference.

We must make note of the fact that color perception is not a capacity that is shared by all animals. Indeed, there are no clear overall phylogenetic trends in its possession. The color vision of primates is highly developed, matched only by that of birds. Among infraprimate mammals, some degree of wavelength discrimination has been cited for certain squirrels (Crescitelli & Pollack, 1965; Michels & Schumaker, 1968), cats (Sechzer & Brown, 1964; Brown et al., 1973), and prairie dogs (Jacobs & Pulliam, 1973). Although few other mammals except primates possess color vision to some degree, many birds, fish, amphibia, reptiles, and arthropods have fairly developed color vision.

It is likely that there has been some incentive for the evolution of color vision, that is, some biological advantage to color perception. There are many instances where animals employ color vision or coloration to their advantage, enhancing their survival capabilities. The roles of color in the mating behavior of birds in which the color of the male's plumage initiates sexual activity, and in the prey-predator relationship of many species of terrestrial animals bear this out. Prey animals often possess some concealment coloration or camouflage, generally limited to nature colors— greens and browns. Of course, if the coloration is effective in protecting the prey animals, it means that it is the predator who possesses color vision. In this sense the use of color for concealment is counteradaptive to the predator's color vision. Clearly, color may be considered as a dimension of the spatial environment, hence the ability to differentiate lights of different spectral compositions is potentially informative. Color vision is thus part of the more general capacity to perceive the composition of surfaces and objects in the environment.

The *preference* for a certain color may play a decisive role in survival. Adult frogs markedly prefer blue to other colored surfaces even when the intensity of the blue surface is considerably less than that of the other colors (Muntz, 1963, 1964). A suggestion as to the biological significance of a blue surface is given in terms of the frog's natural habitat—predominantly green vegetation bordering a blue pond. "Since blue light is effective in guiding the direction of the jump and green light is very ineffective—even less effective than yellow or red—when the frog is frightened it will tend to jump away from the vegetation toward the open space and thus into the water" (Muntz, 1964, p. 119).

THE NATURE OF COLOR

It is clear that many forms of infrahuman life possess some sort of color vision. However, we are dealing with a subjective phenomenon that generally requires a clear and precise discriminative response on the part of the perceiver; hence, much of the following discussion will focus on human color perception.

The color sensations are subjective, phenomenal experiences. However, these are related in consistent and measurable ways to the physical features of the light. In order to consider them, we must first identify the stimulus for color vision. One of the earliest recognized comprehensive treatments of color vision was developed by Isaac Newton. He demonstrated in the seventeenth century that a pinpoint beam of light that is passed through a prism is refracted and split into a number of rays of light of different wavelengths forming the entire visible spectrum (see Figure 13.1). That the different wavelengths are discriminable has been taken to indicate that the perception of color is dependent on the wavelength of light.

Although the main component of a color is generally recognized as the wavelength of the light, for a given color sensation there are actually three psychological dimensions: A color has the attributes of *hue, brightness,* and *saturation.* Hue

Fig. 13.1 *Dispersion of white light by a prism. Due to refraction the white light is split into rays of light of different wavelengths, apparent as different colors. (From Principles of Color Technology, by F. W. Billmeyer & M. Saltzman, Wiley, 1966, p. 9. Reprinted by permission of the publisher.)*

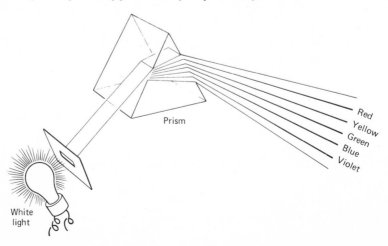

Table 13.1
TYPICAL HUE NAMES ASSOCIATED WITH
SPECTRAL ENERGY BANDS[a]

Approximate Wavelength Region (in nm)	Associated Hue
380–470	Reddish blue
470–475	Blue
475–480	Greenish blue
480–485	Blue-green
485–495	Bluish green
495–535	Green
535–555	Yellowish green
555–565	Green-yellow
565–575	Greenish yellow
575–580	Yellow
580–585	Reddish yellow
585–595	Yellow-red
595–770	Yellowish red[b]

[a] Source: *Color: A Guide to Basic Facts and Concepts,* by R. W. Burnham, R. M. Hanes, & C. J. Bartleson, Wiley, New York, 1963, p. 56. Reprinted by permission of the publisher.
[b] A pure red with no tinge of yellow requires some blue (400 nm). Accordingly, a unique red is "extraspectral" in that no single wavelength produces it.

corresponds to the common meaning of color and varies with changes in wavelength (see Table 13.1). A given color is also specified by its brightness, which varies with physical intensity, and its saturation, or the physical purity of the light. As we noted in earlier discussions, brightness is directly (but not simply) related to the intensity of the light. Generally, the more intense the light, the whiter it appears; decreasing intensity produces a darker appearance. However, for a given intensity, some colors such as yellow appear brighter than colors produced by longer wavelengths, say blue. *Saturation* corresponds to the purity (called *colorimetric purity*) of the wavelength. The addition of other wavelengths, white light, or the addition of gray to a single wavelength reduces its purity and desaturates the color.

COLOR SPINDLE

The relationship between the three psychological dimensions of hue, saturation, and brightness is simplified and represented visually in the *color spindle* or *solid* shown in Figure 13.2. Brightness is shown along the vertical axis, extending from white at the top to black at the base. The vertical line through the middle of the solid represents gray. Saturation is shown laterally with the most saturated colors located on the rim of the central circle and at the midpoint of the vertical distance between white and black. Finally, hue is expressed along the perimeter of the spindle. The conical or tapering shape of the spindle reflects the fact that saturation is maximal

Fig. 13.2 *The color spindle. Hue is represented along the perimeter of the spindle, brightness along the vertical axis, and saturation as the distance from the center of the spindle to its perimeter. (From Psychology: Man in Perspective, by A. Buss, Wiley, New York, 1973, p. 198. Reprinted by permission of the publisher.)*

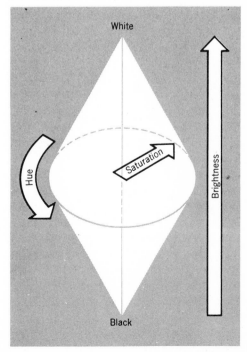

only at moderate brightness levels. In other words, saturation secondarily depends on brightness. The farther from the middle of the brightness axis, either lighter or darker, the less is the saturation of a hue.

There are numerous other ways of expressing and designating color quality. One of the most widely used descriptive systems is based on the fact that lights of appropriate wavelengths—producing so-called *primaries* (colors that do not appear easily reducible into component colors)—may be combined in various proportions to match almost all colors including white (with the possible exception of the "metallic" colors, silver and gold). This is true provided the following conditions are met: The three primaries selected lie far enough apart from each other on the spectrum; no one primary can be matched by a mixture of the other two; and no two of the primaries selected lie opposite each other on the color circle of Figure 13.3. In short, with certain restrictions

almost any spectral color can be specified by the relative contribution of each of three primaries. Procedurally, this method of color specification consists of a quantitative expression of the relative amounts of each primary that must be added to produce a given color sensation. For example, spectral light of a given wavelength, intensity, and purity is shown on one side of a bipartite or divided field, and the viewer adjusts the proportion of the three primaries that are fused on the other side of the field until a match is made. When this is done throughout the spectrum, a set of curves like those shown in Figure 13.4 results. Though many sets of tristimuli are possible, the primaries used in the example cited in Figure 13.4 are a 460 nm blue, a 530 nm green, and a 650 nm red. Based on a tristimulus specification of any color, a general color equation can be stated: $C = xR + yG + zB$, where x, y and z are the coefficients or proportion of the three fixed wavelengths (plotted on the ordinate in Figure

Fig. 13.3 *The color circle. Spectral stimuli from 420 nm to 700 nm are arranged in sequence about the circumference. The circle is arranged so that complementary pairs of colors lie at opposite ends of diagonals drawn through the center at W. Notice that the gap includes nonspectral hues, hues that have no wavelength specification but result from the mixture of spectral hues. (From The Human Senses, by F. A. Geldard, Wiley, New York, 1972, p. 90. Reprinted by permission of the publisher.)*

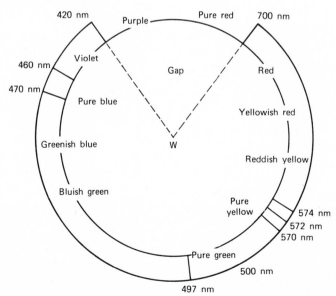

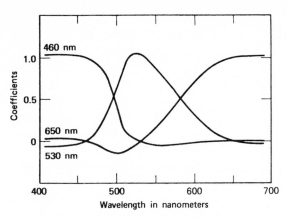

Fig. 13.4 *Trichromatic stimuli for reproduction of spectral colors. The relative amounts of each primary— a 460 nm blue, a 530 nm green, and a 650 nm red— needed to match any part of the visible spectrum are plotted for each spectral color. A negative value indicates that some of that particular primary was added to the spectral color to be matched in order to reduce its saturation to a point where it could be matched by a mixture of the two remaining primaries. (After Wright, 1928: From The Human Senses, by F. A. Geldard, Wiley, New York, 1972, p. 91. Reprinted by permission of the publisher.)*

13.4) whose sizes vary depending on the color to be matched. Thus, for example, equal amounts of red and green are required to match a yellow (roughly at 580 nm).

Of course, color specification is a highly technical matter, one that extends beyond our proper subject. We note in passing, however, that color technologists have available standardized tristimulus spectral combinations whose mixtures are employed to match various parts of the spectrum (see, for example, Judd, 1951 and Graham, 1965).

COLOR MIXTURE

Generally, pure colors of a single wavelength are perceived only under precise laboratory conditions. Most often the light that reaches the eye is composed of a mixture of various wavelengths,

and the dominant wavelength determines the hue experienced. In the preceding section we noted that when lights of two or more different wavelengths are combined, a new color with a different hue is perceived from the mixture. Once the spectral lights are combined the eye cannot distinguish the components; that is, we cannot analyze a color mixture into its component colors by mere viewing. Color experience is a psychobiological product of nervous system excitation, not an inherent property of light energy. The lights themselves are unaffected by the mixture.

Additive Color Mixture

Additive color mixtures concern the addition of the excitations produced by each component color. A number of rules or principles governing the mixing of various wavelengths have been worked out, and the essential phenomena are summarized in the color wheel of Figure 13.5. Every hue has its *complementary* that lies diametrically opposite it on the color circle, which when mixed together in the proper proportion, produces a mixture that appears neutral gray. The following are common pairs of complementaries: blue and yellow, red and blue-green, green and red-purple (note that purple lies within the gap of the color circle—an "extraspectral" region representing hues that have no unitary wavelength specification but can be produced only by mixtures of spectral lights). Mixtures of noncomplementary hues result in color sensations whose hue specifications lie intermediate on the color circle between the hues of the components (see *A* of Figure 13.5). Two such physically different lights, whose spectral compositions differ from a third light but whose mixture produces an apparent match with the third light, are called *metamers* or *metameric* pairs, and the color match is called a *metameric* match (Judd, 1951). If the colors are mixed in equal amounts, the new hue lies on the color circle halfway between the two component colors. If the colors are mixed in unequal amounts, we may gain an approximation of the resultant hue on the wheel by drawing a line

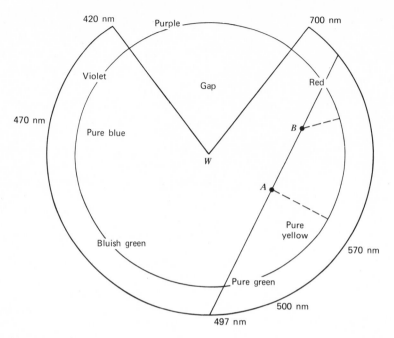

Fig. 13.5 *Additive color mixture on the color wheel. The color of the mixture is indicated by the point lying on the line segment. (A) Equal proportions of red and green produce a yellow hue. (B) About two-thirds of the mixture is red, one-third green; hence, the resultant hue lies closer to the red. The resultant hue in both cases is indicated by the point at which the dotted line reaches the circumference. Notice that the saturation of the hue produced by the mixture lies closer to the center of the color circle; hence, it is less saturated than the saturations of the component hues.*

connecting the two component colors and placing a point on the line representing the proportion in which they are mixed. The location of the point designates the hue and saturation. As *B* of Figure 13.5 shows, the resultant hue of the mixture lies closer to the component that makes the greatest contribution.

The saturation will be less than the saturation of one or both of the component colors. As a rule, the farther away the constituent colors lie from each other, the less is the saturation of the resultant color. This is depicted graphically in Figure 13.5 in that any mixture falls nearer the center (the desaturated region) of the color circle than the components that comprise it. Finally, the brightness of the resultant color will appear as the average of the brightnesses of the two component

colors. Notice that although we have described additive color mixture for only two hues, with certain modifications the above rules hold for any number.

The color circle, although not providing an explanation of any aspect of color perception, provides a good summary of much of the basic phenomena of color mixture. Observe, however, that its use is limited to illustrating experiential aspects of color mixture. For a precise quantitative designation of color, very sophisticated devices and methods must be employed.

There are a number of procedures for showing the additive nature of mixing colors. It is quite simply accomplished by projecting beams of monochromatic light from three projectors onto a

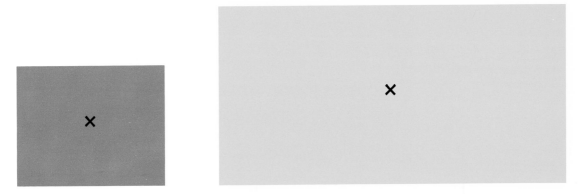

Fig. 13.10 *Negative afterimage and successive contrast. Stare at the fixation cross of the blue patch for 30 sec, then transfer the gaze to the cross of the yellow surface. A supersaturated yellow patch will appear.*

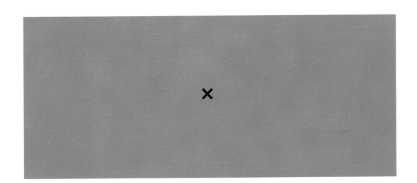

Fig. 13.11 *Desaturation with continued exposure. Cover the right half of the rectangle with a piece of gray paper and stare at the fixation cross for 60 sec. Then remove the gray sheet while continuing to stare at the fixation mark. The left side will appear less saturated than the previously covered right side. (Based on demonstration in Krech & Crutchfield, 1958, p. 1.)*

Fig. 13.12 *Simultaneous contrast. "Shimmering" effects may be seen at the border of the patch and its background because the two colors are complementaries.*

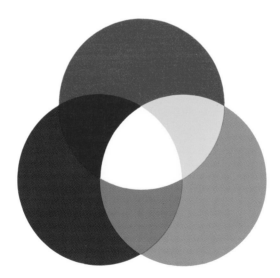

Fig. 13.6 *Color mixture as additions of excitations. The partially superposed projections of red, green, and blue result in: yellow (red and green), purple (red and blue), blue-green (blue and green). The mixture of all three (center) yields white. (From Psychology: Explorations In Behavior and Experience, by Mednick, Higgins, and Kirschenbaum; Wiley, New York, 1975. Reprinted by permission of the publisher.)*

screen, each projector equipped with a different colored filter. The intersection of the beams, shown in Figure 13.6 (see color insert), illustrates the effect of the mixture. Similar sensory effects result when each eye is stimulated with a different spectral light. For example, if one eye is stimulated with a red filter and a green filter is placed over the other eye, the perception of yellow may fleetingly occur.

Another simple means of observing additive color mixture is to employ a color wheel on which discs of colored paper are assembled (Figure 13.7). The colored discs can be overlapped and adjusted so that different sized angular sectors of each color are exposed, thereby varying the proportion of the component colors. When the wheel is rotated rapidly, a completely fused and uniform color is seen instead of the constituent colors. Although an additive method of color mixture is employed here, it is more an addition over time rather than over space.

Fig. 13.7 *A color wheel. Discs of colored paper are cut and assembled on the wheel, overlapping so that different sized sectors of each color are exposed. When the wheel is rotated rapidly, a completely mixed color is seen instead of the separate component colors. The proportions of mixtures can be varied by changing the size of angular sectors of two or more component colors. (Source: Krech & Crutchfield, 1958, p. 59. Reprinted by permission of the authors.)*

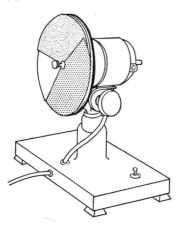

Artists have also used an additive method of color mixture directly on their canvas. A technique called pointillism or divisionism was used by the French Neo-impressionist painters (e.g., Seurat and Signac) in which they did no pallette mixing of the paints; rather, they placed minute but discrete dots of different colored paint on the canvas. When viewed from a certain distance, the discrete dots are not visible as such, but apparently fuse to produce an additive color mixture.

Perhaps the most common example of additive color mixture occurs with color television. Generally, the screen of a color television set is composed of a mosaic of dots, usually red, green, and blue. Because the dots are very small, they cannot be resolved separately by the eye at the usual viewing distance; hence, they are apparently fused or blended together and their joint action—an additive color mixture—results in the perception of a distinct hue. It may not be obvious to the casual viewer, but an apparent patch of yellow seen on a color television screen is composed of small red and green dots. This is consistent with what we have said about additive color mixture.

Subtractive Color Mixture

The principle of the color circle applies to the mixing of colored lights but not to pigments, paints or dyes. In the former case we are combining lights—colored lights *add* their dominant wavelengths to the mixture. It is an additive process in that the effects—receptor activation—of the wavelengths are added together in the nervous system. In contrast, colored pigments selectively absorb or *subtract* some wavelengths striking them and reflect the remaining wavelengths that give the pigment its unique hue.

Subtractive color mixtures are thus based on the fact that the color of an object or surface depends on the wavelengths it reflects. A blue surface appears blue because the surface pigment absorbs or *subtracts* all but the wavelengths of light that appear as blue. Hence, when white light falls on the surface its "blue" wavelengths are predominantly reflected to the eyes of the viewer whereas the other wavelengths are largely absorbed.

Similarly, the result of mixing two pigments involves a mutual absorption or subtraction, canceling the reflectance of all wavelengths but those that the two pigments jointly reflect. As an example of the difference between additive and subtractive mixtures, consider the combination of the complementaries blue and yellow (see Figure 13.8). As lights, the mixture yields gray—a summation of the two spectral regions represented by blue and yellow—whereas as pigments their combined absorption produces the reflection of wavelengths that appear predominantly green. That is, all other wavelengths but those that appear green are absorbed in the combination. In practice it is quite a complex matter to predict accurately the resultant hue from a mixture of pigments because the hue of the combination is highly dependent on the physical and chemical properties of the constituent pigments as well as on the spectral composition of incident light.

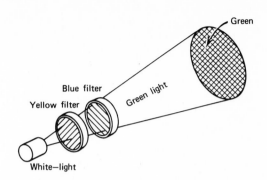

Fig. 13.8(b) *A subtractive mixture of yellow and blue produces green. (Notice that the filters in b produce the same effect as do pigments.) (Source: Lewis, 1963, p. 463. Reprinted with permission of Prentice-Hall.)*

AFTERIMAGES

Chromatic effects of a visual stimulus may persist after its physical termination, in a form called *afterimages*. The usual means of demonstrating afterimages is to have a viewer stare at or fixate on a stimulus configuration or patch for about 30 to 60 sec, after which the gaze is transferred to a different surface. There are two kinds of afterimages. One much less frequent and more fleeting is called a *positive afterimage,* in that the afterimage maintains the same black-white brightness relations and colors as the original stimulus. Positive afterimages most often occur after brief, intense stimulation of the dark-adapted eye. The more frequently occurring *negative afterimage* refers to the persistence of the image beyond the original stimulus but in a reversed state. That is, the image occurs as an afterimage with the black and white and chromatic effects reversed, as in a photographic negative. Figure 13.9 presents an achromatic example of a negative afterimage.

Successive and Simultaneous Contrast

If a chromatic stimulus is fixated on, the afterimage will be in the complementary color of the

Fig. 13.8(a) *An additive mixture is illustrated. Blue and yellow appear gray.*

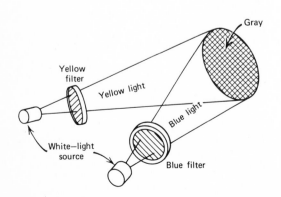

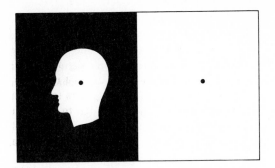

Fig. 13.9 *Demonstration of an achromatic negative afterimage. Stare at the dot in the white profile for about 30 seconds and then shift the gaze to the dot in the white square. You should see a negative afterimage in the white square; that is, a dark profile instead of a white one. (From Color: A Guide to Basic Facts and Concepts, by R. W. Burnham, R. H. Hanes, & J. C. Bartleson, Wiley, New York, 1963, p. 69. Reprinted by permission of the publisher.)*

initial stimulus. This is often called *successive contrast.* Making use of a color's complementary, unnatural color effects may be produced. If a blue patch is fixated on for a minute after which the gaze is transferred to a yellow surface, the surface will appear excessively saturated or "supersaturated." What has occurred is that the afterimage of the blue patch (yellow) has been projected onto a yellow surface. The explanation of this phenomenon is illustrated in Figures 13.10 and 13.11 (see color insert). If the instructions for Figure 13.11 are correctly followed, it will be clear that continual chromatic exposure of a particular region of the fovea produces a loss in saturation of that color. Interestingly, as Figure 13.11 demonstrates, the loss occurs without any clear or immediate perception of a change in saturation. Continuing with the example of color enhancement, during chromatic exposure the region of the retina that is stimulated by the blue stimulus patch becomes adapted, fatigued, or less sensitive to that particular color and it appears relatively desaturated. This is functionally equivalent to making the same retinal area more sensitive to its complementary, yellow. That is, sufficient exposure of a

region of the retina to blue increases the sensitivity of that retinal region to yellow. Thus, when continued inspection of the blue patch fatigues the receptors normally mediating a blue sensation, a yellow afterimage results; if the gaze then shifts to a yellow surface, the additive mixture of the yellow afterimage and the yellow surface makes the yellow surface appear more saturated than is normal.

Similar effects are seen with *simultaneous contrast* or, as it is sometimes termed, spatial induction of the complementary. After continued fixation of a chromatic stimulus patch placed against a neutral or gray background, the edge of the background bordering the patch appears to be tinged with its complementary. This is because with continued inspection the color patch loses in saturation (which coincides with the addition of its complementary). Because the eyes move slightly, even during fixation, the retinal image of the patch is not stationary, and the decreased saturation or slight appearance of the patch's complementary appears at its edges. If the color's complement is substituted for the neutral background, the usual complementary tinge of the patch sums with the chromatic background to produce a simultaneous "supersaturation" at the edges of the patch (see Figure 13.12 of color insert). In many instances visually disturbing effects result from the simultaneous presentation of adjoining pairs of colors that are complementary to each other.

MEMORY COLOR

Within this context mention must be made of the influence of an object's familiarity on its apparent color. This is especially clear when stimuli whose colors are to be matched have distinctive shapes that are associated with objects that typically occur in a single color. The effects of past experience on apparent color are held to be due to *memory color.* Duncker (1939) used cut-outs of a green leaf and a donkey made from the same green felt material. Both stimuli were successively shown bathed by hidden red illumination that was the complementary of the color of the cut-outs; thus each stimulus cut-out reflected the same gray. According to Duncker, past experience with objects associated with these shapes influences their apparent color so that the cut-out of the leaf, typically green, should appear greener than the cut-out of the characteristically gray donkey. This was the result. Matches of the apparent color of each stimulus made on a color wheel indicated that the amount of green required to match the color of the cut-out of the leaf was about twice as much as needed to match the color of the cut-out of the donkey. That is, although both stimuli reflected the same gray light, the cut-out of the leaf, presumably owing to the influence of memory color, appeared to be somewhat greener than the cut-out of the donkey. The obvious conclusion is that previous color and form associations—memory color—does exert an appreciable effect on perceived color. This experiment, in a number of variations, has been repeated and its essential findings confirmed (e.g., see Delk & Fillenbaum, 1965; Epstein, 1967, Chap. 4).

THEORIES OF COLOR PERCEPTION

There have been numerous theoretical accounts of the many diverse phenomena of color perception. However, two main accounts emerge as most coincident with the empirical data. Accordingly, our discussion will be principally confined to them.

The Young-Helmholtz Theory (Trichromatic Receptor Theory)

The phenomena of color mixture, although factual and independent of theory, suggest certain structural, functional, and neural mechanisms of the retina. Because three distinct and disparate wavelengths are sufficient to produce almost all the perceptible colors, it is possible that there are, correspondingly, three sets of receptors (cones) in the eye that respond differentially to different wavelengths; that is, the neural contribution of each set of receptors may vary appropriately for a given spectral light in the environment.

Thomas Young, an English scientist, in 1802 suggested just such a trichromatic receptor theory. Basing his theory on the assumption that there are three different kinds of receptors in the human retina, each sensitive to light of a specific spectral composition, he proposed that when they are stimulated by a given wavelength their neural activity accounts for color experience. This proposal was revived in 1856 by Herman von Helmholtz, who extended Young's initial proposal by postulating a distinct spectral sensitivity curve for each of the three sets of receptors (Figure 13.13) (see Riggs, 1967). Helmholtz modified Young's theory by rejecting the idea that a given receptor for color can be activated by only one wavelength. His original proposal designated receptors not exclusively but *maximally* sensitive to wavelengths that correspond to the hues of

Fig. 13.13 *Sensitivity functions of hypothetical red (1), green (2), and blue (3) receptors. In the original citation type 3 receptors were labeled "violet" but the maximal spectral region lies closer to the blue. (Figure source: Riggs, 1967, p. 3; after Helmholtz, 1866. Reprinted by permission of the publisher.)*

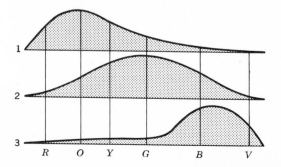

blue, green, and red. In its simplest form the trichromatic receptor theory maintains that only three types of receptors are required for the discrimination of hue. Stimulation by red, for example, produces a chromatic experience specifically due to a strong excitation of the "red" receptors (type 1, in Figure 13.13), together with weak stimulation of "green" and "blue" receptors (type 2 and 3 receptors of Figure 13.13). The result is a red sensation. "Yellow" light stimulates the "red" and "green" receptors and the "blue" very slightly with a resultant sensation of yellow. Accordingly, all the hues resulting from the distribution of spectral lights and their mixtures can be produced by the appropriate proportional contribution of a three-receptor system.

There is strong physiological evidence for the existence of a three-receptor system, supporting the notion of a retinal basis of color vision. Evidence has been reported of the existence of three groups of distinct cones, each set maximally responsive to a different wavelength. Actually, it is three classes of photopigments that are segregated in three kinds of cones. Marks, Dobelle, and MacNichol (1964) directed a fine beam of light on isolated cone photoreceptors of the retinae of monkeys and humans. Utilizing extremely elaborate techniques and equipment, measurements were made of the absorption of light by the pigment of a single cone for different

spectral wavelengths. The major apparatus is called a *microspectrophotometer,* and its aspects are diagramed in Figure 13.14. Simply stated, lights of varying wavelengths but constant intensity were passed through a cone, and the amount of light transmitted at each wavelength was compared with the transmission composition of an identical reference beam passing through a cone-free part of the retina. The difference is assumed to be due to the absorption of some specific wavelengths of light by the pigment of the cone: The more a given wavelength is absorbed by the pigment of a cone, the more sensitive that cone is to light of that wavelength. The results, shown in Figure 13.15, indicate clearly that for cones, peaks of absorption fall into three major groups with maximum absorption at about 445 nm, 535 nm, and 570 nm. Following similar procedures, Brown and Wald (1964) reported maximal absorption at 450 nm, 525 nm, and 555 nm. Though the peak absorption regions are slightly different, likely owing to variations in measuring techniques, nevertheless at least three clear distinct types of receptors can be identified.

Further support for the existence of specific cone pigments has come from the research of Rushton (1962; Baker & Rushton, 1965). By taking into account the difference in the amount of light beamed in and the proportion reflected back from living human retinae after selective absorp-

Fig. 13.14 *Diagram of the components of a recording microspectrophotometer. The beam of a single wavelength is split in two halves, Beam 1 and Beam 2. Both beams are demagnified by inverted microscopes. Beam 2 passes through the cone specimen, whereas Beam 1, the reference beam, does not. The differences in the output of matched photodetectors is a direct measure of the absorption of the cone specimen. (Source: Modified from Uttal, 1973, p. 495; and from MacNichol, 1964a.)*

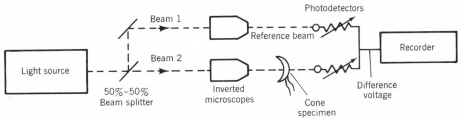

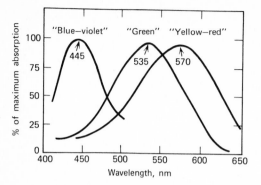

Fig. 13.15 *Curves derived from the absorption spectra for cones of primates. Color vision appears mediated by three types of cone pigments with peaks at 445, 535, and 570 nm. The peak (570 nm) of the "red" curve is in the yellow region but extends far enough into the red region to account for the sensation of red. (Source: Buss, 1973, p. 203; after Marks, Dobelle, & MacNichol, 1964; Brown & Wald, 1964; Reprinted by permission of the publisher.)*

tion of portions of the spectrum, he was able to identify two different cone pigments. He reports the existence of a photosensitive pigment for green called *chlorolabe* and a red pigment, *erythrolabe*. From the two studies noted above (Marks, Dobelle, & MacNichol, 1964; Brown & Wald, 1964) we may assume the existence of the third pigment for blue, *cyanolabe*. Thus, the evidence on pigment absorption indicates that three types of cones are specialized to absorb portions of light over a limited range of wavelengths with a maximum absorption at a particular region of the spectrum.

Employing electrophysiological methods, Tomita implanted microelectrodes into a single cone of a carp retina (see Riggs, 1967, pp. 6–7). Illuminating the cone with various wavelengths enabled recordings to be made of its electrical behavior. This was accomplished for a number of cones, and peak wavelength responses were recorded for the different cones. Again evidence for three types of cones were found. In the carp, peak responses resulted that were characteristic of

a "red" receptor at 611 nm, a "green" receptor at 529 nm, and a "blue" receptor at 462 nm.

These and other data along with the facts of color mixture and matching lend considerable support to a trichromatic receptor theory of color vision, at least at the retinal level (see also Mac-Nichol, 1964a; Sperling & Harweth, 1971).

Opponent-process Theory

A second major theory of color vision is traced to Ewald Hering, a German physiologist (1878) (see Teevan & Burney, 1961). Like the Young-Helmholtz trichromatic receptor theory, Hering postulated three independent receptor types, but his theory differed in that the three classes of receptors were each assumed to be composed of a pair of opponent color processes or neural systems: a white-black, a red-green, and a blue-yellow receptor. Furthermore, each pair is associated with a corresponding pair of unique sensory qualities. The basic scheme is diagramed in Figure 13.16. The positive and negative signs

Fig. 13.16 *Basic scheme for the Hering opponent-process mechanism. The plus and minus signs indicate that each receptor process is capable of two mutually antagonistic responses. (Source: Hurvich & Jameson, 1957, p. 385. Reprinted by permission of the authors and the American Psychological Association.)*

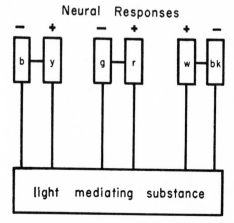

indicate that each receptor is capable of two kinds of physiological and sensory responses that are mutually opposite or antagonistic to each other. That is, a receptor can respond in only one of two possible ways. It follows that either red *or* green, and yellow *or* blue is experienced, but not yellow *and* blue or red *and* green. If one member of a receptor pair is stimulated more than its opponent, the corresponding hue will be seen. If both members are equally stimulated, they cancel each other out (as is the case with mixtures of complementary colors) leaving only gray. Furthermore, members from nonopponent pairs may interact. Thus, for example, stimulation with 450 nm light causes activity in the blue-yellow and red-green receptors: The blue process of the blue-yellow system and the red process of the red-green system react to produce the appearance of violet. The luminance dimension results from the activity of the black-white receptor and contributes to the brightness of the chromatic response.

It is possible to specify what hue will be seen with any given wavelength of light. This has been done, basically as a quantification of the Hering theory, by Hurvich and Jameson (1955, 1957). Because the two members of a receptor process are mutually antagonistic, the magnitude of a given sensory response can be assessed by the amount of the opponent needed to eliminate or cancel the color sensation. According to Hurvich and Jameson, this *null* or hue cancellation method can be used to measure the spectral distribution of the chromatic response. Accordingly, the amount or relative strength of a blue response is determined by the amount of energy of a wavelength appearing yellow that must be added in order to cancel or neutralize the blue sensation. That is, the amount of the blue component is assumed to equal the amount of yellow that had to be added to cancel it. Similarly, the amount of the yellow response is determined by adding just sufficient blue light to cancel the yellow sensation. A similar statement can be made for the green and red response: The amount of red light added

to wavelengths in the greenish region and the amount of green light added to wavelengths in the red region to cancel the appropriate chromatic responses are measures of the amount of green and red response, respectively. The results of these manipulations are given in the *chromatic response* curves in Figure 13.17, which show the amount of each chromatic response that is produced at each wavelength. The fact that a single wavelength, say 520 nm, requires red *and* blue light to cancel the chromatic response indicates that the color has a greenish-yellow appearance. Notice also that red appears at both the long and short wavelengths. That is, some green light must be added at both ends of the spectrum to cancel the chromatic response of red. It also indicates what hue will be seen at each wavelength: At 475 nm, the red-green system equals zero, causing a pure or "unique" blue response; at 500 nm the blue-yellow system equals zero, producing a pure or "unique" green response; at 580 nm the red-green receptor process again equals zero but here producing a pure or "unique" yellow response. At about 600 nm the activity of the red and yellow members produces an orange response. Notice that a yellow response occurs throughout the long wavelengths. It is present in a green of 550 nm and a red of 650 nm. Thus, when red and green are mixed as shown at about 580 nm, the red-green system signals zero and only the yellow response remains.

Thus far we have confined our discussion of color perception to retinal mechanisms. However, there is much neurophysiological evidence of an opponent-type process operating at neural levels beyond the retina. The general finding that emerges from the recordings of neural activity from the ganglion level or the lateral geniculate nucleus is that some cells increase their rates of firing (above a spontaneous or baseline level) for some wavelengths and decrease them for others. Wagner, MacNichol, and Wolbarsht (1960; see also Daw, 1967) found that the ganglion cells of the goldfish gave "off-on" response to stimulation by white light. When single spectral lights were

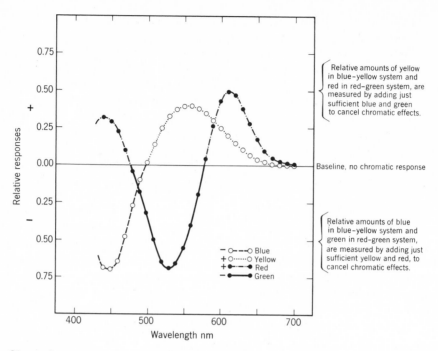

Fig. 13.17 *Chromatic response curves: amount of chromatic response produced at each wavelength as measured by the null method of Hurvich and Jameson. The curves are generated by adding, at each wavelength, the relative amount of the opponent color needed to neutralize or cancel the color sensation. The open dot curve is a plot of the amount of yellow (shown below the baseline level, indicated by the minus values) or blue (indicated by plus values, above the baseline) added to cancel the blue or yellow sensation. As noted in the text these values indicate the amount of blue and yellow response, respectively, at each wavelength. The solid circle curve is a plot of the amount of green (+) or red (−) light needed to cancel the sensation of red or green, respectively. Thus, for example, at 450 nm (violet) about 0.75 yellow is needed to cancel the blue sensation and about 0.30 green to cancel the red. That is to say, a 450 nm light is matched by relative amounts of blue and red. (Source: Hurvich & Jameson, 1955, p. 36. Reprinted by permission of the authors and the American Psychological Association.)*

used, they found that for a given cell an excitatory or "on" response to a band of spectral colors turned into an "off" response to other wavelengths.

DeValois (1965a,b; DeValois, Abramov & Jacobs, 1966) inserted microelectrodes into single cells in the lateral geniculate nucleus of the macaque monkey and recorded the neural activity in response to the presentation of flashes of light of the same intensity but of various dominant wavelengths. Evidence was found of cells that directly increased or decreased their rates of firing in response to lights of any wavelength. However,

evidence was also noted of opponent-type cells whose overall response rates depended on the wavelength of light; they were excited by some wavelengths and inhibited by others and generally showed differing firing rates to different wavelengths. Figure 13.18 provides an example of one such cell. If it is stimulated with long wavelength red light (633 nm), it fires vigorously at the onset and throughout the duration of the light, whereas it is relatively inhibited at the offset of the light. In contrast, short wavelengths of blue or green light produce an inhibition of the cell during the light interval followed by activity at the offset of

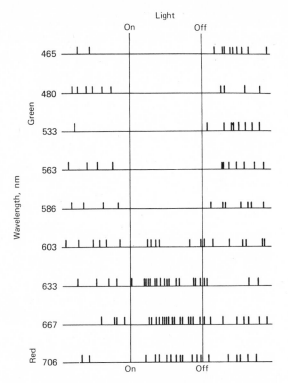

Fig. 13.18 *Responses recorded from a single microelectrode inserted in a cell of the lateral geniculate nucleus of a monkey. The cell that produced this record was classified as an opponent cell because of the opposite actions of the long and short wavelengths. Short wavelengths inhibited the cell, whereas long wavelengths excited it. This opponent cell turned out to be a red-excitatory, green-inhibitory cell (+R −G cell). [The firing before the stimulation (light onset) is due to the spontaneous firing of the cell]. (Source: After DeValois, Abramov, & Jacobs, 1966, 56, 970.)*

the light. Some cells show activity to the same spectral lights that is the reverse of that shown in Figure 13.18 (see DeValois, 1965b, p. 155).

These and other data strongly suggest that there is a correlation between the chromatic response and the post-retinal neural response. Much is yet to be worked out, but it is sufficient to say that the characteristics of a chromatic stimulus are processed and neurally transmitted

along the visual system by means of some opponent-type color coding process. Although a firm resolution between the trichromatic receptor theory and the opponent-process theory cannot be stated, a compromise is possible.

> *All the evidence for the three-color, three-receptor cone system comes up against the earlier electrophysiological evidence for an opponent-color system farther along the visual pathway. Color vision is apparently at least a two-stage process, consistent with the Young-Helmholtz theory at the receptor level and with the Hering theory at the level of the optic nerve and beyond. Each receptor does not have its private route to the brain; three-color information is somehow processed in the retina and encoded into two-color on-off signals by each of the color-sensitive retinal ganglion cells for transmission to the higher visual centers. (MacNichol, 1964a, P. 56)*

In keeping with contemporary thought on color perception, our emphasis has been on the trichromatic receptor and opponent-process color theories. However, there are numerous other theoretical accounts. Two are worthy of some note.

Ladd-Franklin Theory

The Ladd-Franklin theory is an evolutionary theory that employs some concepts from both the trichromatic receptor and opponent theories. Originally Christine Ladd-Franklin (1929) postulated that a basic or primitive black-white achromatic sensitivity evolved into further differentiation, first into a sensitivity to blue and yellow, which at still later stages of evolution became further differentiated into sensitivity to red and green. In support of this, the near periphery of the retina does manifest such chromatic zones or regions. As Figure 13.19 shows, achromatic sensitivity occurs first in the far periphery, blue and yellow zones occur next, and the more central region is required for seeing red and green. The theory supposes that the central areas of the

Indirect Vision

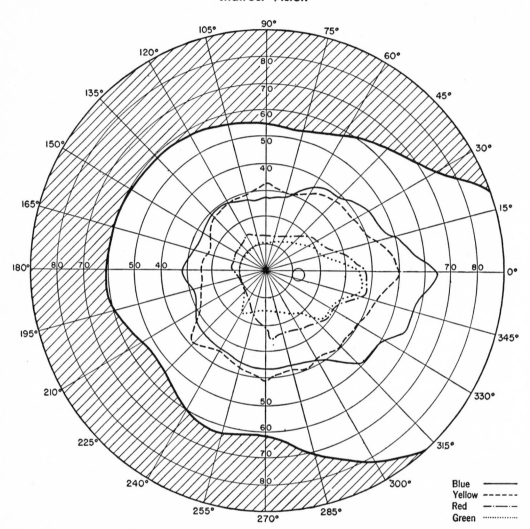

Fig. 13.19 *Color zones of the human retina. The figure shows the portion of the visual field of the right eye within which each of the four basic colors can be seen when the stimulus is a small disc of chromatic light and fixation is maintained on the center of the chart. The distribution of sensitivity to red and green is limited to an area of approximately 20° to 30° about the fixation point, whereas yellow and blue can be seen out to 40° or 50° in the vertical and 50° to 60° in the horizontal meridian. The far periphery is totally color blind. The small area to the right of the central fixation region is the blind spot. (From Foundations of Psychology, by E. G. Boring, H. S. Langfeld, & H. P. Weld, Wiley, New York, 1948, p. 287. Reprinted by permission of the publisher.)*

retina, where all hues are perceived, are the most evolutionarily developed and at the extremes of the retina are found the most primitive receptors responsive to only achromatic light. According to this theory, persons who show red and green chromatic deficiencies, possessing only blue and yellow sensitivity (described in a later section) possess a more primitive level of color vision; the person who is totally color blind, the monochromat, blind to all colors, has a most primitive form of visual ability. However, given the state of known facts on color vision this theory is obviously incomplete. We might also point out the questionable assumption inherent in this theory, namely, that cones are a further evolutionary development than are rods (Walls, 1963). Many forms of life lower on the phylogenetic scale than mammals (lacking cones in most species) are found to possess cones.

The Land Effect

Edwin Land (1959, 1964; see also McCann, 1972), the inventor of the Polaroid camera, has demonstrated the possibility of producing most color sensations by employing only two primaries. One of his methods is as follows. Using black and white film, a polychromatic scene is photographed twice, once with a red filter over the camera's lens, transmitting the long wavelength portion of the visible spectrum, and a second time with a green filter, transmitting a relatively short or middle wavelength band. Next, the film is processed as black and white positive transparencies or slides, and the two slides are simultaneously projected and superimposed on a screen. The slide originally taken with a red filter is projected with a red filter over the projection lens, but no filter is needed for the other slide, which is thus projected with white incandescent light. The resultant projection shows an unusual phenomenon: Nearly the full range of colors in the original scene appears. This suggests, of course, that under certain conditions, fewer than three primaries are needed to produce the usual range of hues. Certainly this cannot be explained only by reference to the classical laws of color mixture, and accordingly Land's chromatic effects have produced some controversy. One attempt has been made to explain Land's hues on the basis of complex applications of induced or simultaneous contrast (Walls, 1960; see also Graham & Brown, 1965, pp. 469–472), but no explanation, including Land's (see Land & McCann, 1971), has met wide acceptance.

DEFFECTIVE COLOR VISION

Although the vast majority of the human population possess normal color vision, a small proportion have some defect. Persons in this latter group match spectral colors with different amounts of primary colors than do persons with normal color vision. Except for those forms based on pathology, defective color vision is inherited. It is recognized as a genetically transmitted sex-linked recessive characteristic and, as such, occurs primarily in males. According to Geldard (1972) about 8% of the male population have some form of color vision defect. Color deficiencies may be divided into three major classes, depending on the number of primary colors required to match all spectral colors. The main forms are termed *anomalous trichromatism, dichromatism,* and *monochromatism.*

Anomalous Trichromatism

Although normal color vision is also trichromatic, the defective or anomalous trichromat requires a different proportion of the three primary colors to match the colors of the spectrum than does a normal viewer. The most common form of dichromatism involves the perception of red and green. As we noted earlier, a yellow color can be matched by the suitable mixture of red and green. Anomalous trichromats, however, require more red or green in the mixture than do normals. The general device used to assess such defects in color matching is a special kind of color mixer that measures the proportions of monochromatic red that must be mixed with monochromatic green to match a monochromatic yellow. Appropriately, it is termed an *anomaloscope*.

Two kinds of anomalous trichromatism may be identified: *protoanomaly* and *deuteranomaly*. The protoanomalous person requires much more red in the mixture of red and green to match a yellow in an anomaloscope, and the deuteranomalous person needs a greater proportion of green in the red-green mixture to match the yellow.

Dichromatism

Dichromats match the spectrum with the appropriate combination of two colors rather than the three required by normal viewers. Dichromats may be divided into *deuteranopia* and *protanopia,* which refer to green and red deficiencies. For both deuteranopes and protanopes, the short wavelength region of the spectrum appears blue and the long wavelength region appears yellow. Moreover, both deuteranopes and protanopes confuse red and green, both colors appearing as desaturated yellow. However, persons who have deuteranopia, the most common form of dichromatism, cannot distinguish green from certain combinations of red and blue, whereas protanopes are relatively insensitive to the long wavelengths of light; that is, much higher than normal intensities of red light are required for a brightness response. Similarly, there is evidence that deuteranopes are less sensitive to wavelengths in the green region (Graham & Hsia, 1954, 1958; Hsia & Graham, 1965).

A third form of dichromatism, which occurs much less frequently than the above two, called *tritanopia,* is characterized by a deficiency in seeing blue and yellow; that is, tritanopes see only reds and greens and confuse yellows, grays and blues. In addition, tritanopes see only a neutral gray in the neighborhood of 570 nm (yellow);

longer wavelengths appear reddish and shorter wavelengths appear greenish (Hsia & Graham, 1965; Geldard, 1972).

Although it is not possible to know how the colors that a dichromat sees compare with those seen by a normal person, some evidence bearing on this issue has been described. Graham and Hsia (1958) reported the case of a unilaterally color-blind subject, a woman who was a deuteranope in her left eye but normal in her right eye. By using color-matching procedures in which different hues could be shown to each eye independently, it was possible to measure the color vision in the defective left eye. The procedure was that for each color presented to her defective left eye she adjusted the color on the normal right eye so that it appeared as the same hue. The results of this color-matching procedure are shown in Figure 13.20. To her defective eye the colors extending the entire spectral range from green to red (502 nm to 700 nm) appeared identical to a single hue of yellow (about 570 nm) as seen by her normal right eye, and all the colors from green to violet looked blue (about 470 nm). The blue-green region (which occurred at about 502 nm) was seen as a neutral gray by the defective eye.

Monochromatism

A third class of persons with a color defect, *monochromats,* match all wavelengths of the spectrum against any other wavelength or a white light. This group could be termed "color-blind." Essentially, they have no chromatic response and usually suffer a reduction in other visual functions. It is likely that they have an abnormality in the number and kinds of cones in their retinae.

Color deficiencies have important theoretical implications for color vision. A reasonable explanation of color deficiencies is consistent with the notion that there are three classes of cones each with a distinct pigment and that one or more of the cones' photopigments is defective or totally

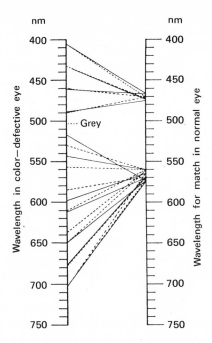

nm

400
450
500 — Grey
550
600
650
700
750

Wavelength in color—defective eye

nm

400
450
500
550
600
650
700
750

Wavelength for match in normal eye

Fig. 13.20 *Results of the experiment with a unilateral color-defective subject. The wavelengths seen by the color-blind eye (left scale) are matched by the indicated wavelengths in the normal eye (right scale). (Source: Graham & Hsia, Science, 1958, 127, 679. Reprinted by permission of the American Association for the Advancement of Science.)*

lacking. That is, there is no absence of actual cones nor are the extrachromatic functions of cones impeded—which is consistent with the fact that the acuity of most color deficient persons, except for the rod monochromat, is at a normal level—but there is an abnormal distribution of cone photopigments. Accordingly, the anatomical distinction between the deuteranopes and protanopes is that each has a set of cones that lacks the pigment of green (chlorolabe) or red (erythrolabe). Other theoretical accounts of color defects are possible, but without a doubt the varieties of color deficiencies must be taken into account by any final theory of color vision.

SUBJECTIVE COLORS

We will end this chapter with a brief commentary on the production of chromatic sensations from essentially achromatic stimulation. We have noted repeatedly that color sensations result principally from the different wavelength compositions of light. However, it is possible to produce some chromatic sensations, called *subjective colors,* from only black and white stimuli. One of the configurations used to demonstrate subjective colors, called "Benham's top," is shown in Figure 13.21. By rotating the disc in a clockwise direction at a rate of 5 to 10 Hz, very desaturated blues, greens, yellows, and reds may appear. When the direction of rotation is reversed, the order of the appearance of the colors also reverses. They can be shown on a black and white television screen when illuminated by monochromatic light. Clearly, neither wavelength variation of the physical stimulus nor differential bleaching of the cone pigments is likely to play a role in the resultant chromatic sensations. It is plausible that the patterns of black and white al-

Fig. 13.21 *Benham's top. When rotated, the figure produces various temporal sequences of black and white. However, subjective colors—desaturated blues, greens, yellows and reds—may appear.*

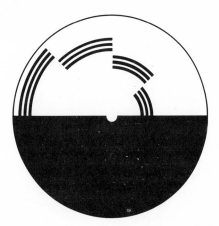

ternations by-pass the contribution of the retina. That is, the step normally performed at the retina is eliminated, and patterns of excitation are set up beyond the retinal level in the optic nerve. This implies that the intermittent stimulation created by rotation of the Benham disc produces a sequence of neural events that simulates or mimics the different temporal patterns of neural activity that normally result from viewing chromatic stimuli. Festinger, Allyn, and White (1971) showed that the sequence of intensity changes over time, produced by the rotation of a figure like that in Benham's top, can also be produced by a stationary pattern of flickering lights. That is, by varying the amount of light emitted as a function of time, reliable color sensations resulted. According to this description, subjective colors are the result of neural stimulation in which the normal cone contribution has been by-passed.

In order to describe the general nature of color vision, color was discussed in terms of its three psychological attributes—hue, brightness, and saturation. These were related to the physical dimensions of wavelength, intensity, and purity. The facts of additive and subtractive color vision were outlined, and these were shown to be involved with many chromatic phenomena such as adaptation, color aftereffects and afterimages, successive and simultaneous contrast, color induction, and memory color.

Two major theories of color perception were outlined, the Young-Helmholtz or trichromatic receptor theory and the opponent-process theory. Evidence bearing on each were summarized, and it was concluded that aspects of both theories are consistent with contemporary research findings. In addition, the Ladd-Franklin theory and the Land phenomenon were noted. Finally, the topics of color deficiencies (anomalous trichromatism, dichromatism, monochromatism) and the perception of subjective colors were summarized. The latter phenomenon indicates that chromatic sensations can result without wavelength variation.

14

The Perception of Form and Shape

Our concern up to this point has been with describing the retinal stimulus and the function of certain basic visual processes. We have not yet said much about the perception of spatial relations occurring within the visual field. Clearly, the perceptual response is different from the reception of a replica of the variegated optic array emanating from the environment. The reflected light that results in the image that is projected on the retina from objects and surfaces in the visual field is far too impoverished to provide the visual characteristics of the world that are experienced. Nor can the structures and known mechanisms of the eye or of the nervous system simply account for organized perception. Rather than a loose aggregation of apparently discrete stimuli, one sees the visual field organized into related units with definite forms and shapes. Perception is thus a constructive achievement involving a set of unifying processes.

Our purpose in this chapter will be to trace the development of the dynamics of form perception beginning with elementary aspects of the processes involved in perceptual organization. We will consider how such processes are elaborated to produce the perception of form, and we will also attempt to isolate some of the specific factors that account for, or contribute to, form perception.

CONTOUR AND CONTRAST PERCEPTION

An enormous number of lateral interconnections among adjacent and neighboring receptor cells exist within the eye and related structures and interact to enable the perception of sharp visual contours. One of the contributions to the understanding of contour perception comes from investigation of the horseshoe crab (more a spider than a crab), *Limulus,* a form of marine life that has existed for millions of years in the same form as a kind of living fossil. The eye of the *Limulus* provides a simple model for analyzing higher visual systems. It is a compound eye consisting of about 1000 ommatidia (see Figure 11.4) that connect to intermediate cells whose axons form the optic nerve. Because neighboring ommatidia partially cover overlapping regions of the visual field, these cells interact when the ommatidia are stimulated by light and the interaction is inhibitory. That is, neighboring units mutually suppress each other (Figure 14.1). This phenomenon is called *lateral inhibition,* and it has been noted to occur in a variety of modalities (see Chapter 4 for a discussion of lateral inhibition in hearing).

When two proximate ommatidia are simultaneously activated, each discharges fewer im-

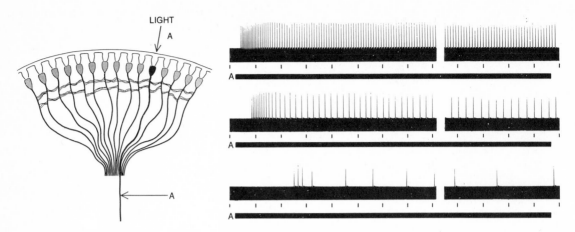

Fig. 14.1a *Rate of discharge of nerve impulses produced by steady illumination of a single receptor, A, in the eye of the horseshoe crab Limulus is directly related to the intensity of the light. The nerve fibers from the receptor are separated by microdissection and connected to an electrode from an amplifier and a recorder. The top record shows the response of A to steady, high-intensity light. The middle record shows the response to light of moderate intensity, and the lower record the response to low-intensity illumination. Duration of the light signal is indicated by the bar. Each mark above the bar indicates one-fifth of a second. (Source: Contour and Contrast, by F. Ratliff, in Scientific American, 1972, 226, 93. Copyright © 1972 by Scientific American, Inc. All rights reserved.)*

Fig. 14.1b *Inhibition of receptor, A, steadily exposed to moderate illumination is produced when neighboring receptors, B, are also illuminated. The beginning and the end of the records show the initial and final rate of impulses by A. The solid bars indicate duration of light signals. The upper record shows the effects on A of moderate-intensity illumination of B. The lower record shows the effect on A of high-intensity illumination of B. The stronger the illumination on neighboring receptors, the stronger the inhibitory effect. (Source: Contour and Contrast, by F. Ratliff, in Scientific American, 1972, 226, 93. Copyright © by Scientific American, Inc. All rights reserved.)*

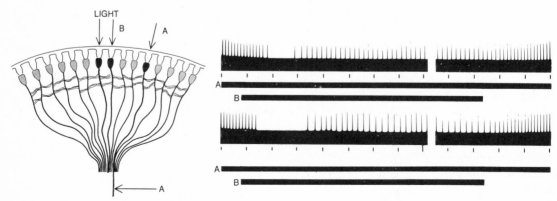

pulses than when a single ommatidium receives the same amount of illumination by itself. The more widely separated the ommatidia, the smaller the mutual inhibitory effect. Thus, flooding the whole eye produces little activity because all cells inhibit each other. However, where there are light-intensity changes, such as those at borders of patterns, interesting and significant visual effects occur. Consider the following demonstration (Ratliff & Hartline, 1959): The *Limulus* eye was illuminated with a "step" pattern (a bright rectangle adjacent to a dimmer one) (see Figure 14.2). Furthermore, the eye was masked so that only a single ommatidium was exposed to the pattern, which was moved to various loci. At each location the frequency of discharge was measured. The result, in terms of frequency of impulses, was a faithful representation of the pattern. That is,

the frequency of response varied according to the position of the step pattern relative to the ommatidium. When the eye was unmasked so that all the ommatidia were exposed to the pattern, the response record from a single ommatidium indicated that the frequency increased on the bright side of the step and decreased near the dim side. This resulted because the stimulated cells nearest the border were inhibited only by excited cells on one side (since the other side was dim and contributed less inhibition). Similar logic explains the decrease in frequency on the dim side: A dimly illuminated area near the boundary is inhibited not only by its dimly illuminated neighbors but also by the nearby brightly illuminated ones. The total inhibition on this region will therefore be greater than that of dimly illuminated neighbors farther from the boundary

Fig. 14.2 *Contour enhancement is demonstrated by letting a "step" pattern of light move across the Limulus eye. Plotted is the discharge frequency of a single ommatidium relative to a control level as a function of the position of a luminance gradient (illustrated in insert). If the eye is masked so light strikes only one ommatidium (illustrated by triangles), a recording of its discharge frequency forms a simple step-shaped curve as the pattern moves along the eye. If the eye is unmasked so that adjacent receptors are also illuminated, the discharge frequency of the single ommatidium is inhibited in varying degrees, as illustrated by the circles. The net effect of the selective inhibition (lower curve) is to enhance the contrast at light-dark borders. (Source: Ratliff & Hartline, 1959, p. 1250, reproduced by permission of the Rockefeller University Press.)*

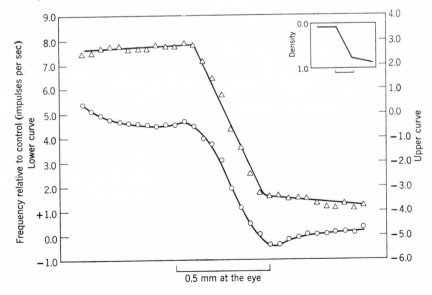

and the frequency response is accordingly less. The net effect of this inhibition by lateral neural connections in the *Limulus* is to enhance the perception of contours by heightening the contrast at light-dark borders.

Border Contrast, Lateral Inhibition, and Mach Bands

The basic features of lateral inhibition are the same for a wide variety of species, hence it is not surprising that a similar reciprocal inhibitory interaction between retinal areas occurs with humans. For example, when looking at a step pattern consisting of a series of uniform bands graded from black to white, as shown in Figure 14.3*a* each vertical band appears to be lighter on the left than on the right side producing a scalloping effect (Figure 14.3*b* and *c*). In fact, however, each band of the figure is of a uniform shade from edge to edge. This is evident when the figure is covered so that only a single band is visible. This subjective contrast enhancement at the contours is called *border contrast*. The enhanced regions—which occur at the points of greatest change in luminance—are called *Mach bands*, after the Austrian physicist-philosopher, Ernst Mach. An explanation of the contrast effect in terms of lateral inhibition at the retinal ganglion cells is outlined in Figure 14.3 *d*. Another example of Mach bands (or rings) is seen in Figure 14.4. When the wheel

is rotated, the black and white portions fuse to produce rings of uniform grays. The result is steady change in illumination, from an initial intense region at *a*, to a less intense region at *d*, with transition points in intensity at *b* and *c*. Though we have described the physical condition of lighting, this is not what is seen. Rather, a bright line appears at *b* and a dark one at *c*. The enhancement of stimulus differences—border contrast—is the result of the luminance from the different regions interacting with each other. One function of these interactions is obvious: It is crucial to perceive the borders, contours, and edges of objects even where there is not much physical difference in the light intensities between the object and its surroundings. The phenomenon of border contrast, by augmenting the difference in the neural firing rates of receptors located at either side of the imaged boundary, enables the perception of the contour and thereby provides a necessary step in the process of pattern recognition (see Brown, J. L. & Mueller, 1965). Moreover, border contrast enhances the formation of discontinuities, which, as we will see in a following section, is necessary to enable the stable perception of form.

Brightness Contrast

Other spatial interactions, in which contrasting regions are juxtaposed, produce *brightness*

Fig. 14.3a   *A step pattern consisting of a series of uniform bands graded from black to white.*

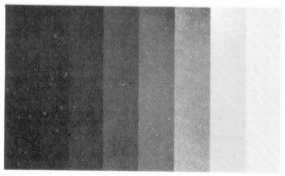

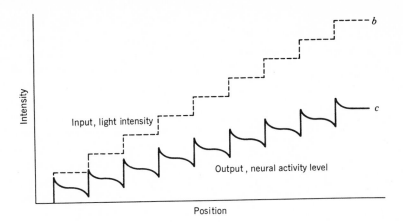

Fig. 14.3b & c *(b) The actual intensity distribution. (c) The brightness distribution. The scallops or furrows seen in 14.3a—the Mach bands—are plotted here. (Source: Buss, 1973, p. 199; after Cornsweet, 1970, pp. 276, 304. Reprinted by permission of the author and publisher.)*

contrast effects. The intensity of relatively large background regions can modify the brightness of smaller enclosed areas. Figure 14.5 illustrates this effect. The intensity of the inner four gray squares are identical in the intensity of light they reflect, yet their perceived brightness differs. That the inner square on the far left appears to be brighter than the one on the far right indicates that the brightness of a region depends on the intensity of its background. In fact, merely increasing the intensity of a surface does not necessarily increase its brightness; some objects may even appear darker when illumination is increased. Although far from clear, some of the quantitative relationships of the brightness of a target region to the intensity of its background have been worked

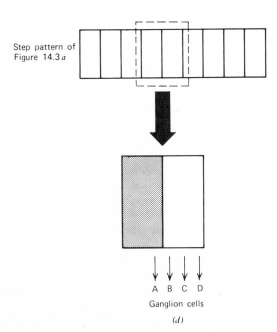

Fig. 14.3d *Lateral inhibition and border contrast. Assume that the lighter of the two uniform bands, shown in the bottom enlargement on the right, results in two units of inhibition to adjacent ganglion cells, but the darker band results in one unit of inhibition. It follows that cell C receives four units of inhibition (two units from B and two units from D), whereas cell B, at the border of the dark and light bands, receives three units of inhibition (one from A, the darker band, and two from C). Thus cell B, stimulated by the border area, is less inhibited than cell C. This means that it will signal the presence of more light and thus accounts for the border's lighter appearance. (From Psychology: Man in Perspective, by A. Buss, Wiley, New York, 1973, p. 200. Reprinted by permission of the publisher.)*

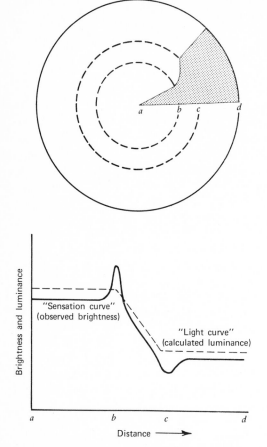

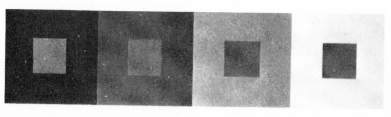

Fig. 14.4 *When the white disk with a black sector is rotated rapidly the result is the physical (luminance) and subjective (brightness) effects, shown by the dashed and solid curves, respectively.*

out (see Wallach, 1948; Heinemann, 1955; Jameson & Hurvich, 1961; Stevens, S. S. 1961).

It is worth noting, in passing, that contrast phenomena are not restricted to the nervous system. A common occurrence is found with the xerographic process, which reproduces only the edges of extended uniform areas. Unless special precautions are taken, homogeneous areas are not copied and appear largely as blank patches. One technique is to cover the original image with a mesh (e.g., a halftone screen) that breaks up the image into a pattern of changes from light to dark. The xerographic copy thus rendered is much closer to the original pattern (see Crovitz & Schiffman, 1968; Ratliff, 1971, p. 154).

The Ganzfeld: Perception In a Homogeneous Field

Usually stimulation from the environment is of a variegated nature with discontinuities of luminance and surface textures. However, when a completely textureless field of uniform brightness, an entirely homogeneous field called a *Ganzfeld,* is viewed, the resultant perception is of an unstructured ambiguous and disoriented environment (see Avant, 1965). There are several means for producing a Ganzfeld, for example, having subjects look into a translucent globe (Gibson & Waddell, 1952) or by having subjects wear ping-pong ball halves over their eyes (Hochberg, Triebel, & Seaman, 1951). Under such conditions, viewers experience

Fig. 14.5 *Brightness contrast effects. Although the intensities of the four inner squares are identical, they differ in brightness. Clearly, the square on the far left appears brighter than the square on the far right. This demonstrates that the perceived brightness of a stimulus varies depending on the intensity of its background. (Source: Cornsweet, 1970, p. 279. Reprinted by permission of the author.)*

an undifferentiated space extending for an indefinite distance. "A diffuse fog," is a representative characterization (Cohen, 1957, p. 406). Such homogeneity—although quite unnatural—occurs from the simplest level of stimulation and produces the simplest possible perceptual experience. When the Ganzfeld surface is illuminated with colored light, subjects generally report that the chromatic quality disappears within minutes (Hochberg, Triebel, & Seaman, 1951; Cohen, W., 1958). The most primitive level of form perception appears in the Ganzfeld with the introduction of a simple inhomogeneity such as a shadow or a gradient of intensity. With further increases in inhomogeneity, using definite contours, a segregation of portions of the Ganzfeld into a figure and a background occurs, and forms, figures, and surfaces may become perceptible. Not surprisingly, the greater the degree of stimulus change introduced, the greater is the perception of form qualities. Further evidence for the necessity of *stimulus change* for form perception follows.

Stabilized Image

The Ganzfeld experience indicates that the visual system is incapable of functioning effectively with invariant or completely uniform stimulation. Normally this is not a problem. As we noted in Chapter 12, the eye is constantly in motion. Even when the eye is fixated on a stationary target, small involuntary movements (drifts, saccades, and tremors) persist. Accordingly, the target image on the retina of the eye is kept in constant motion. However, it is possible to control or cancel the effects of eye movements on the retinal image. Several methods for stabilizing the retinal image exist (see Heckenmueller, 1965; Yarbus, 1967), but the general findings are similar so that we need consider only the following procedure. A contact lens on which is mounted a tiny self-contained optical projector is fitted directly over the cornea (see Figure 14.6). This device is set so that a focused image falls on the retina. Because

the contact lens and projector move with the eye, the image projected onto the retina will not shift over the retina with movement of the eyeball. The result is that the effects of eye movement are eliminated, and the image remains stabilized on the retina. When an image is stabilized on the same retinal location as described above or by one means or another, it soon fades and disappears leaving an unstructured gray field. However, it can be quickly restored by the introduction of such stimulus changes as flickering of the image, changing its intensity level, and by movement of the image after its disappearance.

In many ways the result of stabilizing projections on the retina is very similar to that produced from a Ganzfeld, in that eye movements are rendered incapable of bringing about a changing pattern of stimulation as they normally do. In general, the results of research on stabilized imagery and the Ganzfeld demonstrate that variation and inhomogeneity of visual stimulation is a necessary condition for the formation and maintenance of a visual image.

FIGURE-GROUND DIFFERENTIATION

Perhaps the first and simplest step in the complex dynamics of form perception is the perceptual phenomenon that certain parts of any differentiated visual field stand out in a distinctive manner from other parts. That part that appears as a sharply delineated and distinct shape is known as the *figure*, and the remainder is called the *ground*. This distinction was brought out by the Danish psychologist, Edgar Rubin in 1915 (the present discussion is based on a more recent, 1958 translation). In the simplest case, where there is a total visual field consisting of a black and a white portion, one portion is most likely to be seen as figure and the remaining part appears as the ground (see Figure 14.7). However, it is possible that any well-marked part of the visual

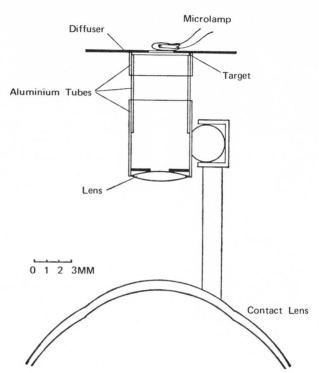

Fig. 14.6 *Stabilized-image device is a tiny projector mounted on a contact lens worn by the subject. The contact lens moves with every movement of the eyeball; so, therefore, does the projector, and as a result the target image is kept fixed at one point on the retina. The entire optical system weighs only 0.25 gram. (Source: Pritchard, Heron, & Hebb, 1960, p. 69).*

field may appear as the figure, leaving the remainder as the ground. There are a number of defining factors in figure-ground differentiation. However, as stated by Rubin, "The following principle is fundamental: if one of the two homogeneous, different-colored fields is larger than and encloses the other, there is a great likelihood that the small, surrounded field will be seen as figure . . . ." (Rubin, 1958, p. 202).

A quantitative approach to the tendency to see a figure as a function of its relation to the total stimulus configuration was made by Oyama (1960). He presented the stimulus pattern shown in Figure 14.8 and instructed subjects to indicate whether the α or β crosses appeared as figure. A trial consisted of continuous viewing for 60 sec; subjects indicated which of the two crosses they

saw by depressing one of two buttons, each designated to represent one of the crosses and each connected to a separate clock. When the angle of the sectors was varied, for either α or β crosses, the result was that the thinner the cross, the more likely it was seen as the figure regardless of whether it was black or white.

Ambiguous Figure-Ground Relationships

The preceding example points to an interesting variation of figure-ground differentiation: the condition where there are two distinct homogeneous regions but neither is enclosed by the other. In addition, both parts share a common contour so that no tendency exists for either part to be seen as figure. Some examples of such labile configura-

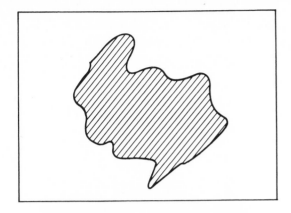

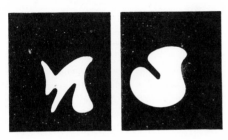

Fig. 14.7 *Simple figure-ground relation. (Source: Woodworth & Schlosberg, Experimental Psychology, 1954, Holt, Rinehart and Winston, p. 404, for bottom two figures; after Rubin, 1921.)*

tions are shown in Figure 14.9. Clearly, these are ambiguous figures. One of the effects is that there is an initial perception of one portion as figure but this is followed by a reversal. In Figure 14.9a one sees alternately a radially marked or concentrically marked cross. If the concentric cross is seen as figure the radial lines form the background. However, when the radial cross is seen as figure, the concentric lines, as part of the ground, do not appear interrupted. As Rubin points out with this example, one has the impression that the concentric circles continue behind the figure. Clearly, the shift in figure and ground in such patterns can be produced by a shift in attention. After a brief period of exposure, the region seen as figure can be determined by the focus of attention. In ordinary commerce we have no difficulty resolving reversible figures. Ambiguous configurations such as Rubin's (Figure 14.9 a and b) or Dali's (Figure 14.9d) or Escher's (Figure 14.9e) are rarely, if ever, confronted—certainly not as natural objects (see Attneave, 1971 and Teuber, 1974, for discussion and some elegant illustrations of reversible figures).

Rubin has identified the main differences between figure and ground as follows:

1. The figure has a "thing" quality, and the contour appears at the edge of the figure's shape. In contrast, the ground has a characteristic

Fig. 14.8 *Stimuli used to examine the role of angle sector on figure-ground perception. (Source: Oyama, 1960, p. 299.)*

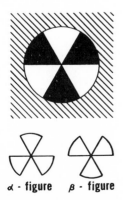

α - figure   β - figure

Fig. 14.9a *Figure-ground reversal. Either a radially or concentrically marked cross is seen. (Source: Rubin, 1958, p. 195.)*

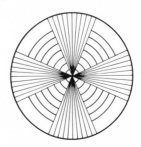

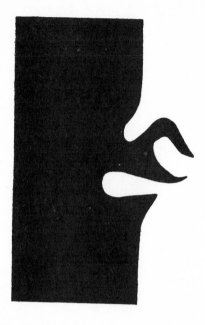

Fig. 14.9b *Reversible figure and ground pattern. Here the two fields have about an equal chance of being the figure, though the white field, being the same in color as the page, is more likely to be seen as ground. (Source: Woodworth & Schlosberg, Experimental Psychology, 1954, p. 404, Holt, Rinehart and Winston; after Rubin, 1921.)*

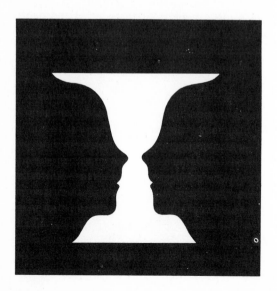

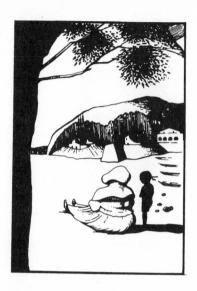

Fig. 14.9d *Reversible figure-ground pattern based on detail from Salvadore Dali's painting "The Three Ages." (Source: Fisher, G. H., 1967, p. 329. Reprinted by permission of the publisher.)*

more like a "substance" and appears relatively formless.

2. The figure appears closer to the viewer and in front of the ground, whereas the ground appears less clearly localized than the figure, extending continuously behind the figure. To these characteristics we must add Coren's (1969) finding that the region perceived as figure shows a greater amount of brightness contrast than when the same area is perceived as ground.

3. In relation to the ground, the figure appears more impressive, dominant, better remembered, and the figure suggests more associations of meaningful shapes than does the ground. As Figure 14.9c shows, the configuration appearing either as profiles or a goblet is easily assigned meaning, whereas the ground in either case is seen as shapeless (see also Figure 14.9f).

Fig. 14.9c *Reversible figure-ground pattern. Either a goblet or a pair of silhouetted faces in profile is seen. (Source: Boring, Langfeld, & Weld, 1948, p. 227.)*

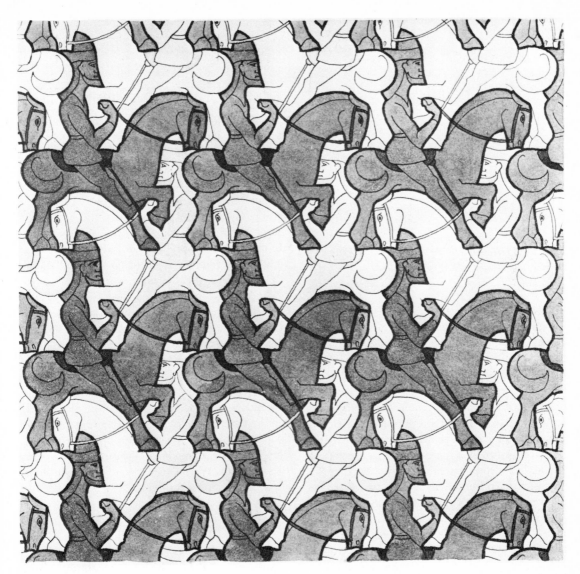

Fig. 14.9e *Reversible figure-ground pattern of procession of horsemen. (Based on woodcut of M. C. Escher, 1971, p. 11, "The Horsemen", Escher Foundation, Haags Gemeentemuseum, The Hague.)*

Figure-ground differentiation is recognized as the simplest step in the perception of form. Hebb (1949) has noted that the figure is seen as a cohesive self-contained unit, standing out from the background. According to Hebb, this occurs prior to and independent of recognition of the figure as a particular figure with properties of association. The former capacity Hebb calls *primitive unity*, and the latter he calls *figural identity*. In addition, evidence for the operation of a fundamental organizing tendency resulting in figure-ground differentiation comes from the reports by von

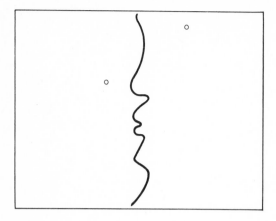

Fig. 14.9f *Reversible figure-ground drawing of profiles formed by the same contour.*

Senden (1960) on patients who have had congenital cataracts removed in adulthood, thus first given sight at maturity. He noted that such patients showed figure-ground differentiation before they could discriminate and recognize different figures (we will return to von Senden's reports in a later section concerning the development of perception). That the unity of a clearly demarcated figure is present in the first visual experience strongly suggests that the figure-ground relation is independent of experience. Further evidence for its primitiveness is that figure-ground differentiation is among the first perceptual experiences to occur in the Ganzfeld when a slight inhomogeneity is introduced. Moreover, many lower forms of animal life demonstrate the capacity to distinguish figure from ground even with minimal visual experience.

The apparent one-sidedness of contours helps to define the shape of an object and enables the perception of distinct entities. Thus, when looking at a cityscape we see the contours between buildings and sky as belonging to the buildings and the sky appears as ground. That is, the contours appear as the buildings' edges. Clearly, the priority of contours in defining the shapes of ob-

jects in the natural environment is an important consideration of figure-ground differentiation.

GESTALT GROUPING PRINCIPLES

Why do some elements of the visual field form the unified figure and others become ground? Clearly, this is a result of some organizing tendency based on certain features of the stimulus array. The study of what factors determine the formation of a figure was made by a group of German psychologists (in particular, Max Wertheimer, Kurt Koffka, and Wolfgang Köhler) at the beginning of this century. The school they founded is called *Gestalt* psychology. "Gestalt" is the German word for "form," "shape," or "whole configuration." Max Wertheimer, recognized as the founder of the Gestalt school, studied patterns of stimuli and observed the manner in which some appeared to be grouped together with figure-like qualities. Aside from the effects of attitudes and past experiences of the viewer, there appeared to be fundamental organizing tendencies to perceive the visual field on the basis of the arrangement and relative location of elements. A set of grouping principles, supported by numerous illustrations, has been described by Wertheimer (1923; based on 1958 translation). Some of these follow.

Nearness or proximity

Grouping may occur according to the distance separating elements. Elements that are closer together tend to be organized or grouped together (see Figure 14.10). The proximity may be of a spatial or temporal nature.

Fig. 14.10 *Due to proximity a row of dots is spontaneously seen as a row of elements in the arrangement ab/cd/ef . . . , not a/bc/de.*

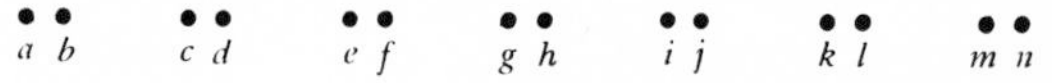

•• •• •• •• •• •• ••
a b   *c d*   *e f*   *g h*   *i j*   *k l*   *m n*

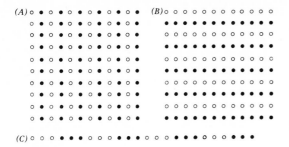

Fig. 14.11 *One sees groups of elements that are determined by the principle of similarity. Thus, in the figure, one sees columns of elements in A, rows in B and groups of O's and ●'s in C.*

Similarity

With the proximity of elements equated, elements that are similar in physical attributes tend to be grouped together (see Figure 14.11).

Good Configuration

The principle of good configuration was stated as a very general organizing tendency, intended to encompass a number of figural characteristics such as continuation, common fate, closure, and symmetry.

CONTINUATION Elements that appear to follow in the same direction, such as along a straight line or a simple curve, are readily perceived as forming a group (see Figure 14.12). All such elements appear to follow in a uniform direction so as to permit the continuation of an aspect of a figure (e.g., a line or curve) whose movement or direction has been established.

COMMON FATE Elements that move in the same direction are grouped together. This is basically grouping on the basis of similarity but applied to moving elements. Thus, if a number of elements are seen in movement, those that appear to be moving in parallel paths tend to be grouped together.

CLOSURE In closure grouping occurs in a way that favors the perception of the more enclosed or complete figure (see Figure 14.13). An interesting phenomenon, involving a completion or closure-type process, may occur across a blank portion of the field to produce a subjective contour. Examples are presented in Figure 14.14. According to Coren (1972), the subjective contour is simply the edge of an apparent plane in depth; the subjective contour serves to simplify a complex two-dimensional array of elements into an easily coded three-dimensional array of meaningful elements.

As is true for all the Gestalt principles of organization, good continuation and closure enhance the perception of a stable environment. The line drawing in Figure 14.15 can be perceived as three discrete shapes, yet the most likely result is that it is seen as two bars, one standing in front of the other, the partially covered bar appearing continuous. (This example of one figure in front of another also suggests a feature of depth and distance perception, which is a topic taken up in detail later.)

SYMMETRY In symmetry priority in grouping is given to the more natural, balanced, and symmetrical figure over the asymmetrical ones (see Figure 14.16).

Fig. 14.12 *The natural organization, due to continuation, is to see acegij and bdfhkl, not abefik or cdghjl. (After Wertheimer, 1958.)*

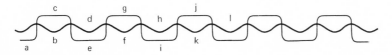

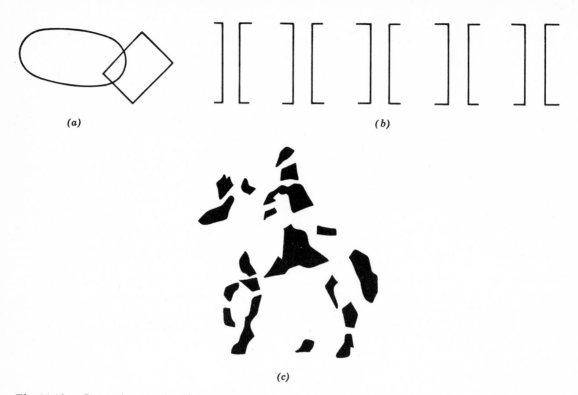

(a)

(b)

(c)

Fig. 14.13a *Due to the operation of closure, one sees two distinct and intersecting shapes, an ellipse and a rectangle, rather than three discrete enclosed areas. (After Wertheimer, 1958.)*

Fig. 14.13b *One tends to see rectangles. In this example, the principle of closure overides proximity.*

Fig. 14.13c *One tends to perceive a completed figure although only fragmentary stimuli are present. (From Psychology: Explorations in Behavior and Experience, by S. A. Mednick, J. Higgins, & J. Kirschbaum, Wiley, New York, 1975, p. 157. Reprinted by permission of the publisher.)*

Fig. 14.14 *Subjective contours produce an apparent triangle on the left and a rectangle on the right. (Based on figures in Coren, 1972. Reprinted by permission of the author and publisher.)*

Fig. 14.15 *At least three discrete shapes is a possible perception of the below line drawing. Good continuation and closure tend to favor the perception of two bars, one lying in front of the other. (Source: Boring, Langfeld, & Weld, 1948, p. 226.)*

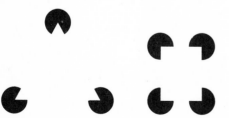

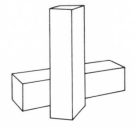

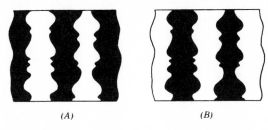

(B)

Fig. 14.16 *The contours of the vertical shapes are identical but in A, one sees the white "columns", and B, the black ones. In both cases organization follows the symmetrical pattern. (Source: Zusne, 1970, p. 116.)*

In one experiment on the characteristics that affect perceptual organization, Beck (1966) showed that perceptual grouping of two-line figures may be influenced by the orientation of the lines comprising the figure. When subjects were instructed to divide the pattern shown in Figure 14.17 into two parts, the division was based primarily on the orientation of the figures; that is, figures with lines oriented in the same direction were grouped together. In the example given, the physical similarity of figures was not an important factor of perceptual grouping.

Wertheimer offers the following summary of the Gestalt principles outined above: ". . . all of these factors and principles point in a single direction: perceptual organization occurs from above to below; the way in which parts are seen, in which subwholes emerge, in which grouping occurs, is not an arbitrary piecemeal and summation of elements, but is a process in which characteristics of the whole play a major determining role" (p. 134-135). Indeed, one of the main tenets of the Gestalt school is that figure quality—the *whole figure*—has its own set of unique properties that are different from merely the sum of the constituent elements comprising the figure.

Figural Goodness

Many of the Gestalt principles stated above along with several corollaries have been codified under the general rubric of the law of *Prägnanz*, or the law of the *good figure,* which refers to the tendency to perceive the simplest and most stable figure of all possible alternatives. However, as used by the Gestaltists, the descriptive term "good," although possessing some intuitive appeal, demands further elaboration. One attempt

Fig. 14.17 *Stimulus pattern used by Beck. When subjects were instructed to divide the pattern into two parts, the division was based on the orientation of the elements: Elements with lines oriented in the same direction were grouped together. In the figure below the elements of A and B appeared to form a group distinct from the elements of C although the elements of B had greater physical similarity to those of C than to those of A. (Source: Beck, 1966, p. 300. Reprinted by permission of the publisher.)*

(A)   (B)   (C)

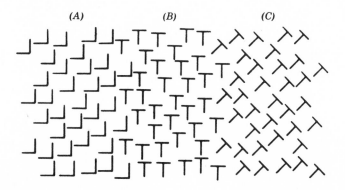

at a quantitative index of the structural properties of figural "goodness" was made by J. E. Hochberg and McAlister (1953). They suggested that figural goodness is inversely proportional to the amount of information necessary to specify a figure. That is, ". . . the less the amount of information needed to define a given organization as compared to the other alternatives, the more likely that the figure will be so perceived" (p. 361). Bearing on this issue is the notion of the *minimum principle* (see Hochberg, 1964). According to this principle, the organization that is perceived from an ambiguous configuration is the simpler one, where simplicity is specified in terms of certain objective physical measures. Stated in another way, the perceptual response that will tend to occur is the most economical response. Accordingly, the good figure is in the Gestalt sense the simpler and informationally economical one. Grouping or organizing the visual pattern on the basis of this principle—that is, on the basis of minimum information—represents an efficient and adaptive mechanism. For example, a closed figure can be more easily defined than an open one—not requiring specification of the gap size and location—and a symmetrical figure can be succinctly described by indicating half of its features because the remaining half is its mirror image. Look at Figure 14.18. Its description is generally of two overlapping rectangles. Alternatively, however, it can be construed as five irregular shapes. In the latter instance more angles, lines, and points of intersections are required to specify the general configuration. Hence, according to the analysis of J. E. Hochberg and McAlister, this is the least likely perception. In contrast, because less information is necessary to specify the configuration as two rectangles, it is the figure most likely seen. Hochberg and McAlister tested this notion of information content and were able to predict which organization of a reversible figure would be seen most frequently. Subjects viewed each of the outline drawings shown in Figure 14.19 (called Kopfermann cubes) separately. Their task was to indicate whether the figures were seen as two- or three-dimensional shapes. The result was that figures that were more symmetrical, as in the case of drawings y and z, were seen as two-dimensional most often. That is, ". . . that figure which possesses the best phenomenal symmetry as a two-dimensional pattern was obtained least often as a cube . . ." (p. 363). A further extension of this was later proposed by J. E. Hochberg and Brooks (1960). Again using line drawings (Figure 14.20) they had subjects indicate whether each was seen as more two- or three-dimensional. They hypothesized that, "The relative tridimensionality of each member of a family of reversible-perspective representations of a given three-dimensional object will be a simple function of the geometrical complexity of the two-dimensional figure . . ." (p. 340). From an analysis of the number of physical features of the drawings—

Fig. 14.18 *Less information is required to specify this figure as two overlapping rectangles (8 line segments and 8 angles) than the alternative construction of five irregular shapes (16 line segments and 16 angles). (Source: after Hochberg, J. E. & E. McAlister, 1953, p. 362. Reprinted by permission of the first author and publisher.)*

Fig. 14.19 *The Kopfermann "cubes" used by Hochberg and McAlister. (Source: Hochberg, J. E. & E. McAlister, 1953, p. 363. Reprinted by permission of the first author and publisher.)*

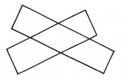

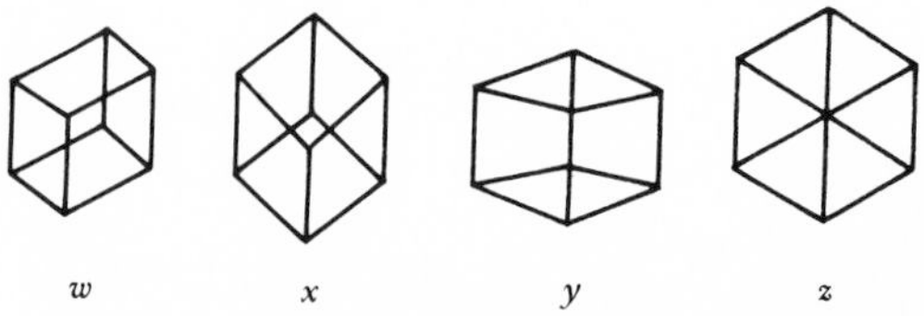

w   x   y   z

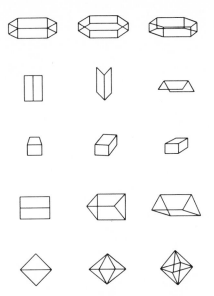

Fig. 14.20 *Reversible stimulus forms that can be seen as two-dimensional or three-dimensional figures. Generally, the first member of each series will be perceived as two-dimensional and the remainder as three-dimensional. (Source: Hochberg, J. E. and V. Brooks, 1960, 78, pp. 340, 348.)*

such as the number of line segments, interior angles, and intersections—they were able to relate the simplicity or complexity of the drawing to its likelihood of being seen as a two- or three-dimensional figure. For simpler drawings (e.g., drawings with a small number of interior angles), the simplest and best organization was in two-dimensions. With increases in complexity a three-dimensional organization was best. In general, they found that as the complexity of the two-dimensional drawing increased, the likelihood of a three-dimensional perception correspondingly increased.

Extensions on the Gestalt theme of figural goodness have been given by Garner (1970) to include redundancy as well. "... there is a direct relation between pattern goodness and redundancy. ... poor patterns are those which are not redundant and thus have many alternatives, good patterns are those which are redundant and thus have few alternatives, and the very best patterns are those which are unique, having no perceptual alternatives" (p. 42).

We now turn to a consideration of some of the factors that affect the perception of form.

MASKING

It is well known that under certain conditions a stimulus is affected by stimuli that occur simultaneously with it and those that immediately precede and follow it. The impairment to the perception of a target stimulus by the presentation of a closely following second *masking* stimulus is called *backward masking*. If the masking stimulus precedes and is close in time to the presentation of the target stimulus, the impairment to the perception of the target stimulus is called *forward masking*. When backward and forward masking occur in an experimental arrangement where the target and masking stimuli fall on nonoverlapping adjacent retinal areas, they are termed *metacontrast* and *paracontrast*, respectively.

Although there are a number of further distinctions that can be made, in general visual masking refers to the phenomenon in which the perception of the target stimulus is obscured by presenting a masking stimulus close in time to a target stimulus. If, for example, a circular disk and a masking ring just circumscribing it (see Figure 14.21) are presented in sequence for a brief duration, when the pause between them, called the *interstimulus interval* (ISI), is at a certain duration, the presence of the disk may not be perceived, or it may appear dimmer or less structured than if shown without the ring. Masking of this sort is maximal when the borders of the masking stimulus are coincident with the borders of the target stimulus; with spatial separation between the masking and target stimulus the masking effect falls off. Other variables that affect masking are the duration and

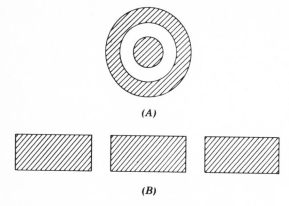

(A)

(B)

Fig. 14.21 *Patterns used to produce masking. In (A) the central disk is the target stimulus and the concentric ring is the masking stimulus. In (B) the central rectangle is the target stimulus, and the two flanking rectangles are the masking stimuli. (Source: Uttal, 1973, p. 443.)*

intensity of the target and masking stimuli and the temporal interval separating them.

It should be noted that although masking suggests the existence of important processes of the visual system, its occurrence is comparatively rare (Uttal, 1973, p. 448).

Though there are a number of current explanations of masking effects, none is completely satisfactory. However, as pointed out by Kahneman (1968), many share the common theme of stimulus persistence: The temporal course of sensory and perceptual events exceeds the course of stimulus events—sensation, or its effects, continues beyond the termination of the physical stimulus. One consequence of this within the context of masking is that brief stimulus events that do not physically overlap in space or in time may be perceived as contemporaneous. Thus, if the pause between the target stimulus and the masking stimulus is of sufficient brevity, say 100 msec or less, the stimuli may be processed at the same time—the image of the target stimulus sums with the image of the masking stimulus—with the result that they do not appear as two different stimuli and the perception of the

target stimulus is impaired (Eriksen & Collins, 1965). Accordingly, masking may be considered to be the result of the temporal summation of physically successive components that appear to be concurrent. However, the precise nature of the interaction between the components—target and masking stimulus—is not well understood.

We must note in passing that the finding that some of the information contained in a briefly flashed stimulus momentarily lingers after the removal or termination of the initiating physical stimulus has implications for problems other than masking. The "trace" amount that remains as a sort of fading image is called an *icon* (Neisser, 1967). Ordinarily, it is not perceptible, but under the proper experimental conditions a surprising amount of the contents in the icon may be recovered (e.g., Sperling, 1960).

It should be emphasized that the issue of masking is a controversial one, and a number of theoretical accounts of masking exist (for ample reviews see Kahnemann, 1968 and Lefton, 1973).

Cognitive Masking

An interesting experiment by Erdelyi and Appelbaum (1973) demonstrated an inhibitory effect on the detectability of simple figures due to the presence of an "emotional" stimulus. The authors termed this disrupting effect "cognitive masking." They flashed (200 msec) an array of eight neutral stimulus items flanking a central stimulus. The central stimulus was either a neutral or an "emotional" figure (see Figure 14.22). The result was that the detectability of the eight neutral stimulus items was inferior when the central figure was an emotional rather than a neutral stimulus. The authors conclude that the ". . . symbolic meaning of portions of a stimulus may disrupt the proceessing of adjacent stimulus components in a single-fixation exposure of the whole stimulus" (p. 59). In a follow-up study by Erdelyi and Blumenthal (1973), the same form of disruption—cognitive masking—occurred when the stimulus items were presented as a sequence of pictures.

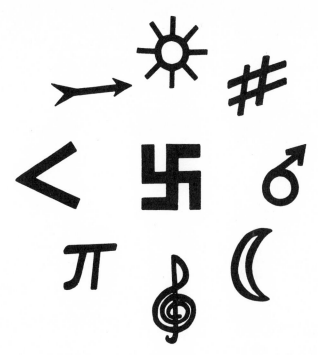

Fig. 14.22 *For this array the emotionality of the central item, a swastika, was assured by presenting it to subjects who were members of a Jewish organization. (Source: Erdelyi & Applebaum, 1973, p. 50. Reprinted by permission of the publisher.)*

The result was decreased retention of items immediately preceding and following an emotional stimulus figure.

Facilitative Interaction

Although the interaction of successive but different visual stimuli may, under the proper conditions, result in masking, one may question whether a similar integrative mechanism will show a facilitative effect on the perception of a stimulus if the two successive stimuli are identical. That is, if the sequential presentation of two *different* stimuli, the target and masking stimulus, interact to produce a reduction in recognition, then it is reasonable to assume that if two stimuli are *identical* their effects on the visual system will summate to produce a facilitative effect on their recognition. An important study by

Eriksen and Collins (1967) illustrates this phenomenon. They presented briefly (6 msec) the dot pattern *a* and dot pattern *b* of Figure 14.23, simultaneously and with a brief pause (from 25 to 100 msec) between them. Notice that each pattern by itself appears to be meaningless. However, when they are properly aligned and exposed simultaneously, the resulting perception is of the nonsense syllable "VOH" of Figure 14.23*c*. The experimental manipulation of sequentially presenting the stimuli was that the identification of the nonsense syllable increased as the pause time between the presentation of the two dot patterns decreased (see Figure 14.24). This study, as with the masking studies, indicates the existence of a temporal summation of stimuli into a composite perception of forms or patterns.

Interestingly, summation of a similar kind occurs even when the interval between stimuli is

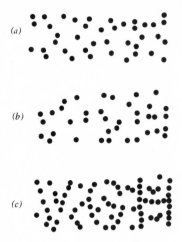

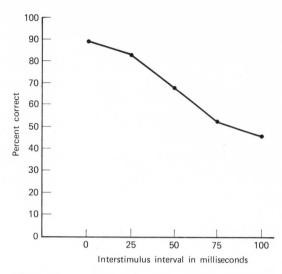

Fig. 14.23 *Stimuli used by Eriksen and Collins. When the upper two dot patterns, a and b, are superimposed or when the temporal interval separating their sequential presentation is 100 msec or less, the likely perceptual result is the bottom stimulus pattern, c, in which the nonsense syllable "VOH" can be read. Notice that in order to minimize the possibility that the nonsense syllable could be guessed from the dots on only one dot pattern, slightly smaller camouflaging dots were distributed over each pattern. (Source: Eriksen & Collins, 1967, 74, p. 477. Reprinted by permission of the American Psychological Association.)*

Fig. 14.24 *Accuracy of nonsense syllable recognition as a function of the pause (interstimulus interval) between the two dot patterns. (Source: Modified from Eriksen & Collins, 1967, 74, p. 478. Reprinted by permission of the author and the American Psychological Association.)*

Fig. 14.25 *Probability of perceiving a word as a function of repeated exposures. (Source: Modified from Haber & Hershenson, 1965, 69, p. 43. Reprinted by permission of the author and the American Psychological Association.)*

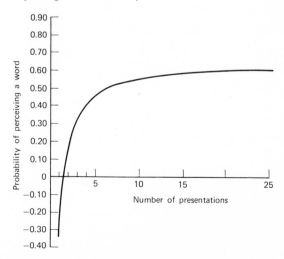

considerably longer than those used in the above study. However, more than two presentations of the same stimulus were employed so that in relation to the above study there was a trade-off between the duration of the interstimulus interval and the number of stimulus presentations. In a provocative study, Haber and Hershenson (1965) flashed seven-letter, three-syllable words at a duration below recognition threshold (from 5 to 35 msec). This was repeated with the same word for a number of times with the result that successive flashes produced increasingly correct recognitions (see Figure 14.25). With a constant exposure duration, the likelihood of correctly perceiving a word increased with the number of repetitions; the word appeared clear and distinct after a number of flashes even though on the first flash it appeared to be blank. The subjects' reports of the stimuli when the stimulus duration was brief are summed up by the authors as follows. The subject

> *. . . was usually unaware of letters or parts of letters on the first flash—the flash was blank. On the second or third flash, with no change in duration, beginnings of letters and sometimes whole letters would appear. After several more flashes, a number of letters would be present—often the whole word.*
>
> *The percept of the word that developed after repetition was in no sense fuzzy, hazy, or the product of a guess. It assumed very clear status, so that S was never uncertain about his report, even though he was unable to see anything a few exposures earlier. These reports were a dramatic demonstration that perceptual thresholds must have been a function of repetition as well as energy and duration of stimulation. (P. 41)*

This positive cumulative effect of repeated exposure has been labeled by Haber and Hershenson (1965) as the "growth of a percept." It should be pointed out that the presentation interval (ISI) between the stimuli was considerably longer in this study than those employed in the study by Eriksen and Collins (1967). Accordingly, the increase in recognition owing to number of presentations in the Haber and Hershenson study and owing to a reduction in the interstimulus interval in the Eriksen and Collins study reflects the operation of fundamentally different summative processes. At any rate, the basic findings of Haber and Hershenson have been replicated and extended by Murch (1969) using very brief interstimulus intervals (see also Standing, Haber, Cataldo, & Sales, 1969). Overall, these studies show the integrative capacity of the visual system over time and the influence of stimulus repetition on form perception. Furthermore, with regard to visual acuity these findings suggest that there is a relation between the pause time between stimuli and stimulus repetition for a constant degree of stimulus recognition. That is, the longer the inter-

stimulus interval employed, the greater the number of stimulus presentations required for recognition.

AFTEREFFECTS

Having shown that even quite brief viewing of an image has an effect (i.e., masking) on subsequent perception, we now turn to the general topic of *aftereffects*. Some aftereffects are quite simple and pervasive. As we noted in the preceding chapter, if one stares at a colored shape for, say, 30 sec and the gaze shifts to a neutral achromatic surface, the shape is still perceived but in a reversed or complementary color. Perhaps the most common and persuasive aftereffect results from inadvertently viewing the very brief but intense light of a flash bulb. In other instances prolonged inspection of a stimulus configuration causes not only a form of stimulus persistence but also creates a measurable distortion in the perception of other figures. Two main classes of aftereffects are *figural* and *shape* aftereffects. But as we will see, there are a number of additional categories.

Figural Aftereffects

An example of figural aftereffects is an often cited demonstration by W. Köhler and Wallach (1944) wherein the contours of shapes are apparently "displaced" from the region adjacent to the site of previously fixated contours. The typical arrangement is shown in Figure 14.26. If the x in Figure 14.26*a* is fixated for 40 sec and then the gaze is transferred to the x in Figure 14.26*b*, the distance between the two left squares in *b* will appear greater than that between the two right squares, whereas, in fact, the distances are equal. Although it is clear that this distortion is caused by the prior inspection of Figure 14.26*a*, there is no fully acceptable explanation of the general

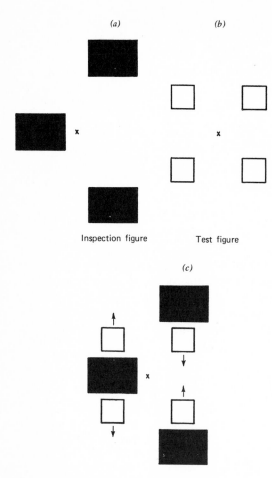

Fig. 14.26 *Inspection or inducing figure (a) and test figure (b) used to demonstrate figural aftereffects. Following the inspection of the fixation* ✗ *in (a) for about 40 sec, fixation of the* ✗ *in (b) results in the two left squares of (b) appearing farther apart then the two on the right. This displacement is schematized in (c). The arrows indicate the apparent displacement. (Source: After Köhler & Wallach, 1944.)*

exposure becomes fatigued, resistant to stimulation, or *satiated*. This causes new figures projected near the satiated retinal area to be apparently displaced from it. Accordingly, the distortion—the shift in apparent location—of the squares in *b* is due to their displacement from the retinal region to which the inspection figures had been previously exposed. Figure 14.26*c* is a schematic of the relation, indicating the appearance of components *a* and *b* of Figure 14.26 if they were combined. It follows from the above that owing to satiation the two left squares are pushed apart and the two right squares are pushed together. It must be noted, however, that this explanation has been seriously questioned in a number of quarters, and its validity is not generally agreed on (see Zusne, 1970, pp. 48–54; and Ganz, 1966, for alternative explanations).

Shape Aftereffects

A second example of aftereffects occurs with changes in the apparent shape of figures. An experiment by J. J. Gibson in 1933 with simple lines illustrates the phenomenon of shape or curvature aftereffects. Subjects wore special distorting prism glasses that displaced the incoming light rays so that straight vertical lines appeared curved. During the course of the exposure, the subjects reported that the extent of the apparent curvature diminished. That is, the straight line curved by the prism glasses began to appear as straight (see Figure 14.27). When the prism glasses were removed, an aftereffect of wearing them occurred: Straight lines appeared curved in the direction opposite to the direction of apparent curvature produced by the glasses. J. J. Gibson and Radner (1937) found that after a period of continuous visual inspection of tilted or curved lines the same aftereffect resulted: Physically vertical straight lines appeared off-vertical (tilted or curved) in the direction opposite to that of the initial inspection. This aftereffect is not restricted to the visual modality. In his original study Gibson (1933) reported that if a blindfolded subject feels along a curved edge for a duration, then

phenomenon. One hypothesized effect proposed by Köhler and Wallach (1944) to account for displacement effects has been termed "satiation." They contend that when a figure has been exposed for a period of time to a given region of the retina, the receptors of the region and of the areas immediately adjacent to the retinal site of

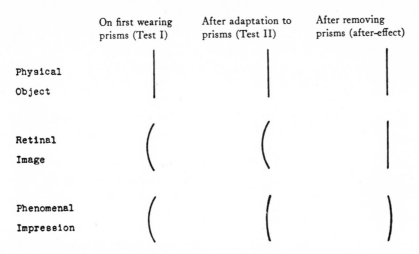

Fig. 14.27 *Schematic diagram of the relations between the physical object, the retinal image, and the apparent perception (phenomenal impression) in the experiment on curvature aftereffects by Gibson. (Source: Gibson, J. J., 1933, 16, p. 7. Reprinted by permission of the author and the American Psychological Association.)*

a straight edge feels curved the other way; in other words, a kinesthetic aftereffect results (see Howard and Templeton, 1966, Chap. 8 for a review of the Gibson-type studies on shape aftereffects).

FEATURE-SPECIFIC DETECTORS

An appealing explanation of aftereffects is that there are specific neural detectors or channels for different features of stimulation—features such as shape, movement, orientation, or color—and that prolonged stimulation by such features causes the appropriate detectors to fatigue. An implicit aspect of specific feature detectors is that paired up with each kind of neural detection unit is an antagonistic one (e.g., horizontal-vertical, left-right, up-down, blue-yellow, etc.) such that the stimulation of one unit causes relative inactivity of the other. However, if one pair is rendered inoperative as from overstimulation, its opponent counterpart detector will be actuated. Thus, continued or prolonged stimulation of a specific

kind of detector eliminates the normal response to the stimulus, and the opposite response occurs. In brief, the contention here is that aftereffects result from reduced sensitivity to a specific class of stimulus features and that this, in turn, is owing to the adaptation or fatigue of specific underlying neural mechanisms. Although this sort of explanation has been proposed by Coltheart (1971) to explain curvature aftereffects, perhaps the first direct report on the aftereffects of specific feature detectors is that of McCollough in 1965. She presented a grating of vertical black stripes on an orange ground for a few seconds, alternated with an identical grating of horizontal black stripes on a blue background (see Figure 14.28). The alternation of patterns lasted for 2 to 4 min. In essence, this served to fatigue or adapt the receptors to edge- or orientation-specific colors. After this exposure she found that a typical observer reported a faint orange aftereffect on the horizontally oriented grating of the black and white test pattern shown in Figure 14.28 and a faint blue-green aftereffect on the vertically oriented grating pattern. Thus, some units of the visual system respond with decreased sensitivity

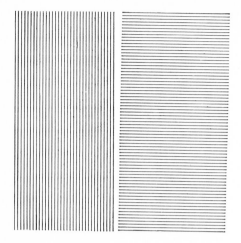

Fig. 14.28 *Black and white test pattern used by Mc-Collough. After adaptation to orange-vertical and blue-horizontal grating patterns, the left half appears blue-green (approximate complement of orange) and the right half appears orange. (Source: McCollough, Science, 1965, 419, 1115, September 1965. Copyright © 1965 by the American Association for the Advancement of Science.)*

to those wavelengths by which they have recently been most strongly stimulated and accordingly, this results in the antagonistic response (orange is approximately the complementary color of blue-green). What is very interesting is that this color adaptation is specific to the orientation of the edges or contours of the pattern. The result that the aftereffects are color sensitive and specific to the orientation of the stripes in the test pattern strongly hints at the existence of feature subunits of the human visual system that are selectively tuned to both color and orientation. This effect for color has been extensively replicated and extended (see for example, Held and Shattuck, 1971; Stromeyer, 1972; Riggs, White, & Eimas, 1974).

Evidence for a number of other specific neural detectors has been reported. The existence of a size-detecting mechanism is suggested by the following study by Blakemore and Sutton (1969). Consider the demonstration illustrated in Figure

14.29, *a* and *b*. The two grating patterns on the right are identical. Focus on the two grating patterns on the left (*a*) for at least 60 sec with your gaze wandering back and forth along the horizontal fixation bar that separates the two patterns. After this period of adaptation, transfer your gaze to the fixation point between the two patterns on the right (*b*). They should no longer appear identical in size. The grating above the fixation point at *b* should appear to have narrower stripes because of the adaptation to the "wide stripe" detectors in the upper retinal region. Similarly, the lower grating pattern of *b* should appear wider because of adaptation to the narrower stripes of the bottom grating pattern of *a*. In other words, the top grating pattern of *a* adapts the wide stripe detectors in the upper part of the retina so that medium stripes produce less of a response from them than from narrow stripe detectors. The opposite effect results from adaptation of the lower part of the retina to the narrow

Fig. 14.29 *Inspection figures (a) and test figures (b) used by Blakemore and Sutton to demonstrate the existence of size-detecting channels in human vision. (Source: Blakemore & Sutton, Science, 1969, 166, 245, October 1969. Copyright © 1969 by the American Association for the Advancement of Science. Reprinted by permission of the authors.)*

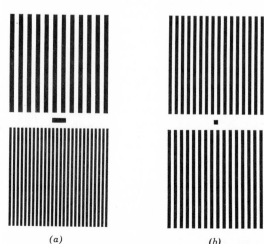

(a)   (b)

stripes. Pantle and Sekuler (1968) have shown that adaptation to a horizontal grating produces no size distortion to a vertical grating, suggesting that size detectors are also orientation specific.

The existence of feature detectors that are movement-specific have also been found. Helper (1968) reported that after subjects alternately viewed green stripes (across a black background) moving up and red stripes against a similar ground moving down, they saw a pink aftereffect when white stripes moved up and a green aftereffect when white stripes moved down. That is, the paired-stimulus attributes of color and motion produced color aftereffects that were motion contingent. Evidence for a different kind of movement-specific detector has been found by Favreau, Emerson, and Corballis (1972). After they exposed observers to repeated alternations of rotating, chromatically tinted spirals (see Figure 14.30)—a red contracting spiral and a green

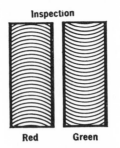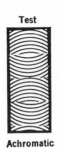

Fig. 14.31 *Inspection and test patterns used to evaluate curvature-contingent colored aftereffects. The red inspection pattern has lines that are convex upward, and the green pattern has lines that are concave upward. After alternate inspection of these two patterns, the subject sees the corresponding curves on the test panels as greenish and pinkish, respectively. (Source: Riggs, Science, 1973, 181, 1170, September 1973. Copyright © 1973 by the American Association for the Advancement of Science. Reprinted by permission of the author and publisher.)*

Fig. 14.30 *When rotated the spiral appears to contract or expand, depending on the direction of rotation. When the rotation ceases, the apparently expanding spiral appears to contract and move in the opposite direction. Similarly the apparently contracting spiral appears to expand and move in the opposite direction of its initial movement. Adaptation to alternations of a red contracting spiral and a green expanding spiral resulted in the appearance of expansion in a stationary red spiral and contraction in a stationary green spiral.*

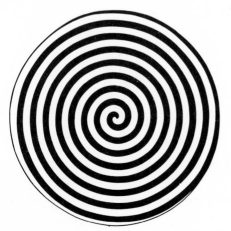

expanding one—the observation of stationary chromatic spirals produced the following: A stationary red spiral appeared to expand and move in a direction opposite that of the moving red spiral, and a stationary green spiral appeared to contract and show similar opponent-type movement. In this case movement aftereffects occurred that were color-contingent. The authors also reported chromatic aftereffects that were motion-contingent. Other studies have shown related variations on the theme of adaptation of color- and motion-contingent aftereffects (e.g., Stromeyer & Mansfield, 1970; Walker, 1972). In addition Riggs (1973) has demonstrated curvature-contingent colored aftereffects (see Figure 14.31), indicating that curvature is a specific feature of human visual perception.

These studies argue that the visual system possesses subunits differentially sensitive to (and thereby, adapted by) specific stimulus features. Some neural evidence has been reported for cortical cell adaptation in the cat that is selective for orientation and size (Maffei, Fiorentini, and Bisti, 1973). However, there are several empirical shortcomings (e.g., Murch and Hirsch, 1972) along with attempts at alternative explanations of feature-specific aftereffects (Harris & Gibson, 1968; Weisstein, 1969). Clearly, the implications of the findings described above are extremely important, but the significant and far-reaching mechanisms mediating feature-specific detectors in the visual system are not yet understood.

Although we have focused on specific feature detectors within the topic of aftereffects, it must be emphasized that they concern matters of great significance for the understanding of many aspects of spatial and especially form perception. As a result, their study has been the concern of many comparatively disparate areas of biological science. For example, attempts to understand the fundamental mechanism of form perception have been made by constructing computer models simulating feature detectors that integrate neurophysiological and perceptual processes. Some of these assume that feature detectors are redundancy-reducing devices that tend to disregard regularities and uniformities and ac-centuate discontinuities or singularities such as contours, edges, and other features with sharp luminance changes. Though the research is in a nascent stage, it has a significant potential for extending the understanding of form perception (see Barlow, H. B., Narasimhan, & Rosenfeld, 1972; Harmon & Julesz, 1973; Harmon, 1973).

Before ending our discussion of feature-specific detectors and aftereffects, notice must be taken of a related figural aftereffect phenomenon. A provocative characteristic of certain aftereffects is that they are not restricted to only those mechanisms and units that are stimulated. Weisstein (1970) has shown that the aftereffects of prolonged exposure to a grating-pattern (i.e., decrease in the apparent brightness of the same kind of grating) occurred to portions of the pattern that appeared to be covered or to lie behind a cube-like drawing (see Figure 14.32). That is, aftereffects occurred not only to those portions of the grating that were visible but also to a portion of the visual field that was blocked from view and thus not stimulated by the exposure pattern, sug-

Fig. 14.32 *Inspection figure (a) and test patch (b) used by Weisstein. After exposure to the inspection figure, subjects had to estimate the apparent brightness of the test patch, which was positioned so that its comparison would be with portions of the inspection field apparently covered by the top plane of the cube-like drawing. Adaptation occurred not only to the visible portions of the grating in (a) but also to those portions blocked from view by the cube-like drawing. (Source: Weisstein, Science, 1970, 168, 1490, June 1970. Copyright © 1970 by The American Association for the Advancement of Science.)*

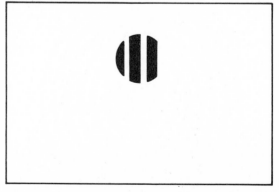

(a)   *(b)*

gesting, according to Weisstein, "... the existence of a neural mechanism which conveys the information 'in back of'." (p. 1489)

PERCEPTUAL SET

As we noted at the beginning of this chapter, perception involves more than the operation of a class of mechanisms concerned with the reception of stimulation at the retina. Indeed, the optical array reflected from the environment—that is, patterns of discrete stimuli composed of lines, dots, and various luminance discontinuities—is insufficient to account for the meaningful structured visual world we experience. The perception of many aspects of the environment is due not only to the biophysical character of the incoming stimulation and the appropriate sensory receptor mechanisms, but it is also due to certain dispositions and existing intentions within the perceiver. There are psychological processes, more specific and tractable than the Gestalt principles described earlier, that play a role in organizing the incoming stimulation toward a meaningful percept. Perception is directed in a particular manner by existing influences such as expectations and anticipations, resulting in a readiness to organize the visual input in a certain way. In other words, the perceiver expects to perceive or is *set* to perceive a particular thing. As Bruner (1957) points out, we more readily organize the sensory input in order to perceive objects that we have frequently experienced in the past.

The influence of set—as a kind of perceptual priming—is well demonstrated by the drawings of Figure 14.33. Depending on whether *a* or *b* is seen prior to *c*, the viewer sees *c* as a drawing of either a young or old woman. In this instance, perception occurs as a consequence of a set, which is caused by the prior inspection of either *a* or *b*.

That perceptual set enables a meaningful perception of labile, fragmentary, or ambiguous stimulation is important, for it is typical for the visual input from the environment to be less than complete. An expectation owing to prior experience as to what "should be there" enables a meaningful interpretation and perception as to what "is there."

Set can be demonstrated in the course of an experiment with relatively little commerce with the constituents of the set-inducing stimulation. Consider the following experiment. Bruner and Minturn (1955) found that, when briefly flashed, an ambiguous stimulus as shown in Figure 14.34 was perceived as a "B" by subjects previously shown four different capital letters and as a "13" by subjects whose immediate prior viewing was four pairs of digits. The tendency to perceive an ambiguous stimulus in accordance with the viewer's experimentally-determined expectation was clear: When the subjects were "set" for a letter, they saw the broken-B of Figure 14.34 as closed; when they were set for a number, it was seen as open.

Many set-related tendencies and influences occur from significant prior commerce with the environment. Such an effect is seen in the following experiment by Bruner and Postman (1949; and repeated more recently by Lasko & Lindauer, 1968). They flashed playing cards (from 10 to 1000 msec) and had subjects name the card exposed. Some cards were normal ones printed in their proper color and suit, for example a red five of hearts, black five of spades; and some were trick or incongruous cards, printed with their suit and colors reversed, for example, a black three of hearts, a red two of spades. The most central finding was that the average recognition threshold (amount of presentation time required for recognition) for the incongruous cards was significantly higher than the threshold for normal cards. Normal cards, on the average, required 28 msec, whereas the incongruous cards required 114 msec—a fourfold increase.

Aside from the direct recognition measures, the authors cite several kinds of set-related reactions to the incongruous cards. In some instances

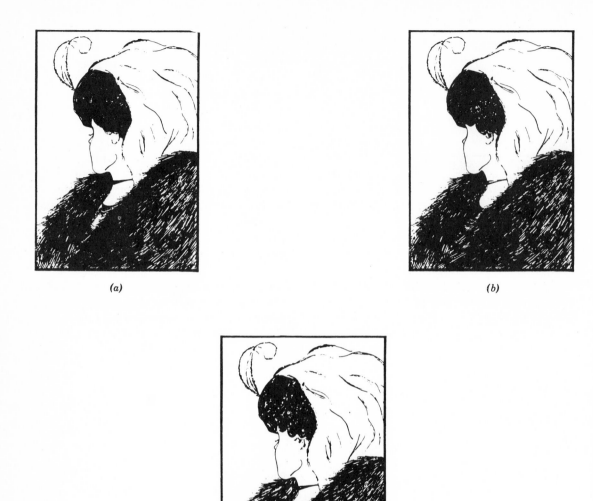

Fig. 14.33 *Whether a young woman or an old woman is seen in (c) can be shown to be due to the viewer's set. If (a) is seen first, the drawing in (c) is seen as of a young woman; if (b) is seen first, (c) appears as an old woman. (Adapted from Boring, 1930.)*

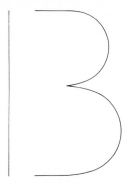

Fig. 14.34 *The "broken-B" stimulus figure used by Bruner and Minturn (1955). Subjects who previously saw letters or digits, first identified the test figure as the letter "B" or the number "13," respectively. (In the experiment the stimulus test figure was 7 mm in height and the curved part of the figure was separated from the vertical line by a distance of 1 mm.)*

a given set *dominated* so that, for example, a red six of spades was seen as a black six of spades or as a red six of hearts: The perception conformed with past expectations about the "normal" nature of playing cards. A second technique for dealing with incongruous stimuli the authors termed *compromise:* The red six of spades was reported as a purple six of hearts or a purple six of spades. A third reaction to stimulus incongruity was called *disruption,* in which the subject failed to resolve the incongruous stimulus in terms of his available perceptual set or expectation and the resultant experience tended to be somewhat bizarre. In the words of one frustrated subject after viewing an incongruous card at an exposure well above his normal threshold, "I don't know what the hell it is now, not even for sure whether it's a playing card." Although not without controversy (see Haber, 1966), the fundamental conclusion of this study and of our brief discussion of set is that perceptual organization may be powerfully determined by expectations built on past commerce with the environment.

FIGURAL ORIENTATION AND FORM PERCEPTION

In most of the preceding material, we have focused on a somewhat sensory analysis of form perception. We noted that form perception is heavily based on certain groupings of contours and that, in turn, the detection of contours can be reduced to the detection of luminance discontinuities that cause neural activity. This level of analysis does not emphasize the operation of cognitive processes involving decisions and corrections on the part of the viewer. However, other views on the nature of form perception do exist.

Rock (1973, 1974) recently proposed that the perceived shape of a stimulus figure involves a level of cognitive processing that requires more than the mere detection of its internal geometry. According to Rock, a major factor of form perception is the perception of the figure's orientation, in particular, the perceptual assignment by the

Fig. 14.35 *The shapes in (a) appear different from those in (b). However, the shapes within each row are geometrically equivalent except that they have been rotated to the right. The upper left shape has been rotated 90° and the bottom left shape, 45°. (Modified from Rock, 1974, p. 81.)*

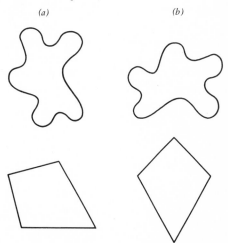

(a)   (b)

observer of the location of the top, bottom, and
sides of a figure. If these are altered in certain
ways, perception accordingly changes. The unfamiliar shapes in Figure 14.35a, look different
from those in 14.35b, yet the shapes in each row
are geometrically equal but shown in different
orientations. Clearly, to the naïve viewer each
shape would be described quite differently.

In addition, it is not the orientation of the
shape on the retina that is crucial to its perception
but, rather, how the shape appears to be oriented
with respect to gravity and to the visual frame of
reference—what Rock calls *environmental
orientation*. The ambiguous shape in Figure
14.36a, viewed with the head tilted 90° to the
right side continues to be perceived as a bearded
profile; similarly, the viewing of Figure 14.36b,
with the head tilted 90° in the opposite direction
still results in the perception of an outline map of
the United States. However, in each case the
orientation of the image of the shape on the retina
is for the reversed perception. Thus, the environ-
mentally upright as opposed to the retinally upright version of the figure is the one recognized.

That shapes are perceived on the basis of
their environmental orientation rather than
retinal orientation is owing to the tendency for
the perceptual system to correct or compensate for
head or body tilt. Of course, the priority of
perceiving things against a perceptually (though
not necessarily retinally) stable and invariant
background or environment has obvious adaptive
significance. It makes more sense for a biological
system to be able to compensate for its own
physical displacements with regard to a stable environment than to perceive the environment tilted
with every tilt of the body.

In this chapter we have attempted to trace
the development of form perception beginning

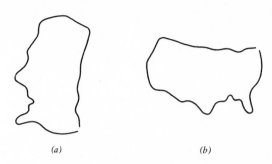

(a)   *(b)*

Fig. 14.36 *The ambiguous figure above can be
perceived as a different shape depending on its orientation. The drawing at (a) looks like a bearded profile in
one orientation and as an outline map of the United
States in another orientation. When viewed with the
head tilted 90° to the right, (a) still appears as a profile;
when the head is tilted 90° to the left, (b) still appears as
a map. The viewer sees the shape that is upright in the
environment rather than the shape that is upright on the
retina. (Modified from Rock, 1973, p. 13.)*

with certain elementary visual features, such as
luminance discontinuities and contours and the
perception of figure-ground differentiation,
progressing to grouping principles and some
specific visual factors (e.g., masking, aftereffects)
that directly affect or contribute to form perception. We have outlined some organizational
schemes (e.g., contour perception, Gestalt principles, perceptual set, Rock's cognitive theory,
and some neural correlates of form perception
such as feature-specific detectors). However, no
single class of explanation is entirely sufficient to
account for the visual ability to perceive form.
Nor is there a general principle that unifies the
many experiences of form perception. Form perception may be understood, at least in part, as
resulting from neural mechanisms as well as being the result of a cognitive, learning-based
achievement.

15

The Perception of Movement

With only a few exceptions our discussion of visual processes thus far has been confined to the perception of static or immobile stimuli by a stationary viewer. However, in the normal course of viewing, there is much movement occurring in the environment. Most organisms of whose vision we have taken note are comparatively mobile and move about in an environment containing a variety of moving objects, objects to be pursued or potentially dangerous objects to be avoided. Clearly, the perception of movement has an important biological utility. To locomote effectively animals must be capable of detecting the relative location, direction, and often even the rate of movement of objects. Perhaps for all species the reception of information about the movement of objects is essential for survival.

The capacity to perceive movement is organized quite early, both ontogenetically and phylogenetically, in that movement perception has been observed in the very young of many species and in animals low on the evolutionary scale (e.g., Schiff, 1965; Bower, Broughton, & Moore, 1970). Additionally, investigations with amphibia (Lettvin, Maturana, McCulloch, & Pitts, 1959) and mammals (e.g., Hubel & Weisel, 1962; Barlow, Hill, & Levick, 1964; Michael, C. R., 1968; Jung & Spillman, 1970; Bridgeman,

1972) give evidence that the perception of movement has a neural basis, that is, there is evidence of directionally sensitive movement-detecting units (see Chapter 11). Boring (1942, p. 594) and, more recently, Gregory (1973) point out that movement perception has evolutionary priority over shape perception. According to Gregory (1973):

> Something of the evolutionary development of the eye, from movement to shape perception, can be seen embalmed in the human retina. The edge of the retina is sensitive only to movement. This may be seen by getting someone to wave an object around at the side of the visual field, where only the edge of the retina is stimulated. It will be found that the movement and the direction of movement are seen, but it is impossible to identify the object. When the movement stops, the object becomes invisible. (P. 91)

The most general condition for the perception of movement is the stimulation of a succession of· neighboring retinal loci by an image. However, retinal displacement does not include all instances where the perception of movement occurs. The movement of a stimulus may be perceived when its image is held relatively sta-

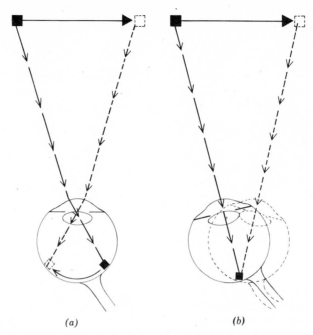

(a)   (b)

Fig. 15.1   *Movement systems of the eye. (a) Image-retina movement system. The succession of images of a moving target stimulus across the retina provides information of movement to a stationary eye. (Source: Gregory, 1973, p. 93.) (b) Eye-head movement system. A moving-target stimulus is tracked by a moving eye so that the image remains stationary on the retina, yet movement of the target stimulus is still perceived. Images that move across the retina are perceived as stationary background stimuli, and images that remain stationary on the retina while the eye moves are perceived as moving. (Source: Gregory, 1973, p. 93.)*

tionary on the retina as in the case where the eyes follow or track a moving object. Here movements of the eye match the target's movement, resulting in a more or less motionless retinal image.

Gregory has identified these as two interdependent movement systems: They are called the *image-retina movement system* and the *eye-head movement system* (see Figure 15.1).

THE IMAGE-RETINA MOVEMENT SYSTEM

The effective stimulation for the perception of movement of a physically moving stimulus, for the image-retina system, is successive stimulation of adjacent retinal loci. Generally, when the eye is held relatively stationary, as during fixation, a succession of images produced by a moving target stimulus shifts across the retina. The movement thus registered is due to the sequential firing of the receptors in the path of the image of the moving stimulus. This sort of movement detection system is well suited to the mosaic of ommatidia found in the compound eye of the arthropod. A neural model of a movement detector coincident with the image-retina movement system is suggested in Figure 15.2 (Schouten, 1967).

EYE-HEAD MOVEMENT SYSTEM

Of course, when we follow a moving target with our eyes, the image of the target remains

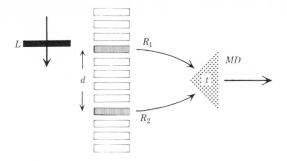

Fig. 15.2 *Neural model of a movement detector. Two retinal receptors, R_1 and R_2, spaced d apart, feed into the movement detector, MD. The movement detector reacts if the light, L, strikes receptor R_1 first and then, after or within a given period of time, t, strikes receptor R_2. (Reprinted from "Subjective stroboscopy and a model of visual movement detectors," by J. F. Schouten, in Models for the Perception of Visual Form, by permission of the MIT Press, Cambridge, Mass.)*

more or less fixed on the same retinal region. In this case, eye movement compensates for target movement, yet the perception of the target's movement still occurs. If the moving target stimulus is tracked against a stationary textured background, a series of velocity signals of the target's background move across the retina. However, the perception of movement still results even when there is no background stimulation. A moving dot of light in an otherwise darkened environment provides sufficient information for movement perception, yet as the eye follows the dot no background imagery shifts across the retina. This means that in the absence of successive stimulation of neighboring retinal elements (i.e., the lack of stimulation of the image-retina system) self-initiated neural signals that effect the rotation of the eyes in their sockets provide information for the perception of movement. That is, some neural mechanism takes account of command signals that move the eyes and relates them to the image on the retina. These neural signals to the ocular muscles commanding the execution of eye movements occur only when the eyes are voluntarily moved.

In the case where a moving target is seen against a physically stationary but textured background, the explanation of the operation of the eye-head movement system relates to the question of why the visual environment appears stationary as we voluntarily move our eyes. Clearly, as we intentionally move our eyes a continuous flow of retinal imagery occurs, yet the visual world continues to be seen as stationary. The answer seems to be that when the eyes voluntarily move, efferent motor command signals or impulses from the brain to the eye muscles are compared with the corresponding flow of images on the retina at a hypothetical center of the nervous system termed the *visual stability center* (Howard & Templeton, 1966, p. 65). The outcome is a perceptual cancellation of apparent movement attributed to the sequential flow of background imagery, that is, a cancellation of the image-retina system. We are thus able to differentiate between movements of the retinal image produced by voluntary eye movements and movements of the retinal image produced by the physical movement of objects in relation to their background. Hence, when the eyes voluntarily move, as during object tracking, the visual field of the target's background remains apparently stable and only physically moving stimuli appear to move. These outcomes are summarized in Table 15.1.

Note that it is not kinesthetic feedback that the eyeball muscles have been stretched in movement that accounts for perceptual stability, but, rather, it is owing to intentional outgoing motor command signals to execute the movements. This perceptual-motor explanation is consistent with the perceptual effects that result from eyeball immobility. If the eye muscles are paralyzed, attempts to move the eyes result in the apparent movement of the total visual field in the same direction as the attempted movement. Here eye movement command signals reach the visual stability center, but are not accompanied by any movement of the retinal image (Howard & Templeton, 1966, p. 66). This explanation of the operation of the eye-head system, attributed to Helmholtz (1962), also accounts for the fact that

Table 15.1

EFFECTS OF RETINAL IMAGE CHANGES AND VOLUNTARY EYE
MOVEMENTS ON THE PERCEPTION OF MOVEMENT[a]

OBJECT	RETINAL IMAGE	COMMANDS TO EYE/HEAD MUSCLES	PERCEPTION
a. Moving	Changes	No	Movement
b. Moving	Stationary	Yes	Movement
c. Stationary	Changes	Yes	No movement

[a] Modified from *Psychology: Man in Perspective,* by A. Buss, Wiley, New York, 1973, p. 207. Reprinted by permission of the publisher.

when the movement of the eyeball is initiated passively, the eye-head system is not properly stimulated and the total visual environment is erroneously seen as in movement. If you close one eye and gently move a finger under the bottom lid of the open eye, moving the eye upward, the visual field appears to move in a direction opposite to the movement of the eye. This occurs because when the action is passively executed, impulses voluntarily directing eye movements are lacking and the eye-head system is inoperative. Thus, with passive movements of the eyeball, the visual field does not remain stable; it is only with voluntary eye movements that cancellation of image-retina movement signals occurs.

Furthermore, the visual world does not appear to move very much as we move our head or body independent of eye movements, indicating that the central nervous system is also capable of taking into account an interplay of visual and vestibular or orientational information in a similar manner.

retinal projection. The perception of the movement of an object in the near-far plane may occur when the approach of the object is signaled by its increasing projected size. (This phenomenon is called "looming" and is discussed in some detail in Chapter 18.) That is, the orderly increase in the projected size of the object on the retina is perceived as a movement toward the observer.

Kinetic Optical Occlusion

As an object moves in space, it systematically covers and uncovers the physical texture of the surface that lies behind it. This differentiated flow of stimulation across the retinal surface is termed *kinetic optical occlusion* by J. J. Gibson (1966). As described by Gibson, there is a *wiping-out* of texture at the leading borders, an *unwiping-out* at the trailing borders, and a *shearing* of texture at the lateral borders of the moving object. That is, the retinal projection of an object moving across a textured background involves ". . . a rupture of the continuity of texture . . ." (p. 203).

THE PATTERN OF RETINAL STIMULATION AND MOVEMENT PERCEPTION

The perception of movement is also mediated by the pattern of changing stimulation in the

APPARENT MOVEMENT

In this context *apparent movement* refers to the perception of movement when there is no corresponding physical displacement of an object in

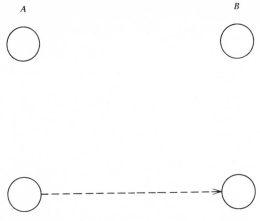

Fig. 15.3 *Strobiscopic movement from two alternately flashing stationary lights, A and B. Depending on the intensity of the light flashes, the physical distance separating them, and the time interval between light flashs, the illusion of movement, schematized in the bottom figure, can be created with two lights flashing sequentially.*

the time intervening between flashes of the lights, and the spatial distance between the lights. The relationships among these three variables have been worked out for a limited range of values and are known as *Korte's Laws.* The set of interrelationships among the three variables—intensity, time, and distance—are outlined as follows: (1) If intensity is held constant, the spatial distance between the lights for optimal apparent movement varies directly with the time interval between lights; that is, if the spatial separation between the two lights is increased, the time interval must also be increased or optimal movement breaks down. (2) If the time interval is held constant, the distance between lights for optimal apparent movement varies directly with intensity. (3) If the distance between the lights is held constant, the intensity for optimal apparent movement varies *inversely* with the time interval separating the two lights.

Motion Pictures

As shown in Figure 15.4, apparent movement from sequentially presented stationary stimuli is not limited to the stimulation from only simple lights. The principles involved in perceiving apparent movement from stationary but intermittently presented stimuli lie at the basis of one of the most familiar and compelling examples of apparent movement—motion pictures. In motion pictures a series of still frames of slightly different photographs are projected on a screen in rapid

space. One of the most convincing instances of apparent movement occurs when two stationary lights, set a short distance apart, are alternately lighted at a certain rate (schematized in Figure 15.3). As light *A* flashes on and off, light *B* flashes off and on, that is, one light is onset just as the other offsets. If the pattern of stimulation is correct, the perception is of simple movement across the intervening space between *A* and *B* in the direction of light *A* to light *B*; that is, a single light is seen moving through the empty space between lights *A* and *B*. This type of movement is termed *strobiscopic* or *beta* (β) movement or sometimes phi, (ϕ). If the rate of alternation is too slow, only succession will be perceived—two lights alternately flashing. If the rate of alternation is too short, the perception of apparent movement changes to one of simultaneity—two lights are perceived flashing, each at a different location.

A number of different kinds of apparent movement can be produced by two flashing lights (see Boring, 1942, pp. 596–597). The most crucial variables determining the nature of the apparent movement are the intensities of the lights,

Fig. 15.4 *Apparent movement with two successive stationary stimuli. When the vertical line A is succeeded by the horizontal line B after an interval of 60 msec, the vertical line will appear to rotate 90° clockwise, as shown by C. (From Foundations of Psychology, by E. G. Boring, H. S. Langfeld, & H. P. Weld, Wiley, New York, 1948, p. 311. Reprinted by permission of the publisher.)*

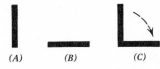

(A)　　(B)　　(C)

succession. Each frame is a view of a slightly different spatial position of a moving object. When this succession of static frames is projected at the proper rate (usually at least 24 different frames per second), movement is perceived. As with stroboscopic movement, the quality of the movement varies with the rate of projection. If the rate is too slow a succession of flickers or at even slower rates, frames of discrete photographs, are seen; whereas, if the rate is too fast, a blur of images is seen.

As noted earlier, once begun a visual image persists for a brief period even though the physical stimulus has ended. In the case of motion pictures when the photographs are shown at the proper rate, the image of each photograph fuses with the image of the preceding and following photograph, thereby producing a perception of steady movement. Thus, the visual system can integrate a series of successive but discrete images producing an apparently continuous visual environment.

In actual practice, the light projected from each frame to the screen by most professional moving picture projectors is interrupted several times prior to the advancement to the next frame. This is necessary because at only 24 frames per second we would still see flicker. To avoid this each frame is usually shown three times. This is accomplished by a shutter arrangement, so that each frame is projected on the screen as three flashes resulting in a frequency of 72 flashes per second. Home movies run on 16 frames per second (48 projections per second), but because they are shown at a lower intensity level there is less of a tendency to see flicker (see Chap. 12). The image produced on the television screen results from a similar fusion principle, although it is technically quite different.

Real Versus Apparent Movement

Though many instances of real and apparent movement are experientially indistinguishable, mention should be made of the fact that there is some controversy over the neural mechanisms that mediate them. Kolers (1963, 1964) contends that the physiological mechanisms underlying real and apparent movement are quite different, and he has identified several disimilarities. In contrast, the more recent research of Clatworthy and Frisby (1973) suggests that real and apparent movement are mediated by the same movement-detecting mechanism. Although not suggesting any resolution of the controversy, Walls (1963) has offered an interesting speculation:

> . . . the close imitation of real movement by apparent movement under the same spatial, temporal, and intensity-conditions presumably has some biological value. What it is, we cannot say. The writer would suggest—most gingerly!—that perhaps when a primitive, stupid vertebrate saw a moving object pass behind an obstacle and emerge again, he could not be trusted to know that it was all one object, and not two different ones, unless he had an automatic means of maintaining the oneness of the object during the moment when it was hidden from him. (P. 362)

THRESHOLDS FOR THE PERCEPTION OF MOVEMENT

Threshold values for the perception of movement vary with many physical and psychophysiological factors other than the actual velocity of a moving stimulus. The threshold varies with target size, luminance levels, the region of the retina stimulated, and the adaptive state of the eye. For example, thresholds for movement are lower for well-illuminated moving stimuli. Under optimal conditions, when stimulating the fovea, the movement of a well-illuminated target of 0.8 cm square seen moving through an aperture of 7.5 × 2.5 cm at a viewing distance of 2 meters is just detected when it moves at a velocity of about 0.2 cm per second (Brown, 1931b; see Spigel, 1965, p. 40).

In contrast, when the velocity of a moving target at 2 meters from the viewer exceeds about 150 cm per second, the object appears as a blur rather than as a target in transit (Boring, Langfeld, & Weld, 1948).

THE EFFECT OF BACKGROUND FACTORS ON THE PERCEPTION OF MOVEMENT

Perhaps one of the most influential variables for movement perception is the field on which a target is perceived. J. F. Brown in 1931 examined the role of the size of the target relative to the size of the field on which it appeared to move. In one experiment observers had to equalize the apparent movement of two sequences of squares that each moved behind a separate aperture. The squares, their spacings, and the size of the aperture of one display were twice the linear size of the other (see Figure 15.5 for an example of the display using dots instead of squares). The subjects adjusted the movement of the squares of the two displays until they appeared to move at the same speed. An equality match occurred when the physical speed of movement of the large squares moving behind the large aperture was set at almost twice the speed of the movement of the small squares. Thus, perceived movement of an object is dependent on the relation of the object to the general structure of the visual field as well as on its physical velocity.

The framework in which the pattern of movement is seen exerts considerable influence on the character of the perceived movement. Parks (1965) demonstrated that when a picture of a figure is moved horizontally behind an opaque cover with a stationary slit that is smaller than the figure, a viewer observing the pattern of stimulation at the slit will see the figure as a whole in the general vicinity of the slit (see Figures 15.6, 15.7). Interestingly, the entire figure is recognized although only a narrow strip

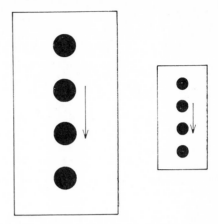

Fig. 15.5 *An endless paper tape moving downward is observed behind each of the two apertures. A row of printed dots is printed on each tape. The size of the larger aperture is twice that of the smaller one; in addition its dots are twice as large and are twice as far apart from each other. The observer must adjust the speeds of the tapes until the dots in the two apertures appear to move at the same speed. The result is that the physical speed of movement of the tape behind the large aperture must be about twice the speed of the smaller for an equality match. (Based on J. F. Brown, 1931 a.)*

of it is visible at any instant. This suggests that the visual system can assemble a set of successive parts that fall on the same retinal region over time into a single unitary form. Along with the shape of the slit, the figure's perceived shape is dependent on the speed at which the figure travels behind the slit. At relatively slow speeds, the figure appears slightly elongated; when moved at relatively high speeds, it appears compressed or condensed (Anstis & Atkinson, 1967; Haber & Nathanson, 1968). In addition, the figure appears displaced in the direction of its movement.

Although the explanation of the perception of a unitary figure viewed under these circumstances remains in dispute, the phenomenon itself is of importance to the understanding of the figural persistence of a visual image, of post-retinal short-term visual storage, and temporal

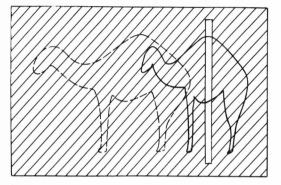

Fig. 15.6 *A sample stimulus and outline of the arrangement for the demonstration of Park's effect. A simple outline figure (dashed line) is passed behind a stationary slit aperture in an opaque screen. At the appropriate speed the figure will be briefly seen in the region of the slit as moving slightly and being compressed (solid line drawing). The compression of the figure increases with the speed of its passage until only a blur is seen. The author termed this example, "Passing a camel through the eye of a needle." (Source: Parks, 1965, 78, p. 146.)*

integration (see Anstis & Atkinson, 1967; Haber & Nathanson, 1968; Hochberg, J. E., 1968; and Rock & Halper, 1969, for differing views).

INDUCED MOVEMENT

What an observer perceives to be in motion is not always in accordance with what is actually in motion. As noted, the perception of movement is strongly influenced by the spatial context or framework in which the moving stimuli are seen. If two lighted figures of different sizes are seen against an otherwise darkened field and only the larger figure is in physical motion, only the smaller one appears to move. The larger moving stimulus is said to *induce* the movement of the smaller one (Wallach, 1959). If a stationary luminous dot is enclosed by a luminous rectangle and the rectangle is slowly moved to the right, the

enclosed dot appears to move to the left. That is, the apparent movement of the dot is induced by the physical displacement of the rectangle. This is outlined in Figure 15.8. In a more familiar example, sometimes the moon appears to race behind apparently stationary clouds, yet clearly it is the clouds that are in physical transit and cover a stationary moon. In general, the smaller and more enclosed stimulus appears to move relative

Fig. 15.7 *Examples of the distorted perception of figures moving behind a stationary slit. (a) The perceived figure appears displaced and compressed in the direction of its movement. (b–g) Slits that are tilted, curved or multiple make moving figures appear tilted, curved or multiple, respectively. (h,i) The shape of the figure and the slit can be interchanged. An "X"-shape figure seen through a vertical-line slit appears the same as a vertical-line figure seen through an "X"-shape slit. (Source: Anstis & Atkinson, 1967, 80, p. 573.)*

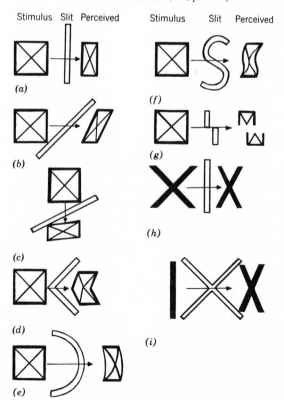

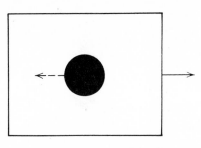

Fig. 15.8 *Induced movement. A luminous stationary dot enclosed by a luminous rectangle is seen in the dark. If the rectangle is physically displaced to the right (solid arrow), the enclosed dot appears to move to the left (dotted arrow). The apparent movement of the stationary dot is induced by the physical displacement of the rectangle.*

to the larger and enclosing stimulus. Perhaps this is so because it is usually small objects that move whereas the larger objects in our environment are stable.

PULFRICH EFFECT

An interesting perceptual distortion of physical movement, known as the *Pulfrich pendulum effect,* may occur when the two eyes are stimulated by different intensities of light. This effect is schematized in Figure 15.9. The pendulum bob is swung back and forth in a straight path in a plane perpendicular to the viewer's line of sight. However, when both eyes are open but one eye is covered with a dark glass or light filter (e.g., one lens of a pair of sunglasses), the pendulum bob appears to swing in an elliptical path arching toward and away from the viewer. According to Gregory (1973) and Enright (1970), this distortion is due in large measure to the fact that the reaction time of the visual system is inversely related to stimulus intensity (see also Riggs, 1971, p. 309). The filter reduces the amount of light reaching one eye, which in turn results in a slight but significant delay in the signals from that eye reaching the brain. That is, at any instant the apparent position of the pendulum bob coded by the filtered eye lags slightly behind the position of the pendulum bob coded by the unfiltered eye. The fact that for the filtered eye the pendulum bob is

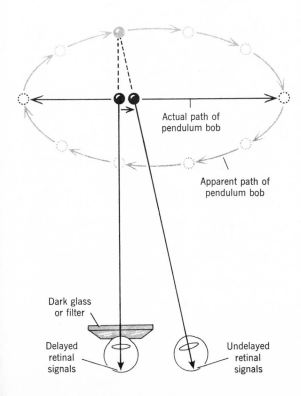

Actual path of pendulum bob

Apparent path of pendulum bob

Dark glass or filter

Delayed retinal signals

Undelayed retinal signals

Fig. 15.9 *Schematic diagram of the Pulfrich pendulum effect. When a pendulum swinging in a straight arc in a plane perpendicular to the line of sight is viewed with a filter over one eye, it appears to swing in an ellipse. This is due to the signals from the eye covered by the filter being delayed. There is an apparent displacement of the pendulum bob away from the viewer when it moves from the filtered to the unfiltered side of the visual field and a displacement toward the viewer when the pendulum bob moves in the opposite direction. (Source: Gregory, 1973, p. 80.)*

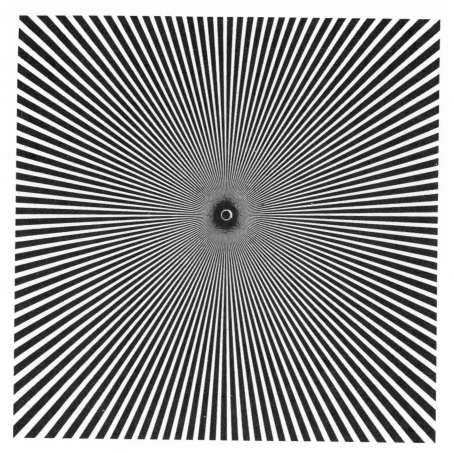

Fig. 15.10 *An example of a geometric pattern that produces afterimages in which motion can be perceived. If the center of the pattern is fixated for approximately 10 sec and then the afterimage is projected on a plain white surface, rotary motion is usually perceived. (Reprinted from "Ways of looking at Perception" by D. M. McKay, in Models for the Perception of Visual Form, by permission of the MIT Press, Cambridge, Mass.)*

seen slightly later in space means that at any given moment the pendulum bob appears at slightly different locations for each eye. The reconciliation of the disparity between the information arriving at the cortex from both retinae is an apparent displacement of the pendulum bob in an elliptical path in depth.

AUTOKINETIC MOVEMENT

An effect similar to induced movement may occur when fixating on a stationary point of light

in an otherwise completely darkened environment. In this condition a spatial context or background is lacking and there is no fixed visual coordinate system to which the point of light may be referred. The result is that a single stationary point of light appears to drift or wander irregularly about, a phenomenon termed *autokinetic movement*. Typically, the point of light appears to make small excursions, but considerable movement is often noted. Though the effect is universal, there are wide individual differences in the extent and direction of the apparent movement, and autokinetic movement has been shown to be significantly affected by social influences (Sherif, 1936).

One explanation offered by Gregory (1973) is based on the fact that there is a variation in the efficiency of the eye muscles to maintain fixation on the point of light. During continued fixation slight tremors of the eyes cause some fluctuation in fixation. Moreover, during prolonged fixation the eye muscles fatigue. In order to compensate for the lack of maintained fixation as well as for fatigue, the eye muscles require abnormal command signals to hold the gaze on the point of light. These abnormal signals are the same sort of signals that normally move the eyes when tracking moving stimuli. According to Gregory (1973):

> We thus see movement when the muscles are fatigued, although neither the eyes nor the image on the retinas are moving. The wandering illusory movements of the autokinetic effect seem to be due to the command signals maintaining fixation in spite of slight spontaneous fluctuations in the efficiency of the muscles, which tend to make the eyes wander. It is not the eyes moving, but the correcting signals applied to **prevent** them moving which cause the spot of light to wander in the dark. (P. 103)

AFTEREFFECT MOVEMENT

A passenger on a stopped train who has gazed at the imagery of a moving landscape for a while sees the landscape appear to move forward so persuasively that he may actually perceive the train as slowly moving backward. A simple illustration of this called the spiral aftereffect was described in Chapter 14. A similar movement aftereffect is shown in the geometric pattern of Figure 15.10. Aftereffect movement is a further example that the perception of movement occurs not only to a pattern of changing stimulation but can occur in its absence.

MOTION-PRODUCED DEPTH: KINETIC DEPTH EFFECT

If a pattern of two-dimensional shadows, such as those created by rotation of a bent wire form, are cast on a translucent screen, as shown in Figure 15.11, the impression is of a rotating rigid object in three dimensions. This phenomenon has been termed the *kinetic depth effect* by Wallach and O'Connell (1953). When the figure is stationary, the shadow of the wire form appears flat, in two dimensions. However, when set in rotation around its vertical axis, the changing shadow pattern is perceived as emanating from a solid rotating object, even though all the movement is imaged on a flat plane. What is occurring is that a sequence of visual images is projected that corresponds to the continuous imagery that normally results from the rotation of an actual three-dimensional object. As a consequence, the visual system interprets the changes in the pattern of shadows in accordance with the occurrence of a rotating three-dimensional object rather than a succession of changing flat patterns.

BIOLOGICAL MOTION

Our discussion thus far has dealt with the perception of movement per se, but one kind of environmental movement warrants specific consideration: the perception of the class of movements by locomoting humans. We quickly recognize whether a person is walking or running, skipping or dancing, and so on. Moreover, we can detect slight deviations from the general norms of these motions. For example, we easily note a slight limp in one's walk, the slower gait of the aged, and we may even recognize (and mimic) a person on the basis of his characteristic posture, style of walk, and pattern of gestures. The complex pattern of movements determining the perception of these Gestalt-like locomotor acts are constructed from combinations of pendulum-type motions that are specific for each type of activity.

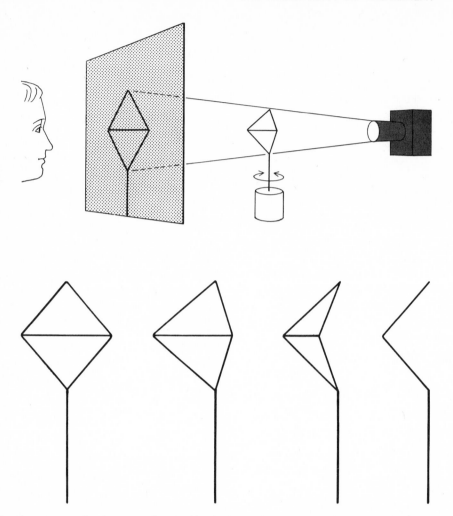

Fig. 15.11 *Arrangement for demonstrating the kinetic depth effect. When stationary, the shadow of a bent wire form looks flat. However, when it is rotated, the changing shadow pattern is perceived as a rigid rotating object in three dimensions. Four different orientations of the wire figure are shown at the bottom. (From Processes of Vision, by U. Neisser, Scientific American, 1968, 219, Pp. 204–205. Copyright © 1968 by Scientific American, Inc. All rights reserved.)*

These complex patterns of motion have been studied and labeled *biological motion* by Johansson (1973).

Johansson has devised a method for directly studying the visual information for perceiving pure biological motion without any interference by the shape of the moving form. In one experiment an actor's movement was recorded on videotape. However, the movement was accomplished in complete darkness and only dots of light placed at 10 main body joints were visible. This effectively eliminated any traces of the visual field background or the actor's body contours (see Figure 15.12). When viewing the kinetic dot configuration shown at *b* of Figure 15.12, the spontaneous perception of a person walking (or run-

(a)   **(b)**

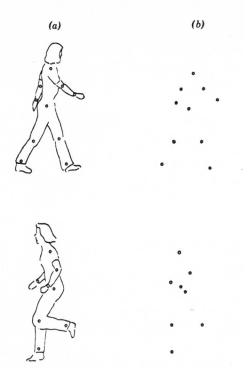

Fig. 15.12 *Outline contours of a walking and a running subject (a) and the corresponding dot configurations (b). After the first one or two steps, subjects viewing the dots of light perceive a walking (top dot configuration) or a running (bottom configuration) person. (Source: Johansson, 1973, p. 202. Reprinted by permission of the Psychonomic Society.)*

ning, bottom figure) resulted even after the actor had taken only one or two steps. Indeed, the effect of the patterns of movement made by the joints was so compelling that subjects could neither combine the moving dots to establish alternative impressions of movement nor could they see the dots merely as a series of unrelated lights in motion. When the motion ceased, the dot configurations did not appear to represent a human form, indicating that it was the pattern of movement that determined the perception of the particular kind of locomotor activity. In short, the general movements of the body when represented by light set at the main joints of the body produce com-

binations of joint interactions that are sufficiently informative to evoke strong and quite identifiable impressions of complex human locomotor activity.

PERCEIVED CAUSALITY IN MOVING STIMULI

Aside from path, direction, and velocity there are other more complex attributes that may be perceived from moving stimuli: They may give the impression of one causing the movement of another. For example, a rolling ball striking a stationary one appears to set the second ball in motion; that is, the movement of the first ball is perceived as causually effecting the movement of the second ball. Michotte (1963) has studied extensively the necessary stimulus conditions for perceiving causality among moving stimuli, and he has found that varying certain of the physical conditions of movement can give rise to different impressions of physical causality in movement.

An outline of the standard apparatus used by Michotte to investigate perceived causality is shown in Figure 15.13A. The viewer sees only a

Fig.15.13(A) *Standard display used by Michotte (1963) to illustrate the form of perceived causality called "launching."*

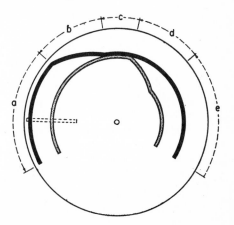

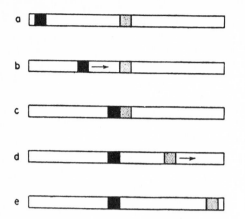

Fig. 15.13(B) *The phases of perceived movement seen in the slot, illustrated in 15.13B, correspond to the interaction of the two arcs as indicated along the perimeter of the arcs in 15.13A. (a) the two squares appear stationary; (b) the black square appears to move toward the gray; (c) the two squares touch momentarily; (d) the black square remains immobile while the gray one moves off; (e) the gray square comes to rest at a distance from the black one. (Source: Krech & Crutchfield, 1958, p. 126. Reprinted by permission of the authors.)*

fixed slot on an aperture shown by the dotted line. Behind the aperture two differently colored spirals or arcs (in this example, black and gray) are drawn on a single disc. When the disc is rotated counterclockwise, the perception of the display produced by the rotating arcs, seen in cross section at the slot, is of two interacting squares that appear to move along the length of the slot. The precise pattern of movement is controlled by the relation of the pathways of the two arcs. Five different phases of movement of the squares are shown along the perimeter of the arc in Figure 15.13A, and these are correlated with the sequence of perceptual events as illustrated in Figure 15.13B. When the basic design shown in Figure 15.13A is employed, subjects report that there is a clear, direct, and almost irresistible impression that the lateral movement of the black square

"causes" the movement of the gray square (as shown in d and e of the figure). Michotte noted that several stimulus variables are critical to the perception of causality: the speed of movement of the black square, the distance it traverses before making contact with the gray square, the duration of contact of the black and gray squares, and the subsequent speed of movement of the gray square after its contact with the black square.

When these stimulus aspects are appropriately varied, a number of different forms of perceived causality are reported. These two are typical: *launching,* in which the black square appears to cause the gray square to move (illustrated by d of Figure 15.13B) and *releasing,* in which the duration of contact between the black and gray square is extended beyond that required to produce the launching effect. In this condition the black square appears to cause a triggering of a latent force of motion residing within the gray square. One of the main stimulus differences between launching and releasing is the amount of time that the black and gray square are held in contact (that is, the length of the arc segment shown by c in Figure 15.13A). When the time delay is comparatively short, launching is perceived; when the delay is long, releasing is seen. Also important to the form of the perceived causality is the relative speed of the two squares: If the black square moves faster than the subsequent speed of the gray square, launching is generally seen. However, when the gray square appears to move faster than the speed of the black square after their contact, releasing is perceived.

A major finding of Michotte's work is that the perception of causality in movement is produced by certain relations between interacting stimuli, in which no actual causal relation between elements need exist. Moreover, different physical interactions of the stimulus elements lead to different impressions of causality.

In this chapter we have described the perception of various kinds of real and apparent movement and outlined several explanations. For the perception of real movement two main interdependent movement systems were identified: the image-retina movement system and the eye-head movement system. Topics and examples of apparent or systematic distortions in movement perception were discussed: thresholds, stroboscopic or phi movement, motion pictures, induced movement, the Pulfrich pendulum effect, autokinetic movement, aftereffect movement, motion-produced depth (kinetic depth effect), and the role of the background and the viewing field or aperture on the perception of the moving stimulus.

Finally, the perception of complex human locomotion and of causality in movement was outlined. In general the discussion of the stimulus events and variables critical to movement perception suggests that the perception of movement is governed by strict spatial and temporal relations between stimuli.

The Perception of Space
I: Spatial Cues and
Constancy

16

We noted earlier that functionally the primary role of vision is to register the spatial arrangement of objects and surfaces in the environment. Indeed, objects are generally seen as solid forms lying at some distance in the terrain. The perception of space in depth and distance presents a most challenging problem: How is it possible that visual space is normally experienced as three-dimensional, yet the retinal layer of rods and cones and the corresponding retinal images are essentially flat two-dimensional surfaces? Part of the answer lies in the character of the stimulation that arrives at the retina. For example, one sees differences in the brightness of different surfaces; objects take up different amounts of visual angle and are seen with varying degrees of clarity; some objects appear to lie in front of, or partially cover other objects. Clearly, the pattern of stimulation contained in the optic array conveys cues and indications about the spatial location of objects that the perceiver uses to "construct" a three-dimensional space.

In this chapter we will describe and discuss these and other stimulus features or cues and attempt to indicate the circumstances and mechanisms in which they are employed for perceiving depth and distance.

MONOCULAR CUES FOR SPATIAL PERCEPTION

A number of spatial cues require only a single eye for their reception. These have been labeled *monocular cues*. Graphic artists employ some of these cues in order to produce the illusion of a three-dimensional space on a two-dimensional canvas.

Interposition

Interposition refers to the appearance of one object partially concealing or overlapping another. If one object is partially covered by another, the fully exposed one is perceived as nearer. Examples of interposition are shown by the simple line drawings of Figure 16.1. When the images are of familiar objects, the effectiveness of interposition for showing relative distance is increased. Figure 16.2 illustrates some curious effects of interposition. Shown are some ambiguous figures in which interpositon provides conflicting information. Relative position is difficult to resolve since both parts of a given figure appear to possess mutually interposing segments.

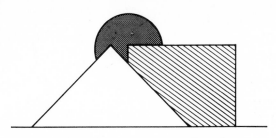

Fig. 16.1*A* *The circle appears to lie behind the rectangle, which appears to lie behind the triangle.*

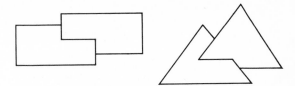

Fig. 16.2 *Interposition provides conflicting cues as to relative position. (Source: Ratoosh, 1949).*

Aerial Perspective or Clearness

Objects whose retinal images are sharp and distinct appear closer than those whose images are blurry or otherwise indistinct. This is due to the fact that dust, water vapor, and other atmospheric chemicals reduce their clarity. Thus, relatively large structures such as buildings appear closer when viewed on a clear day than on a hazy one. Aerial perspective may play a role in spatial perception, particularly when one is viewing over extensive distances. In general, the closer an object is, the clearer are its visual details; more distant objects appear less distinct.

Shading and Lighting

Generally, the surface of an object nearest the light source is the brightest. As the surface recedes from the light, it appears less bright and more darkly shadowed. Observe the bumps and irregular indentations of Figure 16.3, then turn the page around. A convexity-concavity change has taken place. We are accustomed to the source of light coming from above, (e.g., sunlight, ceiling lighting). Thus, when the picture is inverted, the bumps and indentations reverse because we continue to presume an overhead light source. Benson and Yonas (1973) have reported that children as young as three years of age can discriminate concavities from convexities on the basis of shading. Interestingly, chickens, like humans, react to stimuli as if the stimuli were lighted by an overhead source of illumination (Hershberger, 1970).

The appropriate use of gradients of surface shading may provide cues as to the shape of objects (see Figure 16.4). Illumination from a single light source will fall on a three-dimensional object in a consistent pattern. Since those surfaces closest to the light source receive the most illumination, the shape of the object has an effect on the pattern of light and dark areas produced.

Elevation

The horizon is higher in the vertical dimension of the visual field than is the foreground. Accordingly, objects appearing higher in the visual field are generally perceived as located at a greater

Fig. 16.1*B* *Overlapping planes suggest relative depth.*

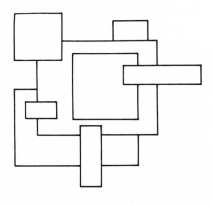

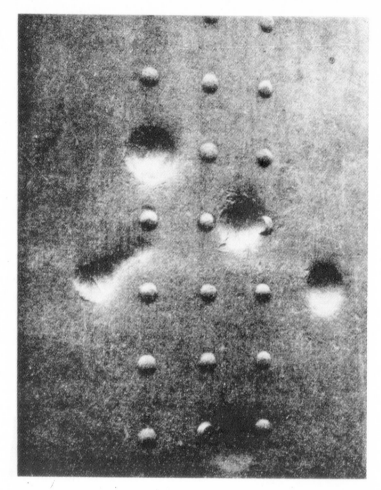

Fig. 16.3 *Light and shade used as depth cues. When the figure is inverted, bumps and pits reverse.*

distance from the viewer than objects that appear lower in the visual field.

Linear Perspective

The illusion of depth on a flat surface can be accomplished by the use of the geometric system of linear perspective. This involves systematically decreasing the size of more distant elements and the space separating them (see Figure 16.5). The image of a three-dimensional object undergoes such a transformation as it is projected onto the retina. A typical example is railroad tracks, as shown in Figure 16.6. The parallel tracks appear to converge at a point in the distance called the "vanishing point." Another illustration of perspective utilizing converging lines is given in Figure 16.7. Observe that the edges that appear farther away are smaller than those that appear closer.

Linear perspective as a precise graphic technique was formalized early in the fifteenth

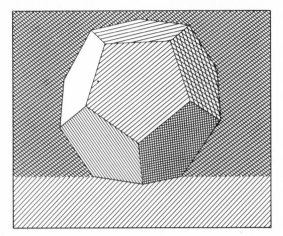

Fig. 16.4 *The pattern of light and dark areas aids the perception of the shape.*

century by the Italian architect and sculptor, Brunelleschi (Janson, 1962). An artist's bizarre use of perspective is given in Figure 16.8. This cue like other monocular cues to depth may appear within a picture or photograph, in which case, of course, the depth effect is somewhat less than would occur if the real scene were viewed. However, the impression of depth in a photograph can be increased by reducing the information that indicates that it is really a flat surface. For example, looking at a two-dimensional picture through a rolled-up paper tube not only eliminates the frame effect but also the binocular cue that the picture is a flat surface. This considerably enhances the depth effect (see Schlosberg, 1941).

Texture Gradients

A form of microstructure, generally seen as a grain or texture, is characteristic of most surfaces. This is obvious in many naturally occurring surfaces such as fields of grass, foliage, and trees, as well as in man-produced surfaces such as roads, floors, and fabrics. As described by J. J. Gibson (1950), the texture of these surfaces possesses a density gradient that structures the light in the

optic array in a way that is consistent with the arrangement of objects and surfaces in the environment. More specifically, when we look at any textured surface, the elements comprising the texture become denser as distance increases. As in linear perspective, the size of the elements and the distance separating elements decrease with distance. Figure 16.9 illustrates some examples of texture gradients. The gradient, or gradual refinement of the size, shape and spacing of elements comprising the pattern of the texture, provides a source of information as to distance. In Figure 16.10a the longitudinal surface *AB* projects a retinal image, *ab*; the latter possesses a gradient of texture from coarse to dense, the coarser elements closer to *a*, the denser elements closer to *b*. The gradient of texture, transmitted in the optic array at *ab*, provides the observer with information that he is viewing a receding surface. Notice that with respect to the eye the change in texture reflected from the surface *AB* is at a constant rate. The frontal surface, *BC*, which is perpendicular to the line of sight, projects a dif-

Fig. 16.5 *The image of the rectangle is shown in perspective on the picture plane. The two dimensional projection of the rectangle ABCD is shown as trapezoid abcd on the picture plane. Clearly, the distances separating the more distant elements of the rectangle. (segment BC) are decreased in their projection on the picture plane (bc). Notice also that since the stimulus pattern for the eye is in two dimensions an infinite number of arrangements in three dimensions (shapes 1, 2, etc.) will produce the same pattern at the eye. (Figure source: modified from J. E. Hochberg, 1964, p. 37.)*

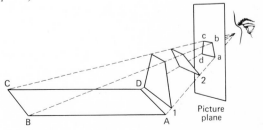

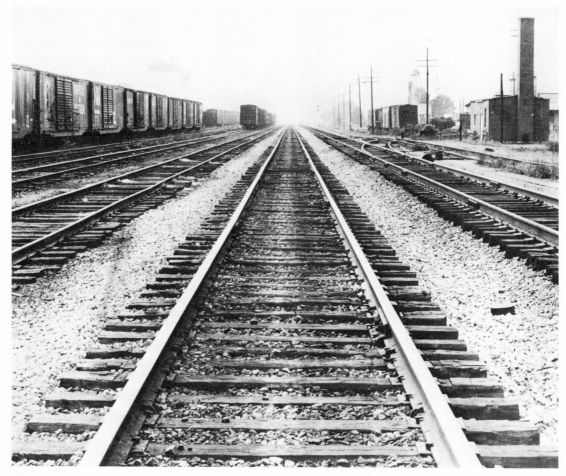

Fig. 16.6 *Perhaps the most common and most striking instance of linear perspective is the apparent convergence in the distance of parallel railroad tracks. Of course, the actual space between the tracks is constant, but the corresponding retinal images and, accordingly, the size of the apparent separation of the tracks decreases with the distance of the tracks.*

ferent sort of image: there is no gradient since all the elements are equidistant from the eye. Thus, the pattern *BC* (which projects a retinal image *bc* in Figure 16.10a) in Figure 16.10b is perceived as a "wall", forming a 90° angle with the "floor" of pattern *AB*. Curvatures, edges, as well as information as to shape and inclination of a surface, are detected from discontinuities in the texture and from texture changes that are not at a constant rate (see Figure 16.11). A number of studies have shown that perceived slant and shape are functionally related to texture gradients (e.g., Flock & Moscatelli, 1964; Winnick & Rogoff, 1965; Kraft & Winnick, 1967).

Texture gradients, along with interposition and linear perspective, are influential de-

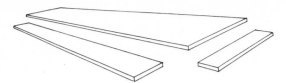

Fig. 16.7 *Planks drawn in perspective. Parts of apparently rectangular planks that are diminished in size appear farther away.*

terminants of perceived size. Neisser (1968) has pointed out that:

> *The gradient of increasing texture density on the retina, corresponding to increasing distance from the observer, gives a kind of "scale" for object sizes. In the ideal case when the texture units are identical, two figures of the same real size [see Figure*

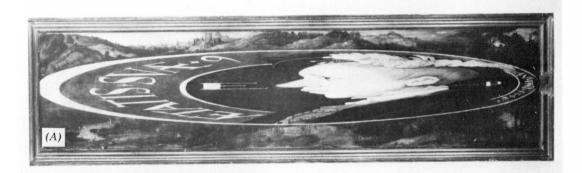

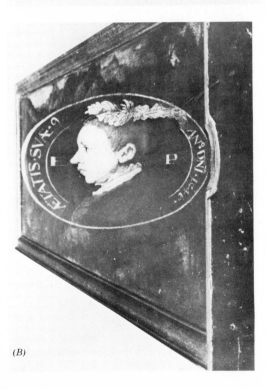

Fig. 16.8 *An artist's bizarre use of perspective. The sixteenth century portrait shown in A was drawn in distorted perspective. When viewed obliquely through a notch in the frame, the distortion is corrected, as seen in B. This can also be accomplished by holding the edge of the page to your eye and looking at the picture in A. (Edward VI, by William Scrots. Reprinted by permission of The National Portrait Gallery, London.)*

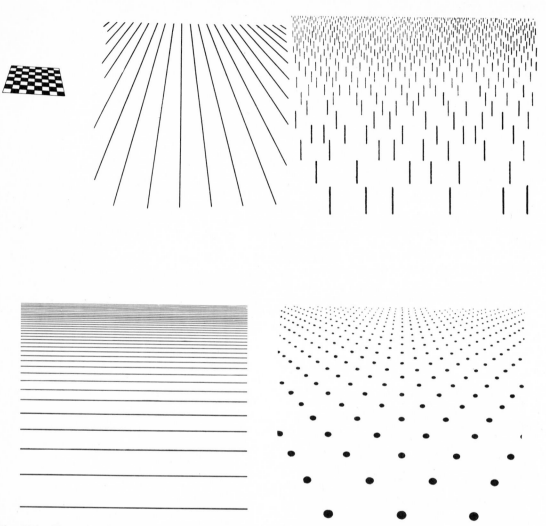

Fig. 16.9 *Examples of gradients of textures. The gradients of texture produce an impression of depth or distance on a flat surface.*

16.12] will always occlude the same number of texture units, regardless of how far away either one may be. That is, the relation between the retinal texture-size and the dimension of the object's retinal images is invariant, in spite of changes in distance. This relation is a potentially valuable source of information about the real size of the object—

more valuable than the retinal image of the object considered alone. (P. 205)

Motion Parallax

Whenever the eyes move in relation to the spatial environment, the retinal imagery undergoes a series of changes. Objects located at different

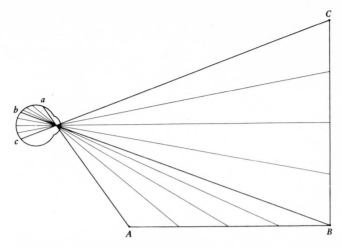

Fig. 16.10a *The optical projection of a longitudinal and a frontal surface. A retinal projection from coarse to dense, ab, is produced by the longitudinal surface AB. A frontal surface, BC, projects a uniform texture to the retina at bc. (Source: Gibson, J. J., 1950, p. 66.)*

distances in the visual field appear to move at different velocities. The relative apparent motion of objects as the observer moves his head is called *motion parallax* (Gibson, J. J. 1950, p. 71). Under certain conditions, these apparent velocity differences contribute to the perception of depth and distance. Generally, when the head moves, elements of the visual field that lie close to the viewer appear to move faster than do distantly located elements; additionally, the relative amount of apparent movement is less for far elements than for near ones. Both the extent and direction of the apparent movement depend on the location of the observer's fixation point.

The way in which motion parallax occurs in one set of conditions is illustrated in the schematic diagram by Gibson (1950) shown in Figure 16.13. What is indicated by the diagram is how the terrain appears to move as an observer gazes

Fig. 16.10b *Another view of the optical projection of above figure. The longitudinal projection, AB is perceived as a "floor"; the frontal projection, BC, is seen as a "wall."*

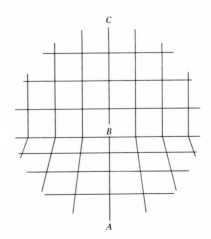

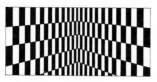

(A) Two receding surfaces meet to form a corner.

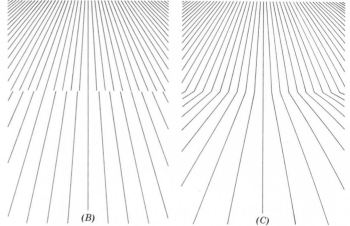

(B)   (C)

Discontinuities in textures: an edge in seen in B, a corner in C.

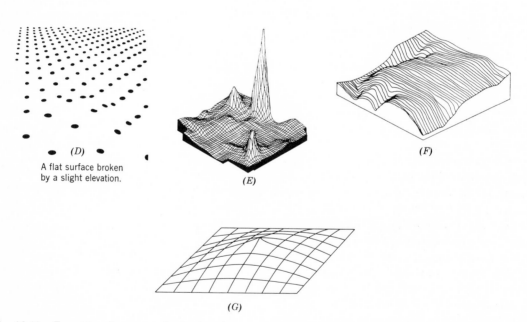

(D)

A flat surface broken by a slight elevation.

(E)

(F)

(G)

Fig. 16.11 *Examples of apparent depth given by texture gradients with discontinuities and texture changes that are not at a constant rate. In E, F, and G, interposition also plays a role in the depth effect. (Source: 16.11G, Békésy & Rosenblith, 1951, p. 1093. Reprinted by permission of the publisher.) (Source: 16.11 E & F, Jenks & Brown, Science, 1966. Copyright © 1966 by the American Association for the Advancement of Science.) (Source: 16.11 B & C: Gibson, 1950, p. 93.)*

out of a vehicle moving to the left. While maintaining fixation at point F, the nearer objects seem to move to the right, in a direction opposite to the observer's motion; whereas objects located beyond the fixation point appear to move to the left in the same direction as the movement of the observer. In addition, objects located at different distances appear to move at different velocities. Specifically, the perceived velocity of an object diminishes the closer it lies to the fixation point, F.

The phenomenon of motion parallax can be simply demonstrated as follows: Close one eye and hold up two objects, such as your fingers, in the direct line of sight, one about 25 cm (10 in) in front of the other. If you move your head from side to side while maintaining fixation of the far finger, the image of the near finger will appear to move in the direction opposite to movements of the head. If fixation is on the near finger, the far finger will appear to move in the same direction as the movements of the head.

This form of differential visual information resulting from movement of the observer is an especially potent source of precise depth and distance information (e.g., Ferris, 1972). Thus,

Fig. 16.12 *The discs appear to lie at different frontal planes. Because each disc covers the same amount of texture surface, they appear to be equal in size but located at different distances. (From the Processes of Vision, U. Neisser, Scientific American, 1968, 219, Pp. 204–205. Copyright © 1968 by Scientific American, Inc. All rights reserved.)*

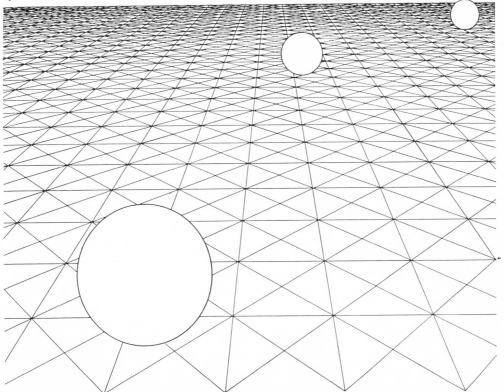

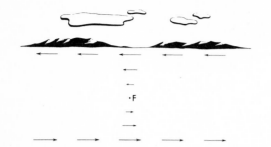

Fig. 16.13 *Schematic diagram of motion parallax when observer fixates a spot on the terrain. If an object located at F is fixated while the observer moves to the left, the image of the nearer objects appear to move to the right whereas farther objects seem to move to the left. The length of the arrows indicates that the apparent velocity of objects in the field of view increases in direct relation to their distance from the fixation point. (Source: Gibson, 1950, p. 124.)*

by noting the direction, extent, and velocity of objects moving in the visual field an observer may gauge their relative distances.

Familiarity

In the discussion of cues used in perceiving spatial features of objects, we have dealt primarily with the information given by the immediate visual cues. However, when viewing familiar objects there is nonvisual information as to the objects' spatial characteristics, such as size and shape, as a result of past experience with similar objects. Although not, strictly speaking, a cue to depth or distance, familiar size may contribute to spatial perception. For example, when familiar objects are judged as to size, it appears to make little difference whether the object, if it is a familiar one, is present during the judgment or not (Brunswick, 1944; Bolles & Bailey, 1956; McKennell, 1960; Churchill, 1962). In other words, we "know" the sizes of many objects in our immediate surroundings and can give reasonably accurate size estimations of them from memory. However, whether or not we utilize this size information, especially for locating objects, is not clear.

There is more than one viewpoint concerning the role of familiarity or memorial information on the apparent sizes of familiar objects when visual and memorial information are both available (C. B. Hochberg & McAlister, 1955). A number of studies suggest that the role of familiarity as a determinant of apparent size is a function of the conditions of viewing. In judging the sizes of familiar objects under ordinary conditions of viewing, it appears that judgments are based on the current visual stimulation (Fillenbaum, Schiffman, and Butcher, 1965). On the other hand, when viewing conditions such as lighting and distance cues are impoverished, familiarity or knowledge of the object's size plays a role in the size judgments (Schiffman, H. R., 1967). Furthermore, realistic representations of familiar objects can, under appropriate circumstances, affect the apparent location of them (Epstein, 1963; Epstein and Baratz, 1964; Gogel, 1965; Ono, 1969; see Epstein, 1967, for a general discussion of this issue). For example, pictures of familiar coins, identical in projected size, but representing coins that differ in familiar size (photographs of a dime, quarter, and half dollar) were observed under cue-reduced, monocular conditions of viewing. Photographs of the coins that represented larger sizes, but that were of the same retinal size, were judged as more distant (Epstein, 1963).

Relative Size

Hochberg (Hochberg, C. B. & Hochberg, J. E. 1952; Hochberg, C. B. & McAlister, 1955; Hochberg, 1964) has argued against familiarity or familiar size as a cue to perceived distance in certain situations. He suggests an alternative cue—*relative size*—to explain the same phenomenon in conditions where more than one stimulus is present for viewing. When two similar or identical shapes of different sizes are viewed simultaneously or in close succession, the larger stimulus will appear closer to the viewer than the smaller one (see Figure 16.14). This explanation does not refer to past experience; rather, it states that in certain situations images of the same shapes but of different sizes are sufficient stimuli for a depth relationship (see Figure 16.15).

Equidistance Tendency

A similar relational cue to distance is that cited by Gogel (1965), who contends that in the absence of effective distance cues there is a tendency for objects in the visual field to appear equally distant to the viewer; furthermore, the strength of this tendency increases as the objects are laterally brought closer to each other in the frontal plane of the visual field. Gogel terms this relationship between the apparent locations of objects the *equidistance tendency*.

Accommodation

We have already described the accommodative mechanism for focusing the lens to form a sharp retinal image. Because different accommodating responses are made for focusing on near and far objects, it is possible that oculomotor adjusting signals from the ciliary muscles (i.e., the degree of contraction) furnish information of a target's spatial location. However, the status of accommodation as an effective source of spatial information has been difficult to evaluate and its role is not agreed on (e.g., Hochberg, J. E., 1971; Wallach & Floor, 1971; Leibowitz, Shiina, & Hennessy, 1972). At any rate, for man it would be of use

Fig. 16.14 *Relative Size. Images of the same shapes but of different sizes may furnish a depth cue. In this figure the larger squares give the appearance of lying closer to the viewer than do the smaller ones.*

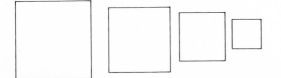

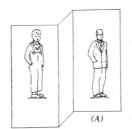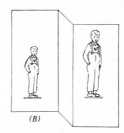

Fig. 16.15 *Reversible "screens" with figures drawn on the panels. In A, relative size is constant and familiar size is varied because normal men and boys are known to differ in their sizes. In B, familiar size is equated for the two boys, but they are of different relative sizes. A more pronounced and stable depth difference occurs with B, hence in this instance relative size is a greater determiner of perceived distance. (The figures in A and B are shown on reversible panels in that either the left or right panel can be seen in depth.) (Source: Hochberg & Hochberg, 1952, 34, p. 111.)*

only for distances up to about 2 meters; for targets located beyond this accommodation is ineffective in furnishing accurate information for the discrimination of distance (Brown, 1965, p. 46; Graham, 1965, p. 520).

BINOCULAR CUES

Although monocular cues furnish a good deal of spatial information, there are cues that require the joint activity of both eyes. We have already discussed some of the structural and functional aspects of binocular vision in an earlier chapter. We now turn to the kinds of spatial information provided by perception with two eyes.

Convergence

Convergence refers to the tendency of the eyes to turn toward each other in a coordinated action to fixate on targets located nearby. Targets located at some far distance from the viewer, on the other hand, are fixated with the lines of sight of the eyes essentially parallel to each other. Because the degree of convergence is controlled by muscles attached to the eyeballs, it is possible that different states of muscular tension for viewing near and far objects may furnish a cue to depth or distance. However, like accommodation, the role of convergent eye movements as a primary source of depth or distance information has been difficult to assess, and the importance of convergence as a spatial cue is not agreed on (see Ogle, 1962; Hochberg, J. E., 1971; Gregory, 1973).

Binocular Parallax

We noted that in higher vertebrates, particularly primates, the two frontally directed eyes receive

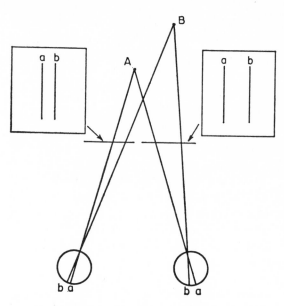

Fig. 16.16*b* *The perception of relative distance of two objects with retinal disparity information. The perception of the relative distance between two lines is due to the slight disparity (difference in separation) of the images projected on each eye, as indicated by the projections in the two boxes. (Source: Ogle, 1962, p. 275.)*

Fig. 16.16*a* *The disparate views of a wedge seen by the two eyes. (Source: Gibson, 1950, p. 20.)*

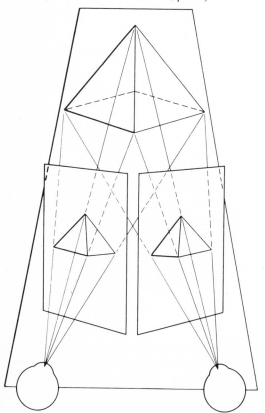

two slightly disparate images of the same three-dimensional scene (see Figure 16.16*a* and *b*). In man this is due to the fact that the eyes are set about 2 to 3 in (5 to 7.6 cm) apart; hence depending on location of the fixation point, the visual field seen by one eye is somewhat different from the visual field seen by the other (see Figure 16.17). This difference in the two retinal images is called *binocular parallax* or *binocular disparity*.

Rather than seeing double images, as a by-product of the disparity of the images projected on each eye, a perceptual process contributing to the experience of depth, called *stereopsis*, occurs. An example of stereopsis is the entertaining depth effect experienced when viewing through a common stereo-viewer. The original stereo-viewer, called a *stereoscope* (see Figure 16.18*a* and *b*), was devised in 1838 by the English physicist,

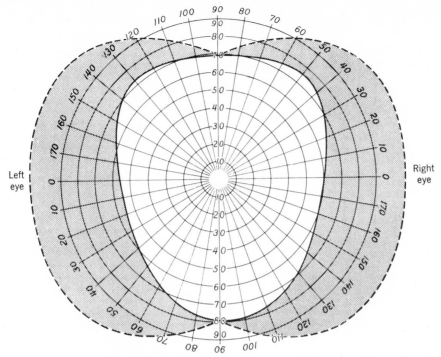

Fig. 16.17 *The visual fields of each eye and the binocular field. (Source: Gibson, 1950, p. 100.)*

Fig. 16.18a *A typical hand-held stereoscope devised to present disparate images to each eye. This type of stereoscope was first designed by Oliver Wendell Holmes in 1861. (From Foundations of Psychology, by E. G. Boring, H. S. Langfeld, & H. P. Weld, Wiley, New York, 1948, p. 303. Reprinted by permission of the publisher.)*

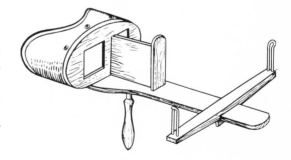

Fig. 16.18b *Stereograms: When appropriately viewed through a stereoscope, each pair of figures is perceived as unitary and in three dimensions. (From Human Perception, by R. H. Day, Wiley, New York, 1969, p. 74. Reprinted by permission of the publisher.)*

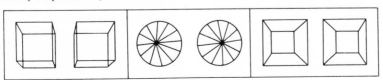

285

Charles Wheatstone, who reasoned that it should be possible to produce a synthetic impression of depth by casting on each eye similar but slightly disparate pictures called *stereograms* (Figure 16.18*b*), representing those views of a single object when observed by the separate eyes (Boring, 1942). When the pictures of the single object are properly paired and shown in a stereoscope, the object appears in depth or as three-dimensional. In short, the stereoscope permits two discrepant but lawfully related images to be projected independently on the two retinae; the typical result is stereopsis, a vivid and compelling experience of a single three-dimensional scene. Within limits the greater the disparity of the two pictures shown in the stereoscope, the greater the impression of solidarity or depth.

Consider the following analysis of the stereoscopic viewing of a wedge (see Figure 16.19).

Fig. 16.19 *Overhead schematic of stereoscopic viewing of a wedge. (From Krech and Crutchfield, 1958, p. 137. Reprinted by permission of the authors.)*

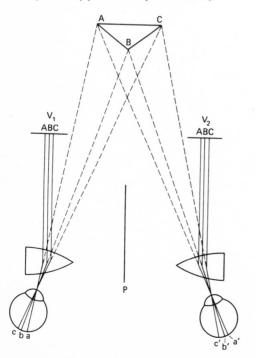

Slightly different pictures of the wedge are presented to the two eyes separately, at V_1 and V_2. The light rays from these pictures are deflected by the prisms so as to appear reflected from the wedge, ABC. The distances between A, B and C differ slightly in V_1 and V_2, as would the retinal images if the observer were actually looking at a wedge. A partition at P, serves to restrict each picture to its own eye. The retinal projections of the surfaces of the wedge, AB and BC, are at ab, a'b' and bc, b'c', respectively. Notice the difference in the retinal projections on each retina owing to the fact that each eye gets a slightly different view. The combination and fusion of these disparate views in the brain produces stereopsis.

Observe also from the figure that the projections of the surface AB are to the nasal part of the retina of the left eye, ab, and to the temporal part, a'b', of the retina of the right eye; similar projections but retinally reversed occur for the surface BC. Thus the left and right visual field are represented on the right and left half of each retina, respectively.

These facts, coupled with the partial decussation of the optic fibers, described earlier (Chapter 11), indicate that the right half of the visual field is represented on the left side of the brain and the left half of the visual field is represented on the right side of the brain. The optical projections to the brain thus reflect a *visual field* rather than a retinal surface.

The common stereo-viewer essentially performs the same function as the stereoscope, in that the viewer is presented with two different pictures of the same scene taken with a stereo camera—a camera that has a double lens, each lens separated by about the same distance as the separation of the two eyes. Thus, two pictures are taken simultaneously. When these are processed, mounted, and each presented by means of a stereo-viewer to the appropriate eye, the images fuse and the striking experience of stereopsis—depth with solidarity of objects—occurs.

In some cases of binocular viewing rivalry between images may occur. This is produced when each eye is presented with quite different stimuli. When binocular rivalry occurs, at one moment the stimuli from one eye may be dominant with a corresponding suppression of the stimuli from the other eye (e.g., see Engel, 1958). Dominance may fluctuate from eye to eye. Though most of the research on stereopsis has been done with the adult human, it has also been demonstrated in the human infant (Bower, 1966b), the monkey (Bough, 1970), and the cat (Fox & Blake, 1970).

A particularly interesting form of stereo-viewing has been devised by Bela Julesz (1964, 1965, 1971). He has termed it *cyclopean* perception because the image on each eye is combined and synthesized in a central visual area of the brain to produce the impression of depth. Julesz used a computer to print out two nearly identical displays of random dot patterns. An example of a pair of patterns is given in Figure 16.20a. The two patterns possess identical random dot textures except for certain areas that are also identical but shifted or displaced relative to each other in the horizontal direction: it is impossible

to see any depth by looking at either half of the pair of patterns. However, when the two patterns are stereoscopically fused, a central square corresponding to the horizontally shifted areas is vividly seen floating above the surround. As indicated in Figure 16.20b, the regions that are shifted differ for the left and right squares of the stereogram. In the left square the shift is to the right, and in the right square the shift is to the left of the horizontal displacement. As a result, there is binocular disparity between elements of texture for this region, and it is perceived as being closer to the viewer than the remainder of the pattern. If the disparity relationship between the left and right squares were reversed, the shifted region would appear as lying farther away from the observer than the random surround. According to Julesz (1964), the pattern matching involved in the depth effect is based on a relatively simple process of finding connected clusters formed by adjacent points of similar brightness.

Another means of experiencing cyclopean perception is to view an *anaglyph* of this sterogram. An anaglyph of Figure 16.20a is

Fig. 16.20a   *Random-dot stereogram. When the images are monocularly inspected, they appear uniformly random with no depth characteristics, but when stereoscopically fused a center square is seen floating above the background in vivid depth. Similarly, when an anaglyph of this stereogram is viewed with appropriately tinted glasses, a center square is seen above the surround. (Source: Julesz, B., Foundations of Cyclopean Perception, 1971, Chicago: University of Chicago Press, p. 21. Reprinted by permission of the publisher.)*

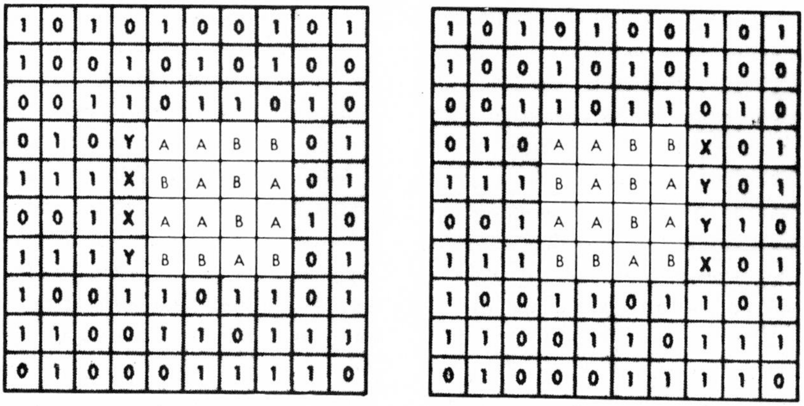

Fig. 16.20b *A schematic diagram indicating the process by which the random-dot stereogram of 16.20a was generated. The left and right images are identical random dot textures except for certain areas that are shifted relative to each other in the horizontal direction as though they were solid sheets. The shifted areas, indicated by A and B cells, cover certain areas of the background, indicated by 1 and 0 cells; owing to the shift, areas become uncovered (X and Y cells) which are filled in by additional random elements. (Source: Julesz, B., Foundations of Cyclopean Perception, 1971, Chicago: University of Chicago Press, p. 21. Reprinted by permission of the publisher.)*

produced by printing the two patterns on top of each other in different inks (usually red and green) to produce a composite picture. When the anaglyph is normally viewed, it yields the impression of a random texture without any clear global shape or contours. However, when viewed through specially tinted filters that allow each eye to sort out a single pattern, the stereo depth effect is perceived.

Some of the findings of cyclopean research with random dot pattern displays are that stereopsis occurs in the absence of depth cues, convergent eye movements, and recognizable or familiar shapes. Indeed, the correspondence and synthesis of objects and patterns in the two retinal projections can be established without actual monocular recognition of contours, patterns, and objects. Hence, contour perception is not a prerequisite for stereopsis.

It should be noted that cyclopean stimulation occurs within a unique set of laboratory conditions in which the monocular and binocular information are separated. Most spatial events are viewed without such restriction. Typically space

perception is accomplished within a complex physical framework furnishing the information for a number of cues, and effective space perception depends on their integration.

THE VISUAL CLIFF

An important experimental analysis of the cues used for the depth perception of a number of animal species has been made by Walk and Gibson (1961). The apparatus used in these experiments is called the *visual cliff*; it is shown in Figure 16.21. A centrally located start platform divides the floor of the apparatus into two sides, each side furnishing different kinds of stimulation. The "shallow" side lies directly over a patterned surface; on the "deep" side the same patterned surface is placed some distance below. Actually, a sheet of glass extends over both the deep and shallow sides for safety and to equate sources of thermal, olfactory, and echo-locating stimulation for both sides. Thus with lighting equalized for

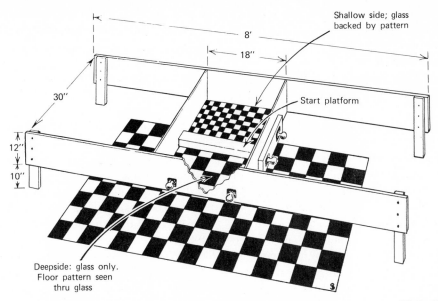

Fig. 16.21 *A schematic diagram of a model of the visual cliff used for small animals. (Source: Walk, 1965, p. 103. Reprinted by permission of the author and the publisher.)*

Fig. 16.22 *The pattern of checks as seen from the start platform of the visual cliff in cross section. On the left side is a patterned surface located near the platform (shallow side). On the right is the same patterned surface placed much farther below (deep side). With an identically textured surface below on the right, the light rays reaching the eyes of an animal located on the start platform will differ in density, a finer density characterizing the surface farthest from the eye. (Source: Walk & Gibson, 1961. Reprinted by permission of the publisher.)*

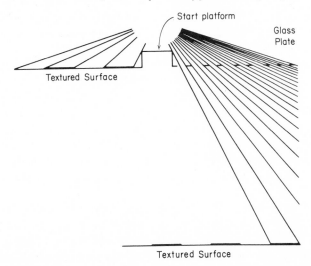

both sides, only intentional visual information is allowed. In the usual situation, an animal is placed on the start platform separating the shallow and deep surfaces (see Figure 16.22). From this position the animal can see the shallow or "safe" side and the deep or "dangerous" side, an edge with a drop-off beyond it that is similar to what it would see if looking over the side of a cliff. A basic assumption of the visual cliff technique is, of course, that a tendency exists for animals to avoid a fall. As an adaptive mechanism preserving the species, it is reasonable to expect that most animals should be capable of depth perception; furthermore, this ability should be effective by the time the organism can locomote independently. The existence of this capacity is demonstrated by a preference for the shallow side. Indeed, based on research with turtles, birds, many species of small and some large mammals, primates, and human infants, there is a strong tendency to avoid the deep side.

A relevant question is: What are the cues used by the animals in making their depth discriminations? One of the main cues examined was a textural one. In one set of experiments, employing a vast range of different animals, a marked preference to descend to the shallow side was shown when the same size stimuli (patterns of checks, as shown in Figure 16.21) were used on the shallow and the deep sides. The deep side thus reflected a more densely textured surface because it was farther away from the animals' eyes than was the shallow pattern. Actually, in this kind of situation there is more information to depth than simply the size of the elements comprising the textured pattern. Binocular cues and the motion parallax that is provided by head movement can contribute additional information about depth. In another study the role of texture size was eliminated by using two different sized patterns of checks. The deep side pattern was composed of larger checks than that used on the shallow side—larger to the extent that they projected the same size retinal image to the organism as did the textural elements of the

shallow pattern. This effectively eliminated the textural size cue. (It should be noted, however, that in certain situations, textural size cues play a significant role in depth avoidance. See Davidson & Whitson, 1973; Walk & Walters, 1974.) In one instance the deep pattern was three times as far from the animal's eyes as the shallow pattern; hence, the checks of the deep pattern were three times as large as those of the shallow pattern. The finding was that descents were significantly to the shallow side. This general result has been shown with species as diverse as goats (Walk & Gibson, 1961) and turtles (Routtenberg & Glickman, 1964).

When monocular animals were tested with this kind of arrangement, textural cues were neutralized, binocular cues eliminated, and only motion parallax served as a cue to depth. The evidence from studies utilizing these conditions indicates rather clearly that monocular rats (Trychin & Walk, 1964; Lore & Sawatski, 1969) and monocular chicks (Schiffman, H. R. & Walk, 1963) make use of motion parallax to discriminate depth. The efficacy of the motion cue was also observed in a 10½-month-old permanently monocular human infant (Walk & Dodge, 1962). It behaved as did normal binocular infants, avoiding the deep side. Similar behavior has been reported with temporarily monocularized infants (Walk, 1968). Adequate depth or distance perception with monocular viewing has also been demonstrated in the following animals: locusts (Wallace, G. K., 1959), frogs and chameleons (Canella, 1936: cited in Walk, 1965), pigeons (Mowrer, 1936), and ducklings (Walk, 1962). It appears that use of only one eye has little effect on the depth perception of most animals. Moreover, motion parallax is a sufficient cue for the mediation of depth or distance perception.

Briefly reviewing our discussion of depth perception, we have noted that systematically eliminating many cues but allowing visual information from the organism's movements is sufficient to mediate depth perception for many species of animals, despite very different optical anatomies. This has been shown with relatively disparate levels of phylogeny (e.g., the locust to human). This serves as an adaptive mechanism: From the standpoint of survival it is of a special significance that most animals be capable of visually detecting a dangerous place such as an edge or cliff—in short, that they be provided with the optical means for detecting a potential loss of support. In this context we might ask, why do animals of any species ever descend to the deep side of a visual cliff? The answer for such behavior in the case of some mammals can be given. It appears that tactual or haptic stimulation, presumably from the vibrissae or whiskers, contributes to this behavior. Research on this matter utilized a modified visual cliff with no starting platform or any other dividing structure in the shallow-deep plane (Schiffman, H. R., 1968, 1970). The shallow side offered both optical and physical stimulation of support, whereas the deep side was only a sheet of invisible glass located above a surface. The latter side thus appeared as an optical void. Animals that were placed directly on the deep or shallow side performed differently depending on the species tested. However, only behavior from deep side placements need concern us here. Day-active chicks when placed on the optical void of the deep side jumped over to the shallow side (Schiffman, H. R., 1968). On the other hand, nocturnal rats and other small mammals, although capable of perceiving depth, did not show this response. That is, when placed directly on the deep side—a surface that offered haptic but not optical stimulation—rats acted indifferently, moving to the shallow side on a chance basis. In short, the day-active chick avoids an optical void even though stimulation of physical support is provided; the rat, however, is generally indifferent to a lack of optical support when physical support, signaled by haptic stimulation, is provided. Thus, some mammalian species may manifest the seemingly maladaptive response of descending to the deep side because the haptic stimulation indicates that there is a source of physical support (provided by

the glass sheet). Indeed, we may consider the locomotor activity of rats and other nocturnal mammals (e.g., kittens, guinea pigs, mice, gerbils, and albino rabbits; see Schiffman, H. R., 1970) to be haptically or tactually dominated, whereas this activity for chicks and perhaps other day-active animals appears to be optically dominated.

CONSTANCY

The pattern of light reaching the visual system from an object undergoes continual changes as the spatial orientation of the object relative to the viewer changes. This can occur both by spatial displacements of the object and by movements of the observer. Accompanying the spatial changes are changes in the distribution of light striking the viewer's retinae; these are seen as variations in the projected size, shape, and intensity. However, in spite of these changes in stimulation, the stable and enduring qualities of the object are perceived.

The book before you does not look rectangular when viewed from one angle and trapezoidal when viewed from another angle of observation: Normally the book is perceived as rectangular from every angle of observation. Neither does a person's size appear to contract or expand very much as he moves away or advances. Yet the laws of spatial geometry dictate certain changes in the retinal image corresponding to the relative displacement of the physical stimulus. Clearly, perception in this instance is based on more than the size and shape of the retinal image. This stability of perception in the presence of variation in physical stimulation is termed *perceptual constancy.*

The fact that perception is linked to the invariant properties of objects—e.g., the actual size and shape—rather than the enormously changing light patterns reaching the visual system has clear adaptive significance: We perceive a world composed of reasonably stable objects with relatively permanent physical properties. Clearly, without the mechanism of constancy, the moment-to-moment variations in stimulation would appear as such—a series of chaotic sense experiences.

BRIGHTNESS CONSTANCY

Brightness constancy refers to the fact that the brightness and color of an object tend to remain relatively constant or stable in spite of changes in the amount of illumination striking it; that is, the perception of an object is relatively independent of its illumination. Thus, we perceive a patch of snow in dark shadow as white or a chunk of coal in sunlight as black. Yet the physical intensity of the light reflected from the surface of the coal may be greater than that from the snow! In some manner we are taking into account information about the general conditions of illumination. In searching for an explanation of this phenomenon, it is necessary to consider the surface property called *albedo* or *reflectance*. The albedo is the proportion of incident light that is reflected (reflected/incident) from an object or surface. Hence, it is independent of the degree of illumination. A sheet of white typing paper may have an albedo of, say 0.80; this means it reflects approximately 80% of the light it receives. If, under ordinary conditions, a part of the paper is placed under dim illumination so that the sheet is not homogeneously illuminated, one still perceives the entire sheet as more or less uniformly bright. The stability of the sheet's brightness occurs because the entire surface of the sheet reflects a constant portion of the light received, even though the amount of incident light may differ for different parts of the sheet's surface.

Relational Properties of Brightness Constancy

In order to utilize albedo, there must be indications of the general conditions of lighting. Accord-ingly, constancy is poor in conditions where the sources of the incident lighting and the background illumination are obscured or lacking, that is, in situations precluding compensation for variations in incident light. If illumination is restricted to the object alone (e.g., by special means of projection so that no light falls on the background) then the perceived brightness of the object will depend entirely on its illumination, and constancy is absent.

We noted in an earlier discussion on brightness contrast, that the brightness of an object, like that of the disc shown in Figure 16.23a, is affected by the intensity of its surrounding annulus or ring. Specifically, the apparent brightness of the disc is a function of the ratio of its light intensity to the intensity of its surrounding ring (see Wallach, 1948, 1963; Heinemann, 1955; Jameson & Hurvich, 1961). However, as demonstrated in Figure 16.23, if both the intensities of the ring and disc are changed by the same proportion, perceived brightness is unaffected. When an observer is required to adjust the intensity of the test disc (at *b*) to match the brightness of the standard disc, rather than setting it at a level for a physically equal match, 180 mL, the adjustment is to 90 mL. That is, the intensity *ratio* of ring to disc of *a* (2:1) is maintained in *b* in order to produce an equal-brightness match. It is as if the overall level of illumination of *a* is halved in *b*. This sort of a fixed proportional change is what occurs in natural settings when the overall illumination changes (Figure 16.24). Normally objects do not appear in complete isolation in the visual field. Thus, since the light that is illuminating an object also falls on regions surrounding it, the ratios of the intensities of light of adjacent objects is invariant in spite of the changes in the absolute intensity of the overall illumination. As a consequence, the brightness of an object seen against a background does not appear to change.

In summary, the important variable for brightness constancy when viewing under ordinary conditions is the ratio of the intensity of light reflected from objects relative to the intensity

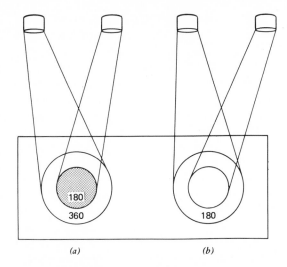

Fig. 16.23 *Sample arrangement for demonstrating brightness constancy as a function of the relative illumination of an area to its background. Each disc and its surrounding ring of light in (a) and (b) is projected on a screen in an otherwise darkened room by a pair of projectors. The intensities of the discs and rings are separately controlled. In (a), the ratio of ring intensity to disc intensity is set at 2:1 (360 mL:180 mL). In order for the disc at (b), with the intensity level of its ring set at 180 mL, to appear as bright as the disc in (a), a setting of 90 mL is required. This shows that the perceived brightness of a disc is affected by the ratio of its intensity to the intensity of its background. Hence, decreasing the incident light of both the disc and ring by the same proportion does not affect its apparent brightness. Thus, within limits, so long as the ratios of the intensities between the discs and their backgrounds remains constant, the two discs appear equally bright in spite of the changes in overall illumination. (Source: Wallach, 1963.)*

of light reflected from the background (with the proviso that the light that is illuminating an object also falls on regions surrounding it). In other words, what is extracted is information about *relative* rather than absolute intensities. When the illumination on a scene is uniformly increased or decreased, the absolute intensities of the images of adjacent objects in the scene may change by different amounts (due to different albedos for dif-

ferent objects), but the ratios of the intensities of their images remain constant. That is, the *proportion* of incident light that is reflected by the stimuli in the scene remains constant. The result is that, within limits, the brightnesses of the objects do not change when there are changes in the overall level of illumination.

An interesting point about the informativeness to the organism of brightness constancy (and which may relate to constancy, in general) has been made by Cornsweet (1970):

> It is relevant to point out that brightness constancy is a manifestation of a **loss** of information by the visual system. No information about the world is gained by constancy, it is merely that absolute intensity information is largely lost. Loss of information, per se, cannot have survival value, but a mechanism that loses any particular class of information may have

Fig. 16.24 *The objects of the scene in B are uniformly illuminated by one-hundredth of the amount of incident light in A. However, since the objects reflect a constant proportion of the incident light (indicated by the albedos or reflectances), the intensity ratios of the chunk of coal to the sheet of paper in the scenes at A and in B are constant (1:9). Accordingly, the objects appear equally bright in both scenes. (Figure source: modified from Hochberg, 1964, p. 50.)*

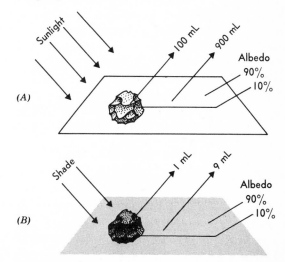

survival value if it is properly related to other aspects of the organism.

> *. . . If the neural circuits in the brain are only capable of processing a limited amount of information, then it may be adaptive to reject, at the periphery, that information which is less important for survival, thereby making the entire central capacity available for the more important information; and it seems quite reasonable that information about relative intensities is more important for human survival than information about absolute intensities.*

> *. . . It is convenient that, with constancy, our perceptions are correlated with a property of objects themselves (i.e., their reflectances) rather than with the incident illumination. (Pp. 379–380)*

The ontogenetic studies (e.g., see Burzlaff, 1931: cited in Woodworth and Schlosberg, 1954) and studies on relatively disparate phyla suggest that brightness constancy is a primitively organized perceptual ability. It has been shown with monkeys (Locke, 1935: cited in Woodworth & Schlosberg, 1954), chickens (Gogel & Hess, 1951), and fish. In the latter instance fish were trained to find food in troughs of a certain color out of a group of different colored troughs (Burkamp, 1923: cited in Woodworth & Schlosberg, 1954). When the illumination was changed, excellent constancy was demonstrated. Increasing the intensity of light did not make the fish go to darker shades nor did decreasing it send them to lighter shades. This finding makes sense on an adaptive basis, for a correction for illumination is even more important for fish than for terrestrial animals, because fish are subjected to large changes in illumination with every movement from one depth to another.

SIZE CONSTANCY

The diagram in Figure 16.25 illustrates some relevant geometrical relations in image formation, such as that the size of the retinal image varies inversely with the distance from which an object is viewed. The size of an object's image on the retina may undergo considerable changes with variation in the object's distance from the viewer, but the size changes go relatively unnoticed in conditions of normal viewing. A man standing 7 meters away looks about as tall as when he stands at 14 meters away although the first image projected on the retina is twice the size of the second. An important fact about the perceived size of an object in normal viewing conditions is that it does not depend solely on the size of the image it casts on the retina. In short, perceived size does not regularly follow retinal size. Indeed, over a considerable range of distances, perceived size is somewhat independent of retinal size. The failure of perceived size to vary with retinal size is owing to the operation of size constancy.

Many variables affect size constancy. Among some of the more important is the familiarity of objects. However, as discussed below, size constancy also occurs with unfamiliar objects. Perhaps of greater significance are apparent distance cues and background stimuli. As shown in Figure 16.26, when properly used they help to effect size constancy in a picture.

Holway and Boring Experiment

A now classic experiment on size constancy by Holway and Boring (1941) provides an examination of several of its influences. In the experiment the observer was stationed at the intersection of two long darkened corridors, as illustrated in Figure 16.27a. An adjustable, lighted comparison disc was placed 10 feet (about 3 meters) from the observer in one corridor; standard discs were placed one at a time at a number of distances varying from 10 to 120 feet (about 3 to 36 meters) in the other corridor. The sizes of the standard discs were graduated so as to cast the same size retinal image at every distance from the viewer's eye. The viewer's task was to adjust the comparison disc so it would look the same size as the

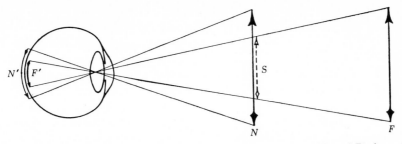

Fig. 16.25 *A schematic diagram showing the relative size of two retinal images, N′ and F′, from the same size objects, N and F, but located at different distances. Object F is twice as far from the eye as object N; hence, its image on the retina is half as large. This is in accordance with the fact that the size of the retinal image is inversely proportional to the distance of the object from the eye. Notice that the smaller retinal image cast by object F could also be produced by the smaller object, S, (smaller by one-half) located at the position of object N. (Source: Boring, Langfeld, & Weld, 1948, p. 232.)*

Fig. 16.26 *Size constancy in a picture. In (a), the near girl was 9 ft from the camera and the far girl 27 ft. The relative distances, and thus the relative retinal heights, are in the ratio 1 : 3. Size constancy is not complete; the distant girl appears somewhat smaller, but clearly not in the ratio 1 : 3, which is correct for the two girls in the photograph. Compare this with (b). The far girl of (a) was cut out of the picture, brought forward next to the other girl, and pasted there with apparent distance from the viewer equal for the two. The size ratio 1 : 3 is now apparent. The right-hand girl looks smaller in (b) than she did in (a), although physically unchanged in size on paper. This is an example of size constancy in a picture with perspective and elevation cues for distance. (Notice that the size constancy of (a) is diminished when the picture is inverted.) (Source: Boring, 1964, 77, p. 497.)*

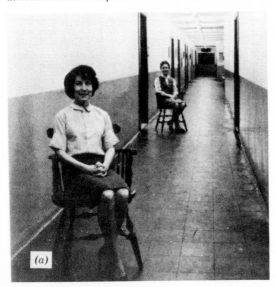

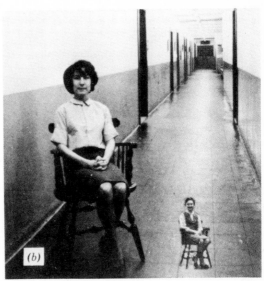

standard disc. There were four experimental conditions: Condition 1 provided binocular observation; condition 2 allowed monocular viewing; condition 3 allowed monocular viewing through a small hole, called an *artificial pupil*, which removed some of the sources of information normally used in distance perception, such as head movements; in condition 4 an even further reduction of distance cues was made by surrounding the standard discs with black cloth creating a reduction tunnel, thereby severely limiting the distance cues originally provided by the floor, walls, and ceiling. The amount of constancy exhibited in each condition is shown in Figure 16. 27*b*. Notice that the top dotted line shows what the judgments would ideally be for perfect constancy: The adjusted size of the comparison disc would be exactly the same size as the standard discs that increased with distance. The bottom dotted line indicates the complete lack of constancy: The adjusted size of the comparison disc would be set to the size of the standard disc at 10 feet (about 3 meters), regardless of the distance at which the standard disc was viewed—in short, a retinal match.

With binocular and monocular viewing (conditions 1 and 2) the achievement of size constancy was excellent. The data suggest that it makes little difference whether one eye or both eyes are used in the task. Both sets of adjustments conform closely to what would be predicted if size constancy were perfect. Artificial restrictions on observation, as in condition 3 in which viewing was through a tiny hole, caused a considerable drop in constancy. Condition 4 presented an even greater loss of distance cues, and the results indicate a greater decrement in constancy. Judgments in the latter two conditions, intentionally less influenced by distance cues, are principally determined by the size of the image projected on the retina. Hence, when the observer could see nothing but the discs surrounded by darkness, their sizes were judged to be about the same at all distances. Constancy had totally disappeared with a complete lack of distance cues.

Later studies using all the above restrictions of visual cues plus screens that cut out all of the visual field except the disks themselves (Lichten and Lurie, 1950; Hastorf and Way, 1952) gave essentially the same results.

Clearly then, distance cues and a visual framework are very important for the operation of size constancy.

Emmert's Law

The retinal size of an object and cues to its distance operate together as a system to determine the perceived size and/or the location of an object. Under certain conditions the apparent size of an object when viewed as an *afterimage* is determined by the distance between the eye and the

Fig. 16.27a *Schematic diagram of experimental arrangement used by Holway & Boring for testing size constancy. The comparison stimulus was located 10 ft from the observer. The standard stimuli, located at various positions from 10 to 120 ft, always subtended a visual angle of 1° (After Holway and Boring, 1941, 54, p. 24.)*

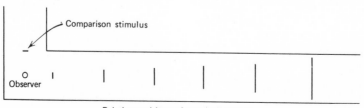

Relative positions of standard stimuli

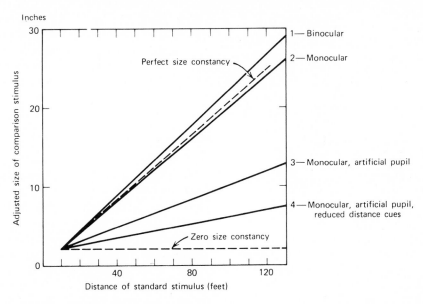

Fig. 16.27b *Results of size constancy experiment. The degree of constancy varied with the amount of visual information. (After Holway and Boring, 1941, 54, p. 34.)*

surface on which the image appears to be projected (see Figure 16.28). This relationship is known as *Emmert's Law* (see Boring, 1942). Specifically, an afterimage will appear larger, the farther away the projection surface appears. In short, the perceived size of the afterimage is directly proportional to the distance of the projection surface from the eye. This is owing to the fact that the area on the retina responsible for the afterimage is of a constant size. As the distance of the projection surface is increased, the size of the object necessary to reflect that constant size must also be increased: Hence, the size of the surface that the afterimage covers is a function of its distance. It is important to note that the apparent size of the afterimage is determined by the *apparent* as well as the actual distance of the projection surface. It has been shown that the utilization of distance cues can affect the size of the afterimage (see e.g., King & Gruber, 1962; Irwin, 1969). For example, if the afterimage is

Fig. 16.28 *Illustration of Emmert's Law. A stimulus object (for example, a black square on a white background) is fixated and briefly inspected at P_2 to form an afterimage. Immediately afterward, the eyes fall upon a surface located nearer (P_1) or farther (P_3). The afterimage will appear to be projected on that surface, and its size will be directly proportional to the distance of the surface from the eye.*

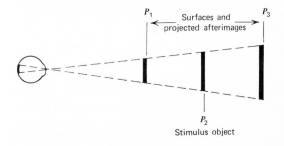

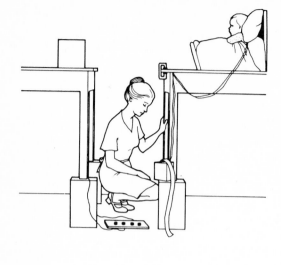

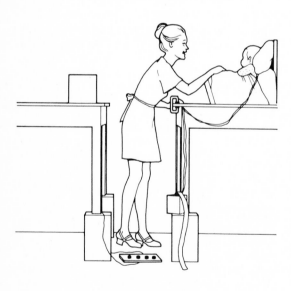

Fig. 16.29 *Experimental arrangement for demonstrating size constancy with infants. The experimental procedure begins with conditioning the infant to respond to the conditioned stimulus. The conditioned response, head turning, closes a microswitch. As shown in the bottom figure, the reward for the conditioned response is a "peekaboo." (From Development in Infancy, by T. G. R. Bower, p. 88. Copyright © 1974 by Scientific American, Inc. All rights reserved.)*

projected on a surface that is made to appear closer (or farther), then the size of the afterimage will appear smaller (or larger). The change in the size of the afterimage likely results from the same mechanisms that produce size constancy.

Size Constancy with Infants

More recent research had indicated that size constancy is possible with human infants between six and eight weeks of age (Bower, 1965, 1966a, 1974). The method of testing for constancy utilized operant conditioning techniques. Very briefly, the experimenter selects some response from the organism's repertoire and delivers some "reinforcement" or rewarding agent contingent on the occurrence of that response. If the reward only follows the occurrence of a particular stimulus, called the *conditioned stimulus* (*CS*), the *response* soon occurs only in the presence of the *CS*. It is then possible to change the stimulus slightly and observe the degree of discrimination of which the organism is capable. In the present experiments the reward was a "peekaboo" from the experimenter. That is, when appropriate, the experimenter briefly popped her head out in front of the infant, smiled and nodded, saying "peekaboo," and then quickly disappeared from the infant's view (see Figure 16.29). The response that was chosen from the infant's repertoire was a turn of the head. As little a turn as half an inch (13 mm) to either side activated a switch and was recorded. In one experiment, the infant was placed in an infant's seat on a table, the "peekabooing" experimenter crouched in front of him, and the *CS*, a white cube 30 cm-per-side, was placed behind the experimenter one meter from the infant's eyes. After the infant had been trained to respond only in the presence of the 30 cm cube at one meter, testing for constancy began and three new stimuli were introduced. They were: (1) a 30 cm cube placed three meters away, (2) a 90 cm cube placed one meter away, and (3) another 90 cm cube located three meters away. The number of responses (head turns) elicited by the *CS* and the three test stimuli were recorded. (During the testing period no peekaboo rewards were given.)

Stimulus 1 was the same size as the *CS* but located three times as far away. If the infant possessed size constancy, this stimulus should have appeared to the infant most like the *CS* and should therefore have elicited the greatest number of responses of the three test stimuli. If only a retinal match were made by the infant, signifying a lack of constancy, then stimulus 3 should have elicited the most responses of the three test stimuli. This follows because although stimulus 3 was three times as large as the *CS*, it was located three times as far away so that it projected a retinal image of the same size as the *CS*. Stimulus 2, three times the size as the *CS*, was also located at the same distance as the *CS*. If the infant was able to perceive distance but did not possess size constancy, then stimulus 2 should have the advantage, in terms of number of responses, over stimulus 1 since it was placed at the same

distance as the *CS*. The various relations between the *CS* and the test stimuli and the results are shown in Figure 16.30. The results indicate that next to the *CS*, the stimulus eliciting the most number of responses was stimulus 1 followed by stimulus 2. In short, the infant responded more on the basis of the stimuli's physical size and distance, than on their retinal size or apparent distance. Further research that controlled for various monocular and binocular cues indicated that motion parallax (Bower, 1965, 1966a) and binocular disparity (Bower, Broughton, and Moore, 1970) provided the necessary information for size constancy.

It should be pointed out that size constancy in the infant is neither perfect nor complete. Rather, it continues to develop with age. Zeigler and Leibowitz (1957), employing a techique similar to Holway and Boring, described earlier, reported that children seven to nine years old demonstrate size constancy to a lesser degree than do adults.

As we have noted with brightness constancy,

Fig. 16.30 *Stimuli and their distances used in size constancy experiment with infants. The conditioned stimulus was a cube, 30 cm on a side, and located one meter away. Test stimuli were cubes 30 or 90 cm on a side, and located one or three meters away. (Modified from Bower, T. G. R., Development in Infancy, p. 89. Copyright © 1974 by Scientific American. All rights reserved.)*

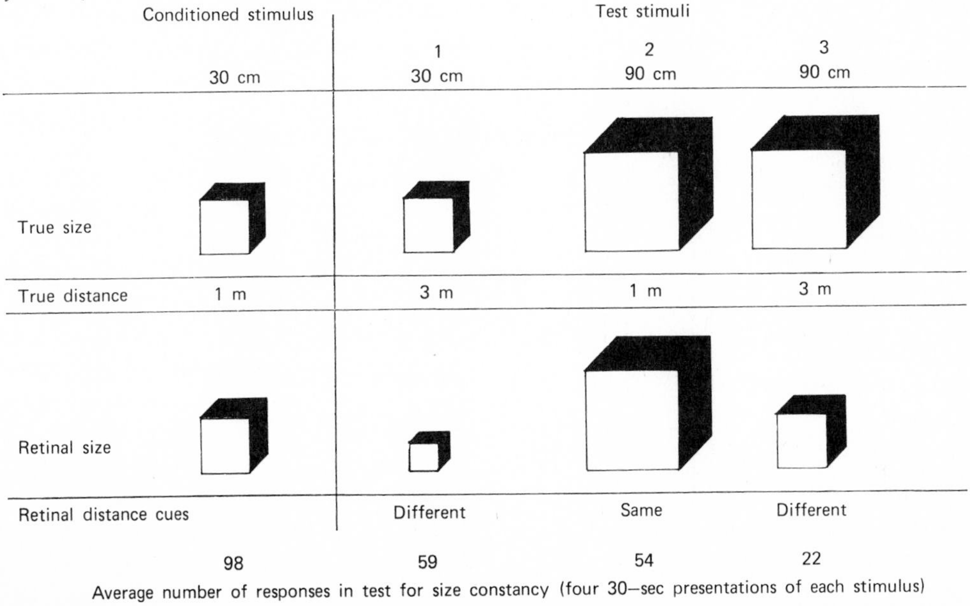

	Conditioned stimulus	Test stimuli		
		1	2	3
	30 cm	30 cm	90 cm	90 cm
True size				
True distance	1 m	3 m	1 m	3 m
Retinal size				
Retinal distance cues		Different	Same	Different
	98	59	54	22

Average number of responses in test for size constancy (four 30—sec presentations of each stimulus) there is evidence that size constancy occurs early in human perceptual development and exists in organisms far below man in phylogenetic development (see Shinkman, 1962; Walk, 1965).

SHAPE CONSTANCY

We have seen above that an object viewed under different conditions of illumination may appear equally bright and an object viewed at different distances with different projected sizes may appear the same size. In addition, an object may appear to possess the same shape even when the angle from which it is viewed changes radically. The latter phenomenon is termed *shape constancy*. A typical window frame or a door appears to be more or less rectangular no matter at what angle it is viewed. Yet geometrically it casts a rectangular image *only* when it is viewed from a certain position directly in front of the viewer (see Figure 16.31).

Experimentally, shape constancy is assessed when a subject estimates the shape of objects such as a circular plate or disc tilted or slanted at an angle. It is found that the estimated shape (illustrated in Figure 16.32), obtained by having subjects draw the shape of a tilted disc or match it against a series of ellipses, is more circular than

the elliptical shape projected on the observer's retinae (Thouless, 1931).

We have noted that the shape of the retinal image changes as the object's spatial orientation relative to the viewer is altered, yet constancy operates to maintain the perceptual integrity of the object's shape. As in the case of size constancy, it is a reasonable assumption that the degree of shape constancy varies with the availability of relevant spatial information as to orientation, such as the tilt or inclination of the object (e.g., Langdon, 1951, 1953; Olson, 1974) or the slant of the surface on which the object rests (Beck & Gibson, 1955). In general, shape constancy varies with indications of the distance and displacement of all spatial aspects of the object. It follows that when visual information as to the object's position relative to the viewer is lacking, shape constancy is impaired or breaks down completely.

Simple shape constancy has been observed in the very young human infant. Using the same operant techniques and general procedures discussed in the section on size constancy, infants between 50 and 60 days of age showed shape constancy. That is, the infants responded more often to the physical shape characteristics of the test stimuli than to the shape of their retinal projections (Bower, 1966a, 1966b). On the other hand, studies on shape constancy in lower animals have

Fig. 16.31 *Shape constancy. Various projected images from an opening door are quite different, yet a rectangular door is perceived. (Source: Gibson, 1950, p. 170.)*

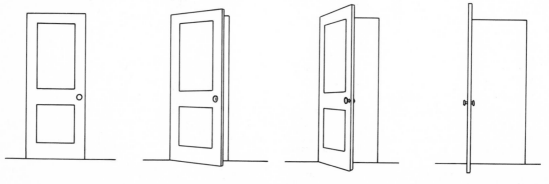

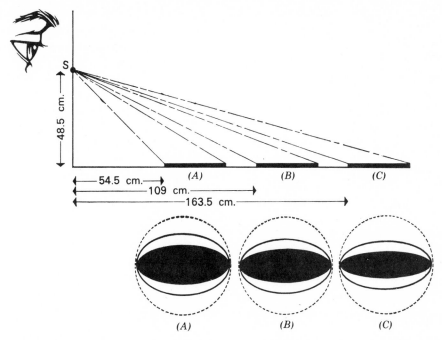

Fig. 16.32 *Shape constancy is shown in the reproduction of the tilted discs, A, B, and C, whose projected shapes are indicated by the black figures. The broken line shows the physical shape, and the continuous line gives the reproduced shape. The reproduced shape indicates that the perceived shape is more circular than the projected shape. (Source: Thouless, 1931, 21, Pp. 340, 343.)*

generally been negative, indicating that it may not be as primitive an ability as brightness or size constancy (e.g., Bingham, 1922; Fields, 1932; also see Forgus, 1966, p. 101). Since it is not clear whether failure to demonstrate shape constancy in infraprimate species is owing to experimental procedures or a lack of capacity, a definitive comment on this matter cannot be given. Clearly, for the visually dominated species— diurnal animals with manipulative dexterity— shape constancy is an important perceptual mechanism, vital to survival.

In closing we must emphasize that constancy effects result from the interplay of numerous factors. An obvious one, which likely plays some role in all the constancies, is the familiarity of the objects in the visual field. That is, past experience may serve to influence the perception of the visual

input in spite of apparent distortions of objects and surrounding stimuli. However, as we have noted, constancy extends to unfamiliar stimuli as well. Perhaps most important for the maintenance of object constancy is the perception of *invariant relations* among the elements of the visual environment.

In this chapter we have identified and described the stimulus indicators and mechanisms that contribute to the perception of three dimensional space. The relevant stimulus features were described under the two main headings of binocular and monocular cues, depending on whether or not the joint function of both eyes is necessary. The monocular cues include such stimulus features and visual processes as interposition, aerial perspective, shading, elevation, linear perspective, texture gradient, motion parallax, familiarity, relative size and accommodation. The binocular cues are convergence and binocular disparity.

Research on depth perception using the visual cliff apparatus was summarized, and it was concluded that a large variety of terrestrial animals possess the visual capability to demonstrate depth avoidance. It was further concluded that information from the cue of motion parallax furnishes a sufficient indication of depth.

Finally, it was noted that objects in the environment are perceived as constant or invariant whereas the conditions of stimulation, such as the physical characteristics imaged on the retina (e.g.,

retinal size and shape) are quite variable. This tendency to perceive the enduring characteristics of objects is called perceptual constancy. The circumstances of occurrence of constancy were discussed and three categories relating to the perceived stability of the brightness, size, and shape of objects were identified. In all cases constancy appears to depend on the context of stimulus features and cues; that is, constancy is relationally determined.

The role that the constancies and cues to depth and distance play in spatial illusions provides some of the material discussed in the following chapter.

17

The Perception of Space
II: Illusions

In the previous chapter we indicated that the relative absence of a spatial context disturbs or reduces object constancy. Similarly, we note here that when cues to space are lacking, are distorted, or are placed in apparent conflict with each other, not only may constancy be reduced but characteristic and quite quantifiable distortions in the perception of the physical environment—illusions—may result.

We have seen in a number of discussions that the stimulation received by the senses bears neither a simple nor an exact relation to the physical environment. Many transformations of the stimulation occur prior to perception. Moreover, numerous visual events contain a potential for perceptual ambiguity, and under certain circumstances they may furnish a distorted representation of the physical environment. It would be an oversimplification, however, to dismiss these phenomena as curiosities, errors of perception, or rare exceptions to perceptual constancy. Not only do they pose many interesting and empirically fruitful problems, but also the study of illusions may furnish clues to the more comprehensive and general mechanisms and principles of perception.

This chapter is devoted to a discussion of illusions, to explaining them, and to showing how understanding them may help to explain some of the general processes of "normal" visual perception.

TRANSACTIONALISM AND THE AMES ILLUSIONS

A provocative theory and a related set of illusions, with particular relevance to constancy and the cues to depth and distance, have been devised by Adelbert Ames (1946). They were an outgrowth of his examination of *aniseikonia,* an optical anomaly in which the image in one eye is larger than the other, resulting in a significant disparity between the images on each eye. This can be simulated with special lenses (see Figure 17.1). However, although optically there is a difference in the size of the two ocular images—with confusing depth cues—persons who are afflicted with aniseikonia perceive the environment in a relatively normal fashion. Objects and surfaces such as floors, walls, and so on appear to be rectilinear although the images on the retina are sufficiently disparate to produce severe distortions. The seeming contradiction between the perception and the optical stimulation led Ames and his colleagues (see Kilpatrick, 1961) to the theoretical notion that experience with specific objects and

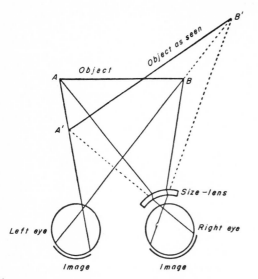

Fig. 17.1 *Simulation of aniseikonia. Special size lenses that produce images in one eye larger than in the other create incorrect and confusing depth cues. [Source: Woodworth & Schlosberg, Experimental Psychology. (rev. ed.), 1954, Holt, Rinehart & Winston, p. 488.]*

surfaces plays a very important role in normal perception. The proponents of this empirical theory, called *Transactionalists,* contend that the perceptual world is, in large measure, constructed from experiences in dealing with the visual environment (Kilpatrick, 1961). Transactional theory is based on the observation that any stimulus pattern that impinges on a single retina could have been produced from an infinite number of objects (see Figure 17.2). Despite the possible perception that might arise from a given retinal pattern, the actual perception is usually quite restricted. Transactionalists attempt to account for this limitation by referring to the learning that takes place during the individual's active interactions with the environment. They argue that owing to a history of interactions or *transactions* with the environment, perceptual alternatives become limited in a way that corresponds closely to the world of real objects. Thus, according to the Transac-

tionalists, we *assume* (and thereby perceive) the world to be stable and organized in a manner that conforms to our past commerce with it.

The Ames illusions are particularly effective in illustrating the role of learning and experience in perception. When observed, generally under quite restricted and contrived conditions (i.e., without information from binocular cues and motion parallax), they suggest that the correspondence between what is perceived and physical reality that is based on assumptions the individual has developed in the course of his environmental interactions can be made to break down. The illusions are most striking when the individual is forced to violate one set of assumptions about the spatial environment to preserve another. Although there are a number of demonstrations, our purpose is well served by considering the two most famous.

The Trapezoidal Window

The dramatic perceptual effects of the rotating trapezoid must be observed to be fully appreciated. The physical device consists of a trapezoidal surface with panes and shadows painted on both sides to give the appearance of a partially turned rectangular window (Figure 17.3). When viewed frontally, it appears to be rectangular in shape but turned at an angle (so long as there are not sufficient depth cues to indicate that it is not turned). It is mounted on a rod, connected to a motor, that can rotate at a slow constant speed about its vertical axis. When the rotating trapezoid is observed with one eye from about 3 meters or with both eyes at 6 meters or more, it is perceived not as a rotating trapezoid but as an oscillating rectangular window reversing its direction once every 180°.

It must be emphasized that in terms of the available stimulus information there are two mutually exclusive perceptual alternatives: an oscillating rectangle or a rotating trapezoid. Indeed, the physical stimuli for the latter perception are present. That the figure is not seen as a rotating trapezoid, the Transactionalists attribute to prior experience and to learning, that is, to the viewer's assumptions about the rectangularity of windows.

> In his past experience the observer, in carrying out his purposes, has on innumerable occasions had to take into account and act in respect to rectangular forms; e.g., going through doors, locating windows, etc. In almost all such occasions, except in the rare case when his line of sight was normal to the door or window, the image of the rectangular configuration formed on his retina was trapezoidal. He learned to interpret the particularly characterized retinal images that exist when he looks at doors, windows, etc., into rectangular forms. Moreover, he learned to interpret the particular degree of trapezoidal distortion of his retinal images in terms of the positioning of the rectangular form to his particular viewing point. These interpretations do not occur at the conscious level; rather, they are unconscious and may be characterized as **assumptions** as to the probable significance of indications received from the environment. A person's perception thus provides him with an awareness not only of the form of the "thing" he is looking at, i.e., "what it is," but also "where it is" relative to his viewing point. (Ames, 1951, Pp. 14–15)

Thus, on this basis, the favored perception of the ambiguous stimulus figure is of a normal rectangular window turned slightly. It follows that if it

Fig. 17.2 *An infinite number of surfaces, differently oriented with regard to the line of sight, may subtend the same visual angle at A as does the square at 1 and therefore may be perceived as a square when accompanying cues to space are lacking. (From S. H. Bartley, in Handbook of Experimental Psychology, edited by S. S. Stevens, Wiley, New York, 1951, p. 924. Reprinted by permission of the publisher.)*

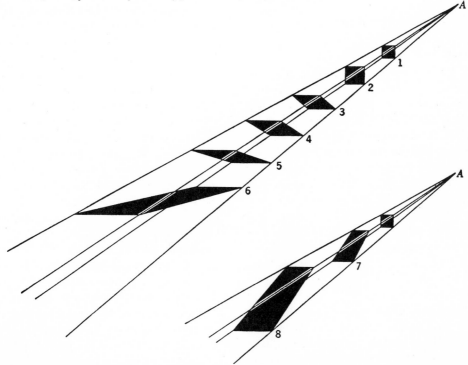

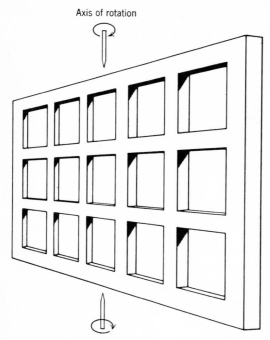

Axis of rotation

Fig. 17.3 *The Ames trapezoid. A rendering of the frontal view (perpendicular to the line of sight) of the rotating trapezoid. (Modified from Ames, 1951, 65, p. 2.)*

is seen as a rectangular window, then the character of its movement must be perceived as oscillation because the continuous array of images could occur only from a rectangular surface that oscillates. The perception of the true motion of the surface, rotation, is inconsistent with the assumption that the figure is a rectangular window. In normal rotation of a rectangular surface, the retinal projection of the farther edge shrinks. Though the retinal image of the actual rectangle may be trapezoidal, "The observer interprets these changes in trapezoidal form as changes of position and interprets the continuing changes of position as a rotation of a rectangular window" (Ames, 1951, p. 15). However, in the case of a rotating trapezoid, one of its sides is *always* longer than the other. Hence, it continuously appears nearer the viewer. This sort of imagery could occur only from a moving rec-

tangular surface when it undergoes oscillation. Hence, it follows that the projection of the apparently nearer long side appears to oscillate back and forth.

In an effort to assess the effect of assumptions about the geometric properties of the environment on the illusory effect of the rotating trapezoid, Allport and Pettigrew (1957) performed a cross-cultural test of the illusion with rural Zulu children (10 to 14 years old) of Natal, Africa. An important reason for choosing this group is that the Zulu culture is virtually devoid of not only windows but also of surfaces with right angles and straight lines as well as many other environmental cues of rectangularity. For example, their huts are round, windowless, and arranged in a circle; their fields follow the contours of the rolling land rather than the rectangular plots characteristic of Western culture. Furthermore, they have no words for "square" and "rectangle," but they do for "round" and "circle."

The rotating trapezoid illusion was presented in four conditions of viewing to two groups of rural Zulu boys, from Polela and from Nongoma, and two urban control or comparison groups, a group of urban Zulu boys and one of urban European boys (Table 17.1). When the illusion was presented under conditions that are optimal for the illusion (condition 4), all groups showed the illusion (i.e., perceived oscillation) to about the same degree. However, in the condition that is marginal for perceiving the illusion (condition 1), where there are more cues for perceiving the true motion (rotation), rural Zulus reported the illusion significantly less than did the urban control groups. From their study the authors conclude:

> *The perception of motion as represented in the rotating trapezoidal window is governed, under **optimal** conditions, by nativistic determinants or by the unconscious utilization of residual (but not immediately relevant) experience, or by both. (Our experiment does not enable us to decide this*

Table 17.1

PERCENTAGE REPORTING THE ILLUSION OF OSCILLATION FROM THE ROTATING TRAPEZOID[a]

Condition	Nongoma Rural			Polela Rural			African Urban			European Urban		
	Yes	No	Uncer-tain	Yes	No	Uncer-tain	Yes	No	Uncer-tain	Yes	No	Uncer-tain
(1) 10′, both eyes	15	85	0	20	70	10	65	35	0	55	45	0
(2) 10′, one eye	70	30	0	80	20	0	95	5	0	95	5	0
(3) 20′, both eyes	40	60	0	85	5	10	80	15	5	80	20	0
(4) 20′, one eye	90	10	0	85	10	5	90	10	0	95	0	5
Totals	54	46	0	68	26	6	83	16	1	81	18	1

[a] Boys 10–14 years of age, N = 20 in each group. Source: Allport & Pettigrew, 1957, *55*, 109. Reprinted by permission of the publisher.

issue.) At the same time, object connotation (meaning) based on closely relevant cultural experience helps to determine the nature of the perceived movement under **marginal** *conditions. (P. 119.)*

It should be added, however, that Zulus do not live in environments completely lacking in outlines that lie perpendicular to each other. Natural objects such as trees, as well as upright people, form right angles with the ground. Accordingly, it is possible that the Zulus tested in the above experiment did not lack rectangular assumptions (Slack, 1959). This would suggest that the small difference between groups in perceiving the illusion in conditions 2, 3, and 4 is owing to the fact that experience with rectangularity was not as lacking with rural Zulus as had been assumed. Further evidence for the role of learning in the perception of the trapezoid illusion comes from a study in which the effects were reduced when subjects were systematically exposed to information about the illusion (Haber, 1965). That is, the perceptual experience of the illusion was modified by controlled experience and by disconfirmatory knowledge of prior assumptions made by the viewer. We will have occasion to return to the role of culture on perceptual illusions.

The Distorted Room

The photograph of Figure 17.4a suggests a view into a specially built room. The interior of the room is usually seen through a small peephole that allows only a monocular view, thereby eliminating a number of depth and distance cues. Under these conditions of viewing, most observers see two men in the windows of an ordinary room, one unusually smaller than the other. It is an illusory perception in that both men are about the same size whereas the room is quite unusual. In fact, the apparently "smaller" man is really located farther away from the observer than the other person. That he does not appear so, according to the Transactionalists, indicates the compelling influence of assumptions about the shape of the environment formed by past experience. They contend that since experience has been with rectangular rooms, the viewer assumes the two men are standing against the usual background of a rectangular room. However, the floor, ceiling, some walls, and even the far windows of the room are actually trapezoidal surfaces as indicated by the outlined structure presented in Figure 17.4b. As shown, the room is carefully distorted so that the window with the "smaller" man is really farther from the observer than the window containing the

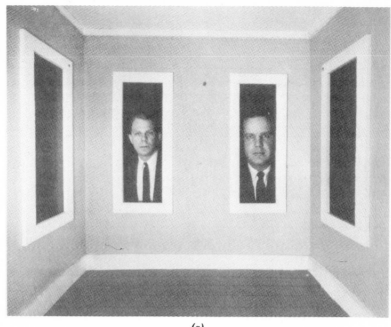

(a)

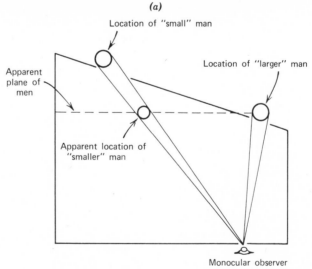

(b)

Fig. 17.4 *Both men in (a) are the same size. The illusion is created by the design of the room as indicated by the floor plan in (b). (From Psychology, by H. C. Lindgren & D. Byrne, Wiley, New York, 1975, p. 231. Reprinted by permission of the publisher.)*

apparently larger person. Similarly, the ceiling and floor are slanted so that the distance between floor and ceiling at the far corner is much greater than at the near corner. Consequently a person physically located in the nearer window appears to fill up the area between the floor and ceiling whereas the more distantly located person fills a smaller portion of the distance between floor and ceiling. In brief, the more distant aspects of the room are correspondingly increased in size so that when seen in perspective the near and far parts appear to be at the same distance from the observer. As in the case of the rotating trapezoid, there are two perceptual alternatives: two persons of similar size at different locations from the observer and standing against a trapezoidal surface or two persons, quite different in size, standing against a rectangular background. The general observation is of a rectangular room with the size of the occupants distorted.

The rotating trapezoid and the distorted room are but two of a series of unusual demonstrations by Ames and his colleagues in support of Transactionalism. However, all point to the same conclusion: Under the proper physical circumstances, past experience is an important factor in determining space perception.

Although there are a vast number of perceptual illusions, the remainder of this chapter will be devoted to a discussion of only a small exemplary group that has been the subject of recent research. In several instances provisional explanations embody comprehensive principles of perception; in almost all cases there is no single acceptable explanation.

THE HORIZONTAL-VERTICAL ILLUSION

A version of the horizontal-vertical illusion, introduced by Wundt in 1858, is presented in Figure 17.5a. The two intersecting lines are equal in length although to almost all observers the vertical line appears to be appreciably longer. If required to adjust the extent of the horizontal line to appear equal in length to the vertical one, a relationship between lines approximately like that shown in Figure 17.5b typically results, with the extent of the horizontal line being over 30% longer than the vertical. The illusory relationship between vertical and horizontal extents is not confined to simple line drawings. Chapanis and Mankin (1967) demonstrated an overestimation in the perceived extent of the vertical dimension using such familiar objects as a building, a parking meter, a nail in a table, and a large tree, all viewed in a natural setting.

Of the numerous attempts to explain this illusion two merit special attention.

Eye-movement Hypothesis

An often cited explanation of the horizontal-vertical illusion stresses the role played by eye

Fig. 17.5a *The horizontal-vertical illusion. The vertical and horizontal lines are the same length.*

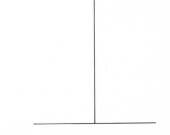

Fig. 17.5b *Apparently equal vertical and horizontal lines. To most observers the horizontal and vertical lines appear equal; however, the horizontal line is over 30% longer than the vertical line.*

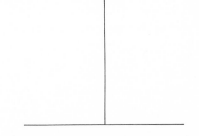

movements. Accordingly, a vertical line appears to be longer than an equal horizontal one because over the same distance vertical eye movements require more effort to make than horizontal ones, and the increased effort is translated into an increase in perceived length. However, H. R. Schiffman and Thompson (1974) have reported that the illusion persists even when a very small illusion figure is flashed at a sufficiently brief exposure time (50 msec) to eliminate the possibility of executing eye movements. Furthermore, Evans and Marsden (1966) have demonstrated that even when the image is stabilized on the retina, by creating an afterimage by a bright light flash, the vertical line of the typical horizontal-vertical figure is perceived as being longer than the physically equal horizontal line.

Visual Field Hypothesis

A different line of attack based on some known optical facts has been taken by Künnapas (1957). The binocular visual field is shaped roughly like an ellipse or oval with the long axis horizontal (e.g., Chaikin, Corbin, & Volkman, 1962). This means that the horizontal dimension of the visual field is considerably longer than vertical dimension. Hence, in viewing the standard horizontal-vertical illusory figure, the vertical line comes closer to reaching the edge of the field of vision—takes up proportionately more of the visual field—than does the physically equal horizontal line (Künnapas, 1957). Research has shown that the perceived size of a line is dependent, within limits, on the size of the background figure on which the line is presented: A line appears shorter as background size is increased (Künnapas, 1955; Rock & Ebenholtz, 1959). Relating this finding to the visual field, we might expect the horizontal line in the illusion to be comparable to the line perceived against a larger background and the vertical line to a line seen on a smaller background. Thus, the vertical line would appear to be longer than the horizontal line because it more fully crosses the visual field

and lies closer to its boundaries than does the horizontal one. Implications of this theory were tested by having subjects view the illusion while tilting their heads 90° (Künnapas, 1958) and by having subjects artificially distort their visual field by wearing specially designed glasses that produced a visual field with the long axis in the vertical direction (Künnapas, 1959). Under these viewing conditions, the ends of the vertical line were located farther from the boundaries of the visual field than were the ends of the horizontal line. The results were consistent with the theory: A reversal of the illusion occurred in that the original horizontal line appeared to be larger than the vertical line.

The visual field theory is inviting, and it has prompted much useful research, but there are aspects of the illusion that cannot easily be explained by it (see Underwood, 1966). For example, Thompson and Schiffman (1974a,b) reported that although the relation between the horizontal and vertical components of the illusory figure and the binocular visual field were held constant, variations in the size and the retinal orientation of the illusion figures produced changes in the magnitude of the illusion. According to Künnapas' visual field hypothesis, the magnitude of the illusion should remain unchanged. Thus, there are sufficient empirical objections to the visual field hypothesis to weaken its generality (see also Avery & Day, 1969).

THE MOON ILLUSION

The moon illusion refers to the phenomenon that the moon appears larger (as much as 1.5 times) when it is viewed at the horizon than at the zenith, although the projected images in both cases are identical. In fact, the moon (as well as the sun) occupies a far smaller fraction of the visible sky than most individuals assume. The angle subtended by the moon is almost exactly 0.5 of a degree (Tolansky, 1964). An object as small as a quarter of an inch (about 6.4 mm) across held 30 in (76.2 cm) from the eye subtends about 0.5 a degree to the eye, yet when it is held in the correct position it is large enough to blot out the image of the moon. (For an interesting general discussion of the moon illusion, see Tolansky, 1964.) A number of attempts have been made to explain this phenomenon.

Angle-of-Regard Hypothesis

Boring (Holway & Boring, 1940; Taylor, D. W. & Boring, 1942; Boring, 1943) proposed that the apparent size of the moon is affected by the angle of the eyes relative to the head. That is, the moon illusion is produced by changes in the position of the eyes in the head accompanying changes in the angle of elevation of the moon. In one task Holway & Boring (1940) had subjects match the moon, as they saw it, with one of a series of discs of light projected on a nearby screen. Viewing the horizon moon, with eyes level, most subjects selected a disc considerably larger than the disc chosen when their eyes were raised 30° to match the zenith moon. Similarly, when a subject lying on a flat table viewed the zenith moon from a supine position, with no raising or lowering of the eyes, or when a subject viewing from a supine position hung his head over the edge of a table, to view the horizon moon with his eyes elevated, the illusion was reversed: The zenith moon appeared larger. This latter effect can also be obtained by doubling over and looking at the horizon moon between one's legs.

Basing his conclusion on a number of years of research on this problem, Boring concluded that the moon illusion depends on raising or lowering the eyes with respect to the head. Mere movements of the neck, head, and body are not causal factors. Findings in support of the notion that visual space is altered with eye movements in the vertical plane have more recently been reported with children (Thor, Winters, & Hoats, 1969).

Apparent Distance Hypothesis

An explanation of the moon illusion based on perceptual factors can be traced to Ptolemy (ca. 150 A.D.), the second-century astronomer and geometrician. He proposed that an object seen through filled space, such as the moon viewed across terrain at the horizon, is perceived as being farther away than an object located physically at the same distance but seen through empty space, as in the case of the moon at its zenith. In brief, the projected images of the moon in both cases are of identical size, but the horizon moon appears farther away. That it also appears larger follows from the relationship known as the *size-distance invariance hypothesis*: If two objects project the same size retinal image but appear at different distances from the viewer, the object that appears farther from the viewer will typically be perceived as larger (see Figure 17.6). The notion of greater distance attributed to the horizon moon is also based on the assumption, elaborated by Robert Smith in 1738 (see Luckiesh, 1965, pp. 173–174), that the apparent shape of the sky is somewhat flattened. Under this assumption, its shape, sometimes referred to as the "vault of the heavens," appears as a semiellipsoid rather than a hemisphere (King & Gruber, 1962). If viewers are asked to point along a line that bisects the arc of the sky from horizon to zenith, they indicate a division that is closer to 30° (Miller, 1943; cited in Kaufman & Rock, 1962a) than to 45° as measured from the horizon (Figure 17.7). Thus, if the moon is perceived on the horizon of a semiellipsoid space, it will appear more distant and therefore, larger than when seen at its zenith.

Kaufman and Rock (1962a,b; Rock & Kaufman, 1962) questioned the method employed by proponents of the angle-of-regard hypothesis in determining the moon's apparent size. They argued that because the real moon is so far away from the observer it appears as a large object but one of indeterminate size. To judge the size of a stimulus of indeterminate size with nearby comparison discs having a visibly specific size is to

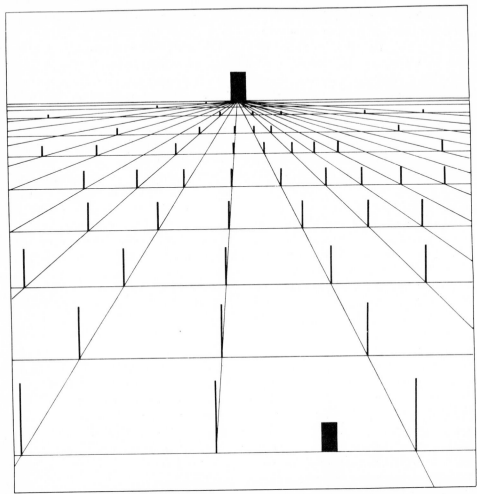

Fig. 17.6 *The effect of apparent distance on apparent size. The black rectangle resting on the horizon appears larger than the one in the foreground, although they are identical in size. This is an example of the size-distance invariance hypothesis. (Source: Rock & Kaufman, Science, 1962, 136, p. 1029, June 1962. Copyright © 1962 by the American Association for the Advancement of Science.)*

ask the viewer to compare things that are essentially incommensurable. Rather, Kaufman and Rock had subjects compare and match against each other two artificial "moons" seen against the sky. This, of course, is fundamentally the same sort of comparison as in the original illusion, though in the original case the two real moons are separated by both space and time. The

technique used by Kaufman and Rock consisted of an optical device that permitted an observer to view an adjustable disc of light (artificial moon) on the sky. Using a pair of these devices, the observer was able to compare a standard disc set in one position (e.g., the horizon) with a variable disc set at another position (e.g., the zenith). The size of the variable disc that was chosen by the

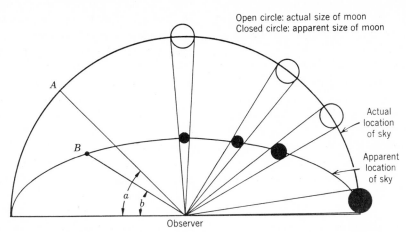

Open circle: actual size of moon
Closed circle: apparent size of moon

Actual location of sky

Apparent location of sky

Observer

Fig. 17.7 *Diagram of the effect of the apparent shape of the sky on the apparent distance and size of the moon. The upper arc indicates the true location and size of the moon at various positions; the bottom arc signifies the apparent locations and corresponding sizes of the moon. Accordingly, the apparent position of the moon is farther from the observer when it is at the horizon than at the zenith. The diagram also illustrates the effect of the apparent shape of the sky on the half-arc angle measures, A and B. The midpoint of the actual arc connecting zenith to horizon is at A and has a half-arc angle, a, of 45°; the midpoint of the perceived arc is at B and its half-arc angle, b, is about 30°. (Source: Kaufman & Rock, Science, 1962 a, 136, p. 955, June 1962. Copyright © 1962 by the American Association for the Advancement of Science. Reprinted by permission of the authors and publisher.)*

observer to match the size of the standard provided a measure of the magnitude of the illusion. The general result was that regardless of eye elevation, the horizon moon was perceived as being much larger than the zenith moon. From a series of studies these authors were able to conclude that the horizon moon appears farther away than the zenith moon, and that this impression of distance is produced by the terrain considered as a plane extended outward from the observer. As we noted, according to the size-distance invariance hypothesis, if two objects have the same projected size but lie at different distances from the viewer, the one that appears to be farther away will look larger (Figure 17.8). It follows from the apparent distance theory of Kaufman and Rock that the apparently farther moon should appear larger. In short, perceived size is a function of perceived

Fig. 17.8 *The size-distance invariance hypothesis applied to the moon illusion. Presumably the horizon moon appears farther away due to the presence of the terrain. The viewer takes apparent distance into account and perceives the more distant horizon moon as larger.*

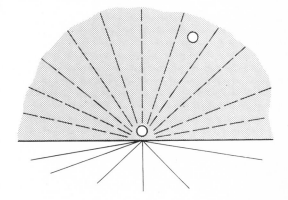

distance; with retinal size constant, the greater the apparent distance, the larger the perceived size.

How are we to resolve these findings with respect to the angle of regard theory? Wallach (1962) has pointed out that proponents of these theories employed two significantly different techniques in their respective research. It is likely that the causes of the moon illusion are of a degree of complexity warranting acceptance of components of both theories. That the matter has not been resolved is evidenced by yet a third explanation.

Relative Size Hypothesis

More recently Restle (1970) has offered an alternative explanation of the moon illusion that does not depend on apparent distance. Rather, it concerns the visual field in a manner similar to the visual field explanation of the horizontal-vertical illusion. The basic assumption of this hypothesis is that the perceived size of an object depends not only on its retinal size but also on the

size of its immediate visual surround. The smaller its boundary or frame of reference, the larger its apparent size. Accordingly, if the moon is judged relative to its immediate surround or bounding surface, then the horizon moon appears to be larger because it is compared with a small space (1°) to the horizon. At the zenith the moon appears smaller because it is located in a large expanse of empty visual space (90°) to the horizon. In this case the moon illusion is considered to be an example of the relativity of perceived size, in that the same object may appear large in one context and small in another. Some role, perhaps subordinate to that of the apparent distance hypothesis, is undoubtedly played by relative size.

THE MÜLLER-LYER ILLUSION

The illusion shown in Figure 17.9, devised by Franz Müller-Lyer in 1889, is perhaps the

Fig. 17.9 *The Müller-Lyer illusion. In both the top and bottom figures the segment on the left appears longer than the one on the right although the left and right segments are the same length. The bottom figure indicates that the illusion persists in spite of the presence of a disconfirming measure. (Source: Gregory, 1970, p. 81.)*

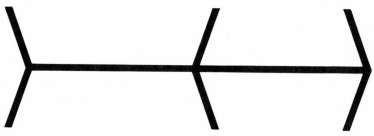

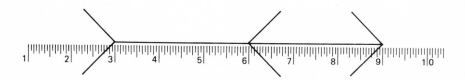

most familiar and researched geometric illusion. Clearly, the apparent length of a straight line is distorted when arrowheads are appropriately added to the ends. Although there are at least 12 theories to account for this distortion (Boring, 1942)—including aesthetic, Gestalt, and eye-movement theories—we will deal primarily with extensions of a perspective-constancy theory originally attributed to A. Thiéry (1896) and Tausch (1954), who proposed that certain stimulus features like the arrowheads of the Müller-Lyer figure are indicators of apparent distance. Recently, the perspective-constancy theory has been conceptually and empirically elaborated by Gregory (1963, 1966, 1968) and Day (1972) to encompass a number of size illusions. In the case of the Müller-Lyer figure, they contend that perspective features furnished by the arrowheads of the figure's lines provide false distance cues. As a consequence, size constancy is inappropriately induced to compensate for the apparent distance of the line segments. The result is a consistent error in the perceived length of the lines.

An example illustrating this is given in Figure 17.10. Drawings of corners and edges in perspective are shown with corresponding outline drawings of Müller-Lyer figures. According to a perspective-constancy explanation, the Müller-Lyer figures as well as the outline drawings are flat two-dimensional projections of three-dimensional shapes in depth, and due to the operation of a size-constancy mechanism, parts of the illustration that appear farther away are perceived as larger. In other words, the mechanism of size constancy compensates for the apparent distance of objects, a compensatory correction that normally occurs for a diminishing retinal image size when distance is increased.

The depth features inherent in the Müller-Lyer figure are largely confined to those of perspective, which is a potent indication of depth or distance. However, a more general statement has been made by Day (1972), termed the *general constancy theory,* in which he argues that if any of the traditional stimulus cues for distance that

normally are utilized to preserve constancy (e.g., binocular and monocular parallax, aerial perspective, accommodation, etc.) are independently manipulated with the size of the retinal image of the object not correspondingly changed, variations in apparent size will result. That is to say, "Illusions occur when stimuli that normally preserve constancy are operative but with the image of the object not varied" (p. 1340). In short, size constancy is brought into play inappropriately.

However compelling the perspective-constancy hypothesis is as an explanation of the Müller-Lyer illusion, it has a number of serious critics. For the most part antagonists argue that the Müller-Lyer illusion can be understood without appealing to apparent depth features. For example, G. H. Fisher, (1967a, 1968, 1970) contends that converging contours per se, not necessarily apparent distance inferences, induce distortions in perceived size. Evidence has been reported that certain apparent-size predictions based on perspective are not generally confirmed (Massaro & Anderson, 1970; Over, 1968); and furthermore, a number of researchers have argued that there exists an alternative class of explanations (e.g., Pressey, 1971; Weintraub & Virsu, 1971; see Hochberg, J. E., 1971, and Rock, 1975, pp. 409–416, for a general discussion of this matter). In addition to these points, there is evidence that a relative lack of experience with perspective cues does not affect the magnitude of the illusion: A cross-cultural study of the Müller-Lyer illusion with adult members of the Banyankole tribe of West Uganda, Africa, reared in a relatively nonrectilinear environment—with a presumable lack of exposure to perspective cues—showed that these individuals were no less susceptible to the Müller-Lyer illusion than were comparison groups of Ugandan and American college students (Davis & Carlson, 1970). The generality of perspective-constancy theory is further questioned by the reports that the Müller-Lyer illusion has been positively demonstrated with the pigeon (Malott & Malott, 1970; Malott, Malott, & Pokrzywinski, 1967), the ringdove (Warden &

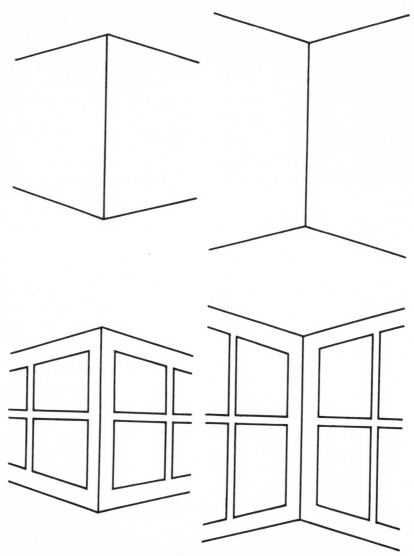

Fig. 17.10 *The Müller-Lyer illusion (top) and perspective drawings of structures whose outlines match the illusion. The bottom left drawing is characteristic of an outside corner of a building—the corner nearer to the viewer. The bottom right drawing suggests the inside corner of a building—the corner away from the viewer. Perspective causes an apparent enlargement of the vertical projection of the farthest corner to compensate for its apparently greater distance from the viewer. (After Gregory, 1973.)*

Baar, 1929), and with fish (cited in Gregory, 1966). Understandably, it is not clear whether these animals are capable of interpreting the arrowheads as perspective cues.

THE PONZO ILLUSION

An example of the Ponzo illusion, devised by Mario Ponzo in 1913, is given in Figure 17.11. Although the two horizontal lines are identical in length, the line located closer to the point of convergence of the two bounding lines appears to be longer. The Ponzo illusion is so closely linked to an explanation based on perspective that it is often referred to as the Ponzo perspective figure. The perspective feature, as applied here, is produced by the bounding converging lines that are ordinarily associated with distance. Accordingly, the perspective cue falsely suggests depth—the line that appears farther away is perceived as larger—thereby producing a size illusion. Evidence in support of perspective as a major factor contributing to the Ponzo illusion has been reported (e.g., Leibowitz, Brislin, Perlmuter, &

Hennessy, 1969). In a study of the factors influencing this phenomenon, Leibowitz and his colleagues had Pennsylvania college student subjects view monocularly and binocularly the actual scene illustrated in Figure 17.12B, from the point at which the photograph was taken. In a second phase, Pennsylvania college students and students of the same educational level but native to Guam were tested with the four two-dimensional pictorial stimuli shown in Figure 17.12. Procedurally, the upper line in the actual scene and in each subfigure of Figure 17.12 was constant while a series of lower lines were individually and randomly presented for an equality match with the upper line. The essential results are given in Figure 17.13. The findings for Pennsylvania students, in general, indicate that the magnitude of the Ponzo illusion is dependent on the presence of a context of cues to depth: The greater the context—the more the photographs simulate the real scene—the greater the magnitude of the illusion. Figure 17.13 indicates that the upper of two lines, when shown alone (D), is slightly overestimated. This is likely due to the cue of elevation. The addition of converging lines (A) produces an

Fig. 17.11 *A version of the Ponzo illusion. The two horizontal lines are equal (Devised by M. Ponzo in 1913.)*

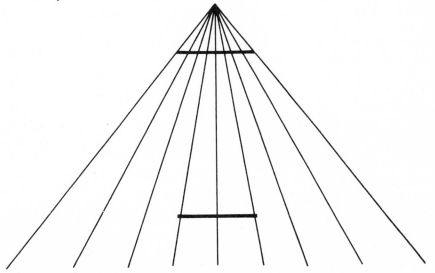

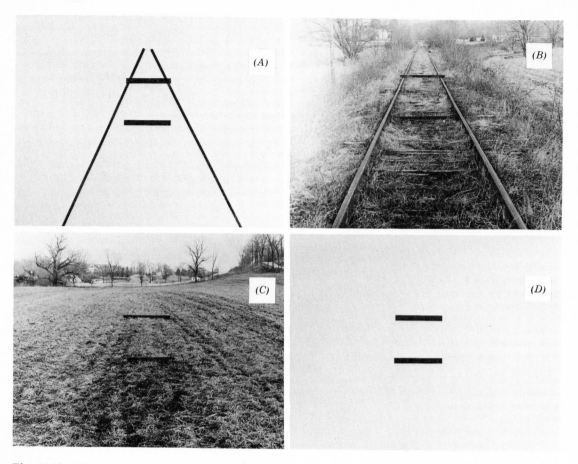

Fig. 17.12 *The stimuli used in the study by Leibowitz, Brislin, Perlmuter & Hennessy. The extent of the horizontal lines in all figures is the same. (Source: Leibowitz et al., Science, 1969, 166, p. 1175, November 1969. Copyright © 1969 by the American Association for the Advancement of Science. Reprinted by permission of the author and publisher.)*

illusion value of approximately 10% (percentage overestimation of the upper line). When the two horizontal lines are shown against texture cues (*C*), a 20% illusory effect obtains, and the addition of perspective cues such as railroad tracks (*B*) results in about a 30% illusion. However, the greatest illusion resulted from the actual scene. In this condition subjects were required, in effect, to judge which line subtended the larger visual angle.

The comparison between the illusory effects of the Pennsylvania and Guam students is rele-

vant to an empirical analysis of the origin of the Ponzo illusion. Although the students from Guam were matched in age and education level to the Pennsylvania students, they had spent their entire lives on the island of Guam, which has a unique sort of terrain. According to the authors, the vistas on Guam are quite short due to hilly formations and tropical plant growth and except for one short spur, there are no railroads. Since inhabitants of Guam do not ordinarily view the kind of topography indicated in the photographs

(*B* and *C*), it is a reasonable expectation, according to the perspective-constancy notion, that Guam students should not show the effects of the context provided by the cues to depth to the extent that the Pennsylvania students do. The results, shown in Figure 17.13, bear this out. Whereas the overestimation of the horizontal line nearer to the apex of the figure (*B*) was slightly over 30% for the Pennsylvania students, the magnitude of the illusion for the Guam students was only about 18%. This study is important in showing that the more the two-dimensional photograph approximates a representation of a three-dimensional scene—the more spatial cues to depth are available—the larger the magnitude of the illusion. It also indicates the importance of experience with topographical factors in the visual environment in determining the use of spatial cues.

An additional factor in the magnitude of the Ponzo illusion has been reported by Leibowitz and Pick (1972). They found a significant difference in the illusion by two different populations in Uganda. Urban university students produced results similar to those of the Pennsylvania college students, whereas subjects who dwelled in rural regions had significantly lower illusion values. For both groups of subjects the environmental ecology was the same, but the history of exposure to *pictorial depth*—two-dimensional printed material such as photographs, movies, and television—was quite different. This suggests that experience with pictorial depth is a prerequisite to perceiving illusions of depth in a two-dimensional surface (see also Kilbride & Leibowitz, 1975). The same point has also been made by Deregowski (1972) who argues, based on his examination of cultures relatively deprived of pictorial depth experience, that the perception of depth in a flat picture requires learning.

As we noted with size constancy, the magnitude of the Ponzo illusion follows a developmental trend. The Ponzo illusion has been shown to increase rapidly with age from childhood to adolescence, after which it remains stable through adulthood, and then decreases in old age (Leibowitz & Judisch, 1967; Farquhar & Leibowitz, 1971). In addition, student subjects,

Fig. 17.13 *The magnitude of the Ponzo illusion for the various conditions of the experiment by Leibowitz et al. (1969). The magnitude of the illusion represents the percentage overestimation of the upper member of the pairs of horizontal lines shown in the preceding figure. (Source: Leibowitz et al., Science, 1969, 166, p. 1175, November 1969. Copyright © 1969 by the American Association for the Advancement of Science. Reprinted by permission of the author and publisher.)*

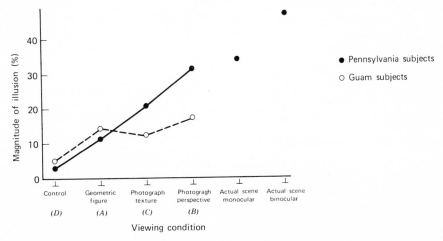

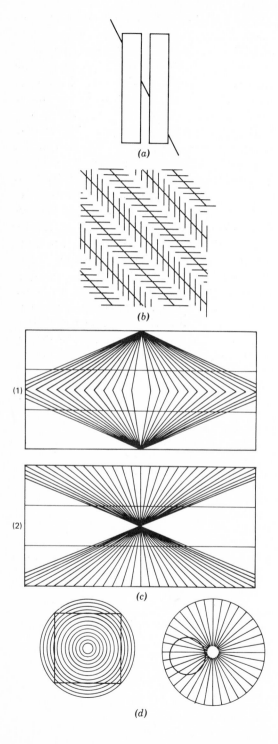

(a)

(b)

(1)

(2)

(c)

(d)

under the effect of hypnotically-induced age regression, gave results on a test of the Ponzo illusion that were more typical of younger ages (to which they were hypnotized) than of their own chronological ages (Parrish, Lundy, & Leibowitz, 1968).

A number of reviews have pointed out that no single theory accounts for the major geometric illusions (e.g., Over, 1968; Hotopf, 1966; Coren & Girgus, 1973). Indeed, there is no consensus that geometric illusions constitute a single class of effects. However, a form of perspective-constancy theory has been implicated as an explanation for a number of other geometric illusions (see Figure 17.14), and it appears to encompass a significant portion of the empirical findings (for a perspective-constancy explanation of the Poggendorff illusion, see Gillam, 1971; for the horizontal-vertical illusion, see Segall, Campbell, & Herskovits, 1966 and Schiffman & Thompson, 1975; see Gregory, 1963 and 1973, for a perspective-constancy explanation of the other illusion figures). Though a reasonable anticipation is that geometric illusions are multiply determined, at this stage a form of perspective-constancy hypothesis provides a useful if preliminary explanatory model.

Fig. 17.14a *The Poggendorff illusion. The segments of the continuous diagonal line appear to be offset when interrupted by the vertical rectangles. (Proposed by J. C. Poggendorff and described by Zöllner in 1860.)*
Fig. 17.14b *Zöllner's illusion. The pattern of short lines causes the parallel lines apparently to converge and diverge. (Devised by J. Zöllner in 1860.)*
Fig. 17.14c *(1) Wundt's illusion. The horizontal parallel lines appear to bend toward the middle. (Proposed by W. Wundt in 1896.) (2) Hering's illusion. The horizontal parallel lines appear to bow apart in the middle. (Proposed by E. Hering in 1861.)*
Fig. 17.14d *The concentric circles and spokes cause an apparent distortion in the inner square and circle, respectively. (After Orbison, 1939.)*

AMBIGUOUS AND IMPOSSIBLE FIGURES

There are a number of figural organizations (quite similar to those of figure-ground, described earlier) with inherent depth characteristics that may be ambiguously perceived with respect to their principal spatial orientation. After a brief period of inspection of any of the drawings shown in Figure 17.15, there is a spontaneous reversal in its spatial orientation. With continued inspection the reversal may occur periodically. The reversal occurs because there is insufficient stimulus information in the configuration to assign to it a completely stable and unitary orientation in depth. Attneave (1971) has referred to the class of figures characterized by ambiguous and equivocal depth information as *multistable* figures. For example, in the case of the Necker cube two simple three-dimensional organizations of a cube in depth are about equally possible: It can be seen as projecting upward *or* downward in depth but not both ways at the same time. In general, when the available depth information is of such a degree of ambiguity as to equally (or nearly equally) favor two or more different depth interpretations, alternative perceptions may be induced by the same figure.

So called "impossible" displays, such as those shown in Figure 17.16, are disturbing as well as confusing to most observers who attempt to see them as depicting three-dimensional objects (see Deregowski, 1969, for a report on the "trident" stimulus). This is because such displays

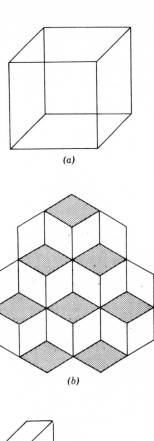

(a)

(b)

(c)

Fig. 17.15a *The Necker cube. After a brief fixation the cube spontaneously reverses in depth. (Based on a rhomboid figure devised by L. A. Necker in 1832.)*

Fig. 17.15b *The figure reverses so that either six or seven cubes are perceived.*

Fig. 17.15c *Schröder's staircase. The figure reverses from a staircase to an overhanging cornice (Devised by H. Schröder in 1858.)*

Fig. 17.15d *Either end of the series of rings may be seen as the near or far end of a tube.*

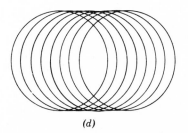

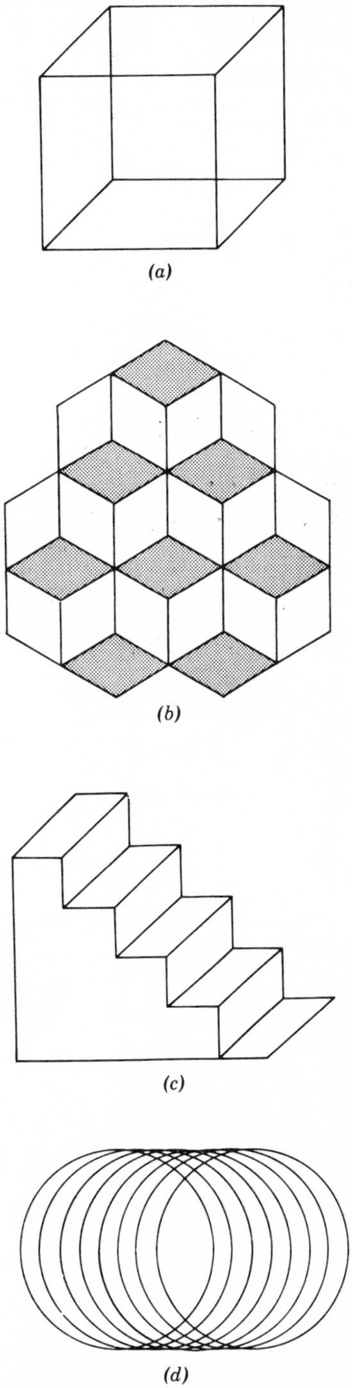

(d)

Fig. 17.15 *Examples of "Ambiguous" figures.*

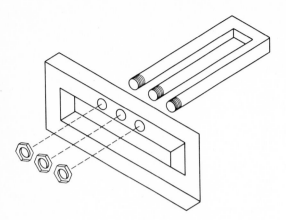

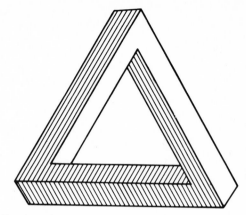

Fig. 17.16a *An "impossible" construction. The three-pronged figure is called a "trident." (Source: North American Aviation's Skywriter, Feb., 18, 1966, Braun & Co., Inc.)*

Fig. 17.16b *An "impossible" triangle. (Source: M. C. Escher, 1971; Penrose & Penrose, British Journal of Psychology, 1958, 49, p. 31.)*

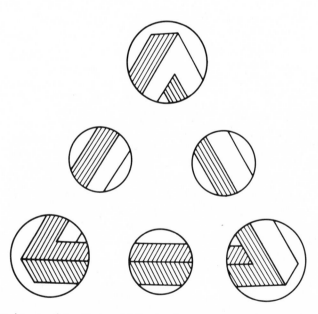

Fig. 17.17 *When isolated parts of the "impossible" triangle are seen, they appear as simple drawings of angles and line lengths in depth. However, when the figure is viewed as a whole, apparently depicting a three-dimensional object, the depth interpretations assigned to the isolated features are in conflict with each other. (Source: After Lindsay & Norman, 1972, p. 25.)*

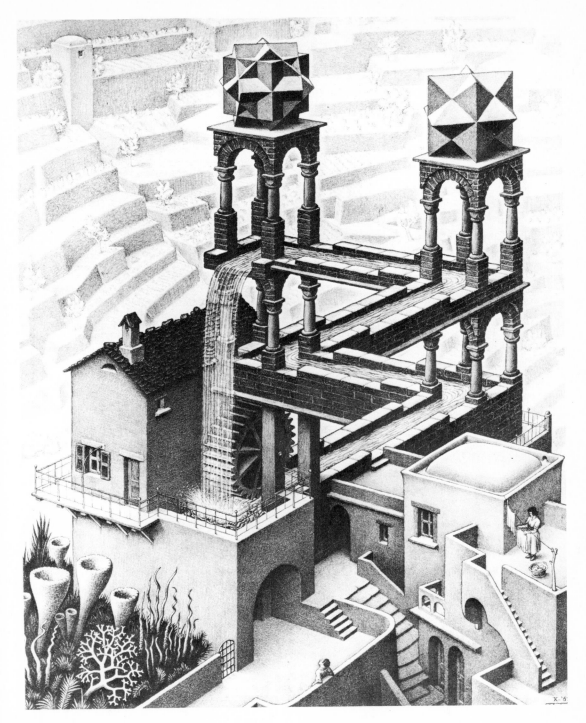

Fig. 17.18 *"Impossible" scene drawn by M. C. Escher (1971). According to Escher the figure above incorporates the triangle of Figure 17.16b. (Source: Escher, 1971, 76, "The Waterfall," Escher Foundation, Haags Gemeente-museum, The Hague.)*

contain inconsistent and contradictory sets of depth information that cannot individually be suppressed. Clearly, when viewed as a collection of individual linear segments and angles they appear as reasonable depictions of parts of a simple three-dimensional object in depth (see Figure 17.17); that is, the segments are "locally interpretable" (Simon, 1967). However, when globally seen as unitary objects, the depth characteristics of the individual features appear to be in conflict with each other and the figures appear spatially "impossible." Thus, the depth interpretation individually assigned to each part cannot be extended to the figure as a whole (see Hochberg, J. E., 1968).

Some of the remarkable graphic drawings of the artist M. C. Escher (1971; see especially M. L. Teuber, 1974), utilizing contradictory depth cues, are fascinating examples of impossible three-dimensional scenes (see Figure 17.18).

This chapter has introduced a variety of visual illusions and their explanations within the context of some of the general principles of space perception. In this sense the present chapter is a continuation of the preceding one.

The Ames series of demonstrations was posed and explained by the Transactionalists, who contended that assumptions about the sizes and shapes of objects are created by past experience with similar objects. The horizontal-vertical illusion, although quite compelling, does not lend itself to a simple class of explanations. However, a number of illusions, such as the moon, Müller-Lyer, and Ponzo, were explained in terms of a general perspective-constancy hypothesis, attributable to R. L. Gregory (1963) and R. H. Day (1972). This notion contends that, owing to the spatial context, portions of certain illusion figures are seen as flat two-dimensional projections of three-dimensional shapes in depth. Accordingly, owing to the compensatory operation of a size-constancy mechanism, parts of the illusion that are apparently farther away appear larger. Although not totally supported by the research literature, some version of a perspective-constancy notion provides a useful, though tentative, model for illusions that possess some inherent depth features.

Finally, figures with ambiguous or contradictory depth information were discussed. It was concluded that the perceptual ambiguity in some figures (e.g., the Necker cube) is owing to the fact that their inherent depth indicators equally favor two or more perceptual organizations. So-called "impossible" figures were described as owing to the merging of incompatible depth cues within the same figure. When these depth features are viewed in isolation, they are easily interpretable; but when they are perceived together so as to appear as a unitary pictorial rendering of a three-dimensional object in depth, the total configuration appears to be spatially impossible.

Studies of relevance to space perception in general were cited on cultural differences in the perception of illusory figures. These suggest that spatial perception may be partly organized on the basis of ecological and experiential factors typical of an individual's culture.

18

The Development of Perception

The problem of whether the ability to perceive spatial features of the world is a totally acquired capacity, completely dependent on experience and learning, or whether it is based wholly on innate, genetic factors predetermined by the way the sensory apparatus is constructed has long been a matter of philosophical inquiry and has had a great deal of influence on psychological research and theory. (There are numerous accounts of the history of this issue: in particular see Hochberg, J. E., 1962; Pick & Pick, 1970; or Pastore, 1971.) This issue—often referred to as "empiricism versus nativism"—can be traced back to the writings of seventeenth and eighteenth century philosophers and nineteenth century scientists. Historically, the nativist approach, proposed by Descartes, Kant, Mueller, and others, asserts that perceptual abilities are inborn. More recently, the Gestalt school has also supported a form of nativist position (Wertheimer, Max, 1958). As we noted, Gestalt psychologists claim that the organization of the perceptual world is governed by tendencies and principles that are innately determined. On the other hand, the empiricists, who include Hobbes, Hume, Locke, Berkeley, and Helmholtz, and more recently the Transactionalists, maintain that perception occurs through a learning process—from commerce and experience with the environment. Although it has a great effect on psychology, both as a philosophical and as an empirical disagreement, the empiricism-nativism issue has been impossible to resolve. Most contemporary psychologists hold that some forms of perceptual capacities and mechanisms are available soon enough after birth to preclude a strict empirical interpretation of the genesis of perception. Similarly, that experience plays some necessary or useful role for perception (for example, that it may modify some genetically endowed sensory mechanism) is not seriously questioned by most psychologists. As a contemporary controversy, the genesis of perception is largely one of emphasis with respect to the interaction of innate and learned factors (see Vernon, 1970). Moreover, the experiential and genetic factors are so intimately related that there are few experimental treatments that allow for independent manipulation of either variable. Finally, to a behavioral science, strict dichotomies and mutually exclusive alternatives such as empiricism versus nativism are to be avoided. It is possible to study and identify the variables that control and affect the perception of space without recourse to the learned-innate issue. As Fantz (1965a) puts it:

Perception is innate in the neonate but

largely learned in the adult! This is
presented partly as a resolution which is as
good as can be found, and partly to point out
that no real solution is possible. It is perhaps
best to be content with determining the
various developmental factors that influence
various stages of phylogenetic and
ontogenetic development, and to give up the
attempt to prove either nativism or
empiricism. (P. 400)

It is of considerable interest to study the perceptually naive organism in order to learn what it
perceives of the normal world, as well as how and
when these perceptual abilities develop.
Psychologists investigating the occurrence of
many forms of perceptual activities have gathered
a fund of knowledge that tells something about
the origin and the developmental course of perception. Indeed, we have already encountered a
number of such instances in various contexts, but
in this section it will be our primary focus. Specifically, what are the basic perceptual abilities of
the individual? When and how do they develop
and what variables govern their operations?

DEVELOPMENT OF THE PERCEPTION OF SPACE

Restriction Studies

A number of studies concerned with the development of spatial perception have been reported in
which animals were reared from birth in a light-
restricted environment. The assumption of such
studies is that if an animal reared without light
experience manifests efficient spatial perception
on emergence to the light, then this ability is
likely unlearned. In general, the results of restriction studies are difficult to interpret precisely, but
some findings, trends, and leads emerge.

One of the earliest systematic and well-controlled studies on visual deprivation was reported
by Lashley and Russell in 1934. They reared a
group of rats in total darkness from birth to 100

days of age and also maintained a comparison
control group of light-reared rats. On the day of
the animals' first exposure to light, the experi-
menters accustomed the rats to orienting in visual
space by placing each rat on a jumping stand and
allowing it to practice jumping a short gap to a
target platform on which food was available (see
Figure 18.1). After a short training period at a
constant distance, accustoming the rats to gap
jumping, the distance between the jumping stand
and the target platform was varied over a range
extending from 24 to 40 cm. The animal's accuracy in perceiving distance was measured by
the force of its leaps toward the target platform.
The force of the jump was recorded by the swing
of a pointer attached to the jumping stand that
was set into motion by the animal's leap. The
results were that the dark-reared as well as the
control group of light-reared animals exhibited a
high correlation between the force of the jump
and the distance of the target platform. In brief,
the rats regulated their leaps in accordance with
the actual distance. It would appear that little, if
any, light experience is required in order for the
rat to gauge depth accurately.

It should be pointed out that the use of the
jumping stand necessitated some practice and
experience in the light. Thus, a conclusion based

Fig. 18.1 *Jumping stand apparatus for the Lashley
and Russell (1934) experiment. (Source: Krech &
Crutchfield, 1958, p. 139. Reprinted by permission of
the authors.)*

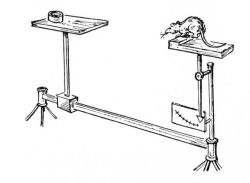

on complete light deprivation cannot be made on the basis of the Lashley and Russell experiment. However, the visual cliff apparatus, described earlier, enables the testing of depth perception with no prior training or light experience: Animals can be dark-reared and tested immediately on emergence to the light.

On the visual cliff apparatus, the rat has been shown to discriminate depth when light deprivation has been maintained for 30 days (Carr & McGuigan, 1965), 90 days (Walk, Gibson, & Tighe, 1957; Nealey & Edwards, 1960; see also Tees, 1974), and 125 days but not beyond (Nealey & Riley, 1963; Walk, Trychin, & Karmel, 1965). However, rats that are light-deprived for 10 months will show depth discrimination on the visual cliff after a month of light experience (Nealey & Riley, 1963). It appears that depth perception is an ability requiring no training in the rat. In fact, infant rats have demonstrated depth perception shortly after their eyes opened (Lore & Sawatski, 1969; Bauer, 1973). Similar findings have been reported for monkeys (Rosenblum & Cross, 1963), hamsters (Schiffman, H. R., 1971), ungulates (Walk & Gibson, 1961), and chicks (Shinkman, 1963). The observation that the chick can locomote, accurately peck (e.g. Cruze, 1935) and manifests depth discrimination almost immediately after hatching indicates the innate origin of depth perception for this animal. These capacities coupled

with the chick's innate use of shading, indicated earlier (Herschberger, 1970), stresses the unlearned character of the chick's perception.

However, some studies, in which animals were raised directly on the deep side of a visual cliff, have questioned the innateness of depth perception. The general results for rats (Kaess & Wilson, 1964) and chicks (Tallarico & Farrell, 1964; see also: Seitz, Seitz & Kaufman, 1973), presented in Table 18.1, indicate that rearing conditions can influence descent behavior. A reasonable conclusion is given in the statement by Kaess and Wilson (1964):

> While visual experience, as shown by the previous research, is not a requirement for the appearance of cliff-avoidance behavior, and while it is possible that the initial response to a visual cliff may invariably be that of avoidance, the present results show that the continuation of this behavior pattern very much depends upon the type of previous experience with visual patterns. (P. 152)

That is, with biased experience an innate behavior pattern can be modified.

In studies similar to the extended duration of dark-rearing for the rats, rabbits (Raskin & Walk, 1963) and kittens (Walk & Gibson, 1961; Walk, 1966), dark-reared for four weeks, did not discriminate depth on the visual cliff upon emergence to the light. However, with light experience normal depth discrimination did

Table 18.1
DIRECTION OF MOVEMENT ON THE VISUAL CLIFF AS A FUNCTION OF REARING CONDITIONS FOR RATS AND CHICKS

	Place of Descent			
	Rats[a]		Chicks[b]	
Rearing Conditions	Shallow	Deep	Shallow	Deep
Shallow	15	3	28	11
Deep	6	12	15	19

[a] Modified from Kaess & Wilson, 1964.
[b] Modified from Tallirico & Farrell, 1964.

develop. Furthermore, the general results from studies that restricted light to infant monkeys for various periods of time are that detrimental effects on guided spatial behavior, depth perception, visual acuity, and discrimination are a matter of length of light deprivation (Fantz, 1965a, 1967; Riesen, Ramsey, & Wilson, 1964; Wilson & Riesen, 1966). For example, monkeys dark-reared less than 10 days manifested depth discrimination when tested on the visual cliff (Fantz, 1965a); animals dark-reared for longer durations showed lack of depth perception (Riesen, Ramsey, & Wilson, 1964). It appears that there are striking species differences in the duration of dark-rearing that can be administered and still enable the proper development of space perception. Although there have not been systematic studies on this matter, it seems plausible to assume that nocturnal animals (e.g., the rat) can tolerate more extended periods of light deprivation without producing deficient space perception that can day-active animals (e.g., the chimpanzee). No doubt, the extent of the deficiency depends on the task or response assessed.

However, initial perceptual deficit may not be directly or only a matter of lack of visual experience, in that light deprivation can produce oculomotor defects and retinal degeneration (Riesen, 1950, 1961, 1965). Riesen (1970) has reported that there is impaired protein metabolism and decreases in the number of ganglion cells in the retina with increases in the duration of light deprivation in a number of experimental animals, including rats and chimpanzees. Moreover, there is histological evidence of retinal atrophy attributable to light deprivation (Riesen, 1965; Rasch, Swift, Riesen, & Chow, 1961).

These results can be extended to other perceptual modalities. For example, the tactual stimulation experiences of a chimpanzee's limbs was restricted from age 15 weeks to 31 months by encasing them in cardboard tubes (Nissen, Chow, & Semmes, 1951). After 31 months (which corresponds approximately in age to a three- to four-year-old child) of restriction, the chimpanzee was unable to master a very simple tactual discrimina-

tion task that required, on the basis of pressure stimulation, the discrimination of the two hands (i.e., a turn of the head to the side, left, or right of the hand that was stimulated). In general, the chimpanzee showed deficient tactual sensitivity, although his performance on visual discrimination tasks, involving the perception of size, form, and depth, was about normal.

Some of the research of Hubel and Wiesel (1963), cited earlier, points out the complex interactions of genetic and experiential factors. They have reported that the innate mechanism underlying the perception of movement, for example, requires appropriate stimulation to continue proper functioning. Kittens reared without patterned light for two months showed no activity in those cortical cells that normally react to movement. The indication, of course, is that the neural response was disrupted due to the extended duration of disuse. Although visual experience is not necessary for the initial organization and functional connections of nerve cells subserving certain aspects of space perception, some patterning of light is required to maintain those perceptual abilities that develop from innate structures (see also Riesen & Aarons, 1959).

There are a number of criticisms that can be leveled against deprivation and restriction studies. We noted that an effect of light deprivation may be an initially unobserved but significant anatomical change in the visual system leading to a degree of neural deterioration and oculomotor abnormality that precludes a clear examination of the role of experience. In addition, visual deprivation may not only result in restricted experience but may unpredictably alter the normal course of visual development producing confounding effects such as excessive arousal to novel stimulation, the development of abnormal competing habits, and the disruption of, and interference with unlearned visual preferences. (See Fantz, 1965a, 1967 for a discussion of these points; see Hinde, 1970, pp. 471–481 and Gibson, E. J., 1969, pp. 233–252 for brief discussions of the effects of light deprivation).

However, with respect to depth perception,

the following summary is warranted: Although there are clear species differences in the duration to which light deprivation can be maintained without producing a deficit in space perception, the evidence, in general, supports the conclusion that the depth perception of a number of species of animals requires no direct prior training although some light stimulation is necessary for its continued maintenance.

Restored Vision with Humans

Experimental manipulations such as dark-rearing are not possible with humans. However, a number of clinical observations have been reported in which otherwise normal individuals, functionally blind from birth because of congenital visual defects such as cataracts of the lens (a condition that eliminates pattern vision allowing only clouded patches of light), have had their vision surgically restored (von Senden, 1960; Gregory, 1966; Pastore, 1971).

Since 1728, when the first scientific citation on the effects of restored sight was made by the operating surgeon, Cheselden, a number of successful operations have been reported (see Pastore, 1971, for a history of restored vision). Although the reports are fragmentary, and for the most part have been unsystematically gathered and informally rendered, there is some concurrence on the effects of restored vision. Generally, the newly sighted person does not "see" much at first. Basically, he perceives unitary shapes against a background—that is, he perceives figure-ground organization—and he can fixate, scan, and follow moving figures. Although he may differentiate between objects, there is difficulty in identifying and recognizing an object as a member of a class of objects (von Senden, 1960; Hebb, 1949; London, 1960).

The fact that reasonably effective figural identification and recognition occur only after a lengthy and laborious period of experience and training has been interpreted to indicate that these abilities are acquired rather than innately determined, and it has been incorporated into a decidedly empiricistic theory of perception (Hebb, 1949). However, we cannot directly compare the behavior of the visually naïve but otherwise sophisticated adult with that of the completely naïve infant. The blind adult with his store of knowledge accruing from his other senses is a very different organism from an inexperienced infant. In addition, there may have been some neural degeneration in the adult due to disuse of the optical system so that indications attributed only to the role of experience are unwarranted. Observations of the effects of vision restoration, although of some interest and suggestive of the role of learning a newly acquired sense, do not provide any straight-forward conclusions (see Wertheimer, 1951, for a critique of restored vision).

Enrichment Studies

If lack of experience can produce perceptual deficiencies, it is of interest to consider whether enriched or extra forms of experience produce corresponding increases in perceptual abilities. Indeed, it has been argued in the case of the rat that early extra experience in the form of continued exposure to certain stimuli produces a subsequent increase in certain perceptual capacities (e.g., Hebb, 1949; Hymovitch, 1952; Forgays & Forgays, 1952; Forgus, 1955; Forgays & Read, 1962; Lavalee, 1970). This is especially relevant with studies in which various forms have been presented in the immediate rearing environment, and these forms have been later used in a discrimination task (e.g., Gibson & Walk, 1956; Forgus, 1954, 1956, 1958).

In one of an extended series of studies by Walk, Gibson, and their colleagues, a group of experimental rats was reared in cages that had cut-outs of circles and equilateral triangles fastened to the cage walls (Gibson, E. J. & Walk, 1956). On reaching adulthood (approximately 90 days) the experimental group and a nonexposed control group were trained to discriminate between the triangle and circle. The performance of the experimental group was consistently superior to that of the control group, suggesting that prolonged visual experience with stimuli may facilitate later discrimination of the stimuli. However, that facilitation was to specific forms was questioned by subsequent research. When only one stimulus form was present in the experimental rats' cages, facilitation of the experimental group's performance on a later two-form discrimination task occurred regardless of whether the previously exposed form was selected as positive or negative (Walk, Gibson, Pick, & Tighe, 1958). Furthermore, when initial cage exposure was to an equilateral triangle and a circle and the subsequent discrimination task was between an isosceles triangle and an ellipse, the experimental group was again superior to the control group (Gibson, Walk, Pick, & Tighe, 1958). These researchers have also noted that the mode of presentation of the figures during rearing was a critical variable (Gibson, Walk, & Tighe, 1959). When figures painted on a flat background were hung on the cage walls in place of the cut-outs (the latter are figures in relief with edges, hence they possess more three-dimensional and depth cues than do painted figures), the original findings were not replicated (Walk, Gibson, Pick, and Tighe, 1959). The conclusion offered is that whatever learning had taken place during the early exposure period was not specific to the stimulus patterns used; rather, it served to draw attention to those articulated visual cues that were employed in the subsequent discrimination task. It is likely that the depth edges of the cut-outs rendered them more attractive, attention demanding, and discriminable than the flat painted figures. From these studies it appears that the benefit of early and prolonged exposure to specific forms is of a general nature, reflecting "attention getting" effects (Gibson, E. J., 1969).

Biased Stimulation

When the total stimulus presentment is completely under experimental control, as with many sensory-physiology studies, specific and predicta-

ble aspects of the stimulus exposure may produce coincident changes in perception. Indeed, some of these studies, using very selective or biased rather than enriched stimulation, indicate that changes in cortical organization may result from early and carefully controlled stimulus exposure (e.g., Hirsch & Spinelli, 1970; Shlaer, 1971). For example, kittens were raised from birth until 10 to 12 weeks of age with special mask devices that completely controlled their visual experiences; one eye was exposed only to three black horizontal lines and the other eye to three black vertical lines (Hirsch & Spinelli, 1970; see also Muir & Mitchell, 1973). The effect of this visual experience on the distribution of orientations of receptive fields (i.e., an area of the visual field in which light stimulation produces an impulse discharge in a given neural cell) was striking: Neurons with elongated receptive fields (i.e., neural cells activated by elongated stimuli) in the visual cortex were either horizontally or vertically oriented and lacking in oblique or diagonally oriented receptive fields (unlike normal kittens who possess manifold receptive field orientations). Cortical neurons with horizontal fields were activated only by the eye initially exposed to the horizontal lines; similarly, neurons with vertical fields were activated only by the eye exposed to the vertical lines. The authors' words best describe the study's relevance to our discussion: "The change in the distribution of orientations of cortical unit receptive fields that we found when kittens were raised with both eyes viewing different patterns demonstrates that functional neural connections can be selectively and predictably modified by environmental stimulation" (p. 871). Similarly, the cortical neurons of kittens, reared in a spherical, planetarium-like environment lacking straight line contours and having only point sources of light, were subsequently highly sensitive to spots of light but not to straight lines (Pettigrew & Freeman, 1973). This was in marked contrast to the cortical neuronal activity of normal animals in the presence of straight line stimulation.

These findings led other researchers (e.g., Freeman, Mitchell, & Millodot, 1972; Freeman & Thibos, 1973) to propose that modification in the organization of neurons in the human visual system can be induced by early abnormal visual input. For example, it was suggested that uncorrected ocular astigmatism, if present during a critical period in the development of the visual system, can alter neuronal connections and permanently modify the brain (see also Annis & Frost, 1973). It has also been suggested that the early visual environment and experience play an important role in developing and modifying the optical characteristics of the eye and may influence the development of ocular abnormalities such as myopia (Young, 1970).

In this context notice should be taken of the studies with rats that indicate that an increased (or decreased) perceptual input of patterned stimulation to the infant can also produce physiological and biochemical changes in the adult (e.g., Singh, Johnston, & Klosterman, 1967; Volkmar & Greenough, 1972). This occurs with other modalities as well: Increased tactual stimulation (from handling) to the infant rat has been shown to eliminate the behavioral effects of early malnutrition (Levitsky & Barnes, 1972).

THE DEVELOPMENT OF OBJECT AVOIDANCE: LOOMING

An object hurled at a person in his direct field of view will produce an automatic avoidance reaction. The perception of an approaching object—signaling an impending collision—is of obvious biological significance to an organism. The complex spatial and temporal information that specifies an imminent collision with an environmental object is called "looming" (Schiff, 1965). Basically this information occurs from an accelerated magnification in the field of view of a shape or silhouette. The magnification of the form occurs with a rate of expansion that causes it to

loom up as it approaches, that is, to fill the visual field. The apparatus employed to study this phenomenon in the laboratory consists of a point source of light from a shadow-casting device that projects the silhouette of an object onto a projection screen (see Figure 18.2). By the appropriate placement of the object between the light and the screen, the projected shadow can be made to undergo continuous expansion or contraction. Expansion or magnification of the shadow results in the impression of an object approaching at a uniform speed. Contraction or minification yields the impression of an object receding into the distance. Notice that nothing actually approaches the animal; the physical information simulates something approaching or receding. Research with this arrangement has been performed with fiddler crabs, frogs, turtles, chicks, kittens, adult and infant monkeys, and adult and infant humans. Crabs responded particularly to magnifica-

Fig. 18.2 *Shadow-casting apparatus. (Source: Ball & Tronick, Science, 1971, 171, p. 819, February 1971. Copyright © 1971 by the American Association for the Advancement of Science.)*

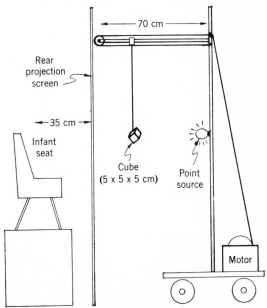

tion by running, flinching, or flattening out. Frogs reacted most often by jumping away from an expanding image. Chicks also responded to magnification with avoidant behavior: flinching, "back-pedaling," crouching or squatting, and hopping. Although their reaction was less consistent and conclusive, kittens also responded to image magnification (Schiff, 1965). Three species of turtles reacted to magnification of a circular image by withdrawal of their heads into the shell (Hayes & Saiff, 1967). Both adult and infant (five to eight weeks) monkeys rapidly withdrew in response to the looming form, leaping to the rear of their cage (Schiff, Caviniss, & Gibson, 1962). Alarm cries often accompanied the retreat of the younger animals. On the other hand, the optical projection simulating a receding form produced exploratory rather than avoidance or alarm reactions.

In a study by Ball and Tronick (1971) with 24 human infants ranging in age from two to 11 weeks, the responses to a symmetrically expanding shadow of a cube were various avoidance activities (e.g., moving the head back and away from the screen, bringing the arms toward the face, stiffening of the body, fear vocalizations). These responses did not occur for asymmetrical expanding shadows that produced the impression of an object approaching the infant on a miss path (in which case the infants showed tracking rather than avoidance responses) nor for a contracting shadow. These results were observed in all infants regardless of age and were not different from the results obtained when real objects were used rather than silhouettes. Similar results have been reported with six- to 20-day-old infants. The responses observed consisted of the eyes open wide, movement of the head back, and both hands moving between object and face (Bower, Broughton, & Moore, 1971).

The functional utility of an avoidance reaction to the optical information indicating a rapidly approaching object is clearly adaptive: Avoidance prevents collision. That the perception of imminent collision and its avoidance occurs in a number of animal species, both vertebrate and invertebrate, and occurs in several species at very early ages, indicates that learning does not play a major role in the phenomenon (Schiff, 1965; Ball & Tronick, 1971).

SPACE PERCEPTION OF THE NEWBORN HUMAN

In this section we will deal primarily with some of the perceptual capacities and mechanisms of infant organisms that are functional with minimal spatial experience. For the most part the focus will be on the newborn human, but where appropriate, comparative data will be included.

We have pointed out that the newborn of many species of infrahuman animals meaningfully perceive a significant portion of their environment with little or no experience. Does this extend to the human infant? Empiricists have held that the newborn human sees merely an undifferentiated blur—that the newborn's visual world is, in the words of the nineteenth century psychologist, William James (1890), ". . . one great blooming, buzzing confusion" (p. 488). However, the findings indicate otherwise.

That the very newly born can respond to his perceptual world is dramatically illustrated by a study in which an infant girl was tested for spatial localization three minutes after birth (Wertheimer, Michael, 1961). As the infant lay on her back, the click of a toy "cricket" was sounded next to the right or to the left ear. Fifty-two successive trials, each consisting of a click, were performed. The response recorded by two independent observers was whether the eyes moved to the infant's right, left, or at all. On most of the trials on which eye movement occurred (18 of 22), the eyes moved in the direction of the click. Notice that when the experiment was over the subject was only 10 minutes old! The importance of this study is that it indicates that some spatial features of stimulation—spatially separated auditory signals—are picked up and are capable of guiding behavior, and that the perception of certain spatial features of direction (i.e., a rudimentary form of auditory localization) are likely innate. It also suggests a coordination between auditory space and visual space.

Direct evidence on this matter with somewhat older infants has been reported more recently. Infants 30 to 55 days of age showed distress on hearing their mothers speak to them while her voice was displaced in space (Aronson & Rosenbloom, 1971). In the experimental arrangement, the mother was located in a room with a window that directly faced the infant. The infant viewed his mother but by use of a stereo amplifier system heard her voice emanate from 90° to the right or left of his midplane. The results—that the infants perceived and reacted to this spatial discrepancy—indicate that auditory and visual information is perceived within a common space.

In recent years there have been numerous well-controlled laboratory experiments performed on the perception of the newborn. These experiments suggest that there are a number of adaptive forms of behavior manifested in infancy. We can only sample from these. A series of pioneer studies of early infant perception, particularly visual preference and attention, has been made by R. L. Fantz based on his research with lower animals. (The term "preference" is used here to refer to systematic behavioral differences in responding, and it should not carry motivational connotations.) Initially, Fantz devised a visual preference task with newborn chicks (Fantz, 1957, 1961). Chicks were presented with a large group of small objects on a wall of the testing chamber, each enclosed in a clear plastic pecking container, connected to an electrical circuit that automatically recorded the number of pecks directed toward it in a specified period of time. To exclude any prior experience, the chicks were hatched in darkness and tested on their first exposure to the light. The most striking finding was a preference for "roundness." When presented

with eight stimuli of graded angularity, ranging from a sphere to a pyramid, the subjects pecked 10 times more often at round than at angular objects (Fantz, 1957). The preference for roundness extended to three-dimensional forms (e.g., a sphere over a flat circular disk) (Fantz, 1958). Furthermore, among circles, one-eighth in (3.2 mm) diameter stimulus was preferred to other sizes. The preference for roundness persisted when other stimulus characteristics such as color, contrast, texture and orientation of form were varied (see Fantz, 1967). Fantz interprets these initial pecking preferences as an adaptive behavior geared toward natural food sources whose physical features for chicks are likely to be round, relatively small, and three-dimensional in shape (e.g., grain or seed).

Fantz's procedure for human infants was similar to the preference technique used with chicks. An illustration of a form of the visual preference apparatus is shown in Figure 18.3. Generally, the infant is placed on its back in a small hammock crib inside a test chamber so that it must look up toward two panels, which have pairs of contrasting stimuli. The experimenter records the movements of the infant's eyes to determine which of the two panels the infant looks at more often and for a longer duration. Such differences indicate not only the discriminative capacities of the infant, but they also suggest what sorts of stimuli attract the attention of the newborn. By appropriate variation in the kinds of stimuli presented to the infant, it is possible to learn a good deal about early infant perception.

In one experiment, 30 infants, from one to 15 weeks of age, were shown four pairs of test patterns (Fantz, 1961). The paired patterns and results are shown in Figure 18.4. In terms of looking time, the more complex pairs drew the most attention (although the preferred level of complexity varies with age; see Hershenson, 1964 and Brennan, Ames, and Moore, 1966). Furthermore, the relative attraction of the members of a pair depended on the presence of a pattern difference. Thus, there were strong preference dif-

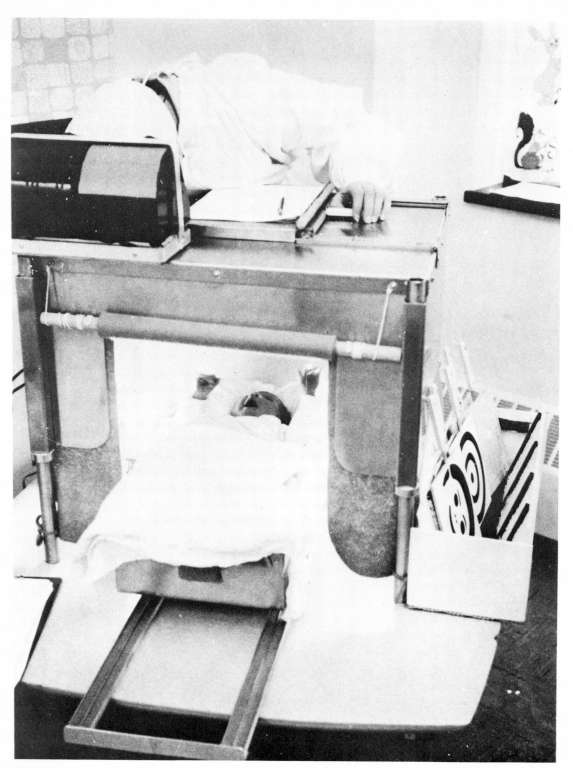

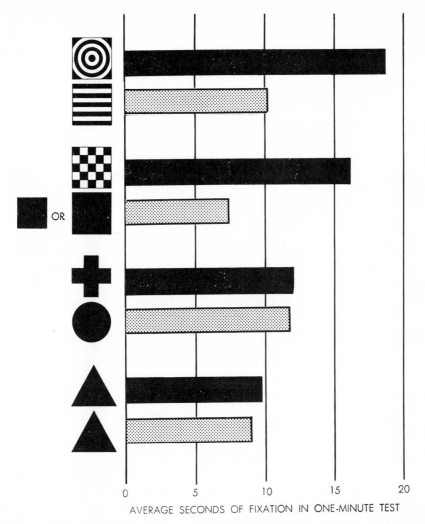

AVERAGE SECONDS OF FIXATION IN ONE-MINUTE TEST

Fig. 18.4 *Pattern preference is shown by infants' reactions, measured by fixation time, to various pairs of patterns (shown on the left) presented together. The more complex pairs received the most attention, and within each of the pairs differential interest was based on pattern differences. (The small and large plain squares were used alternately.) These results are for 22 infants in 10 weekly tests. (From the Origin of Form Perception, R. L. Fantz, Scientific American, 1961, 204, p. 70. Copyright © 1961 by Scientific American, Inc. All rights reserved.)*

Fig. 18.3 *Chamber for measuring visual preferences in infants. The infant lies on a crib in the chamber, looking at stimuli placed in panels at the ceiling. The experimenter peers through a peephole and records the attention given each object. (Source: Fantz, Science, 1963, 140, Pp. 296–297, April 1963. Copyright © 1963 by the American Association for the Advancement of Science.)*

335

ferences between the stripes and bull's eye and between the checkboard and square but not between the other pairs. Since these preferences were shown at all of the ages tested, the role of learning appears to be minimal.

When pattern was compared to color and brightness, pattern appeared more attractive (Fantz, 1961, 1963, 1966). In one experiment with infants 10 hours to five days old and two to six months old, six flat test objects were employed. Three objects had a pattern: a schematic face, a bull's eye, and a patch of newsprint. Three were plain patches: red, yellow, and white. The response measure was the duration of the first fixation of each stimulus. The results are given in Figure 18.5. More than half of each group preferred the schematic face.

The preference for facial patterns was further examined with three patterns that were the size and shape of a head (Fantz, 1961, 1965*b*). One pattern had a schematic face, a second had the same features but in scrambled form, and the third pattern had the same amount of black and white area but in two solid sections. The three objects were paired in all possible combinations and shown to 40 infants, ranging in age from four days to six months. The results were

that the schematic face was preferred over the other two patterns by almost all infants. Fantz's results are clear in that visual attention is controlled by some primitive distinguishing properties such as pattern over color. Because the stimulus features of face-like patterns may have adaptive significance, it is tempting to consider the proposition that representations of the human face are innately recognized. Consider first, however, the stimulus complexity of a face. It contains figure-ground differences, contours, boundaries, edges, brightness contrast, shading, and so on, each of which may be an attractive or attention-demanding feature of the stimulus independent of its structural relation. Furthermore, attention to face-like patterns over abstract forms has not been shown by all investigators for all ages (Hershenson, 1964; Kagan, 1970). Although the evidence indicates a looking preference for face-like patterns in the infant, precisely what features of the pattern are critical for the preference is not clear. Moreover, whether it develops as a Gestalt-like abstraction through experience with faces (Lewis, 1969; Kagan, 1970), or through a gradual extraction of differentiated features (see Gibson, E. J., 1969, pp. 347–356) is unresolved.

In order to make more precise statements

Fig. 18.5 *Visual preferences of newborn and older infants for black-and-white patterned discs over plain and colored discs, presented randomly and repeatedly for the length of the first fixation. (Source: Fantz, 1966.)*

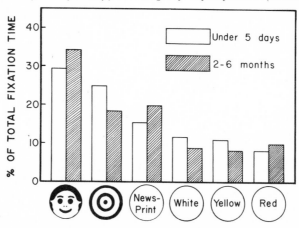

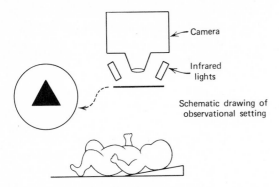

Fig. 18.6a *Arrangement for measuring ocular orientations of the infant. (From W. Kessen, in Early Behavior, edited by H. W. Stevenson, E. H. Hess, & H. L. Rheingold, Wiley, New York, 1967, p. 153. Reprinted by permission of the publisher.)*

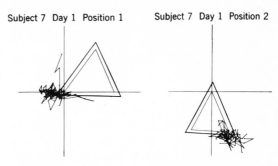

Fig. 18.6b *Sample records of ocular orientations for a subject in the experimental group. The outer triangle represents the outline of the solid, black, equilateral triangle presented to the experimental subjects. The inner triangle refers to a hypothetical one, described below. (From W. Kessen, in Early Behavior, edited by H. W. Stevenson, E. H. Hess, & H. L. Rheingold, Wiley, New York, 1967, p. 174. Reprinted by permission of the publisher.)*

about the perceptual world of the infant—particularly about which features of a stimulus attracts the infant's attention—a series of studies was performed that focused on the relation between aspects of the visual display and ocular orientations of the infant. Salapatek and Kessen (1966; also see Kessen, 1967) exposed a black equilateral triangle on a white field to a group of newborn infants (see Figure 18.6a). The triangle was 8 inches (20.3 cm) on a side and was located

approximately 9 in (22.9 cm) from the infants' eyes. Infrared marker lights (invisible to the infant subject) were placed behind the triangle so that a camera could continuously record the exact orientation of the center of the infants' pupils. A control group of 10 infants was similarly tested with a homogeneous black surface. The results were that the experimental group manifested more

Fig. 18.6c *Sample record of ocular orientations for a subject in the control group who viewed a homogeneous black field. The triangle on each record is a hypothetical one formed by the location of the infrared lights. See text. (From W. Kessen, in Early Behavior, Edited by H. W. Stevenson, E. H. Hess, & H. L. Rheingold, Wiley, New York, 1967, p. 173. Reprinted by permission of the publisher.)*

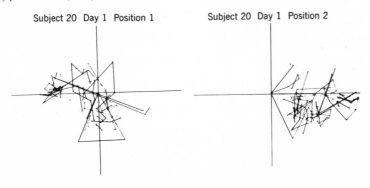

concentrated orientations, and the locus of their ocular fixation was particularly toward the vertices of the triangle (see Figure 18.6*b*&*c*). Most experimental infants tended to fixate on a single vertex though not necessarily the same vertex on different trials. Infants in general did not scan the sides of the triangle. The tendency by infants to direct their fixations toward a limited portion of a figure was supported by subsequent research with various geometric figures (Salapatek, 1969). The important findings from these studies are that the newborn can select and maintain focus on a relatively circumscribed feature of a visual pattern and that certain aspects of contour and boundary are the features that control the infant's attention.

CONCLUSION

With respect to the perceptual capacities so far described, infant animals of a number of species appear competent. The perception of form and pattern, features of space (e.g., depth) and events in space (e.g., looming) appear early both in evolution and in age, suggesting that little if any learning may be required for their appearance. In the section on constancy it was noted that there exists a fair degree of phylogenetic continuity in the vertebrate phylum. Moreover, constancy appears relatively early in those species that possess it. However, the role of learning for size constancy in the human infant is unclear, though it is known that the newborn human infant is capable of forms of learning (e.g., Lipsett, 1967; Siqueland & DeLucia, 1969). Indeed, the findings of the Bower experiments (e.g., 1974), in which infants as young as two months manifest size constancy, do not necessarily rule out learning factors since in two months a good deal of spatial experience transpires.

Eleanor Gibson (1970) has argued that the development of perception is an adaptive process. The findings support this. Clearly the capabilities for effecting guided locomotion, detecting the in-

formation required for avoiding edges, drop-offs, obstacles and missiles, and the perception, on the basis of a unitary feature (e.g., size constancy), that the world is organized into objects with fixed properties are highly adaptive in the sense that for survival animals must ". . . somehow discover where to go, what to seize, and what to avoid" (p. 100).

It has not been our goal to materially add to the resolution of the nativism-empiricism issue. However, we have outlined a number of perceptual capacities and mechanisms whose development, building upon their innate organization, provide the important foundation for the immense number of perceptual experiences that will subsequently confront the organism. It is the interaction of innate mechanisms and these experiences that is necessary for perceiving an orderly and meaningful environment.

In this chapter we discussed the emergence and development of spatial perception. In an effort to identify the origins and the developmental course of perceptual abilities, various experiential and genetic factors were discussed. Studies bearing on the capacity to perceive depth by perceptually naïve and visually restricted animals were outlined. It was concluded that the depth perception of a number of species of animals requires no direct experience or training although some photic stimulation is necessary for its continued maintenance.

Research on the effects of biased stimulation administered to the young of cats and humans suggests that the organization of receptive fields and functional neural connections within the visual system can perhaps be selectively and predictably modified by environmental stimulation. That is, if only certain forms of stimulation are available to an animal during a critical period in the development of its visual system, there may be perturbed and/or modified neuronal connections of its visual system and the visual brain.

A number of studies were described in which the young of many species of vertebrates and invertebrates showed avoidance reactions to the optical information that specifies imminent collision with a rapidly approaching object—that is, to looming. It was concluded that learning does not play a significant role in reactions to looming. This same conclusion can be reasonably applied to the perception of certain features of space and form, to depth, and to constancy.

Finally, the space perception of the newborn human infant was assessed. It was noted that the newborn human infant can respond in a number of meaningful ways to much of its perceptual world. The human infant shows discriminative reactions to certain stimulus configurations and shows preferences for some stimuli over others. It was noted that the newborn human can select and maintain focus on a relatively circumscribed portion of a visual display; in addition, certain features such as contours and boundaries affect the newborn human infant's attention.

In much of the research discussed in the preceding chapter, processes of perceptual development were assessed by the measurement of limb or body-part movement. In particular, an animal is seen to ward off a quickly approaching object (looming) or it extends its limbs toward a shallow rather than a deep surface (depth perception) by bodily movements. It is apparent that such processes involve an important motor component. Accordingly, a discussion of perceptual development requires a consideration of the basis of perceptual-motor coordination.

Normal visually guided spatial behavior generally involves a motor response—intentional limb extension or other self-produced locomotor response—to the pattern of optical stimulation. A question critical to the present discussion is: What is the functional relationship between sensory feedback resulting from self-initiated movement and normal perceptual development? An important series of experiments utilizing a biased sensory input have been performed by Held and his colleagues to study the development of visually guided spatial locomotion. Held and Hein (1963) raised kittens in the dark until they attained a level of motor maturity sufficient to perform the experimental task; this was between eight and 12 weeks. At testing, the kittens were

paired off and given three hours of daily light exposure in the "carousel" apparatus shown in Figure 19.1. The members of pairs of kittens were assigned respectively to an active (A) and a passive (P) movement condition. Kitten A was placed in a neck harness and body clamp that allowed it to move in a circular path within a cylinder whose inside surface was painted in vertical stripes; kitten P was similarly harnessed but restricted to a gondola whose movements directly varied with those of kitten A. The carousel was devised to provide identical optical and motion stimulation to each member of a pair. By means of a yoke arrangement, the self-produced locomotor activity of kitten A controlled the activity of its mate, kitten P. In brief, the apparatus provided equivalent optical and movement stimulation to each member of a pair, but the movement was active and self-produced for kitten A and passively imposed for kitten P.

The behavioral tests selected for assessing the effect of active versus passive movement experience included a *visual-placing* test (the automatic elicitation of a visually mediated extension or reaching out of the paw as if to prevent collision when the animal is moved toward a surface), blinking to an approaching object, and depth perception on the visual cliff apparatus.

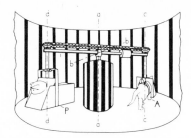

Fig. 19.1 *Carousel apparatus for equating motion and consequent visual feedback for an actively moving (A) and a passively moved (P) kitten. Movements are about the axes labeled a—a, b—b, c—c, and d—d. (Source: Held & Hein, 1963, 56, p. 873.)*

Differences between active and passive kittens occurred on all tests. The onset of the visual-placing and blinking responses occurred earlier for the active than for the passive kittens. The difference between the active and passive animals on the visual cliff test is shown in Table 19.1. The active kittens uniformly performed like normally reared animals, whereas the passive animals gave little evidence of depth discrimination. However, these visual-motor deficiencies of the passive kittens were readily remedied; after 48 hours of free movement in an illuminated room, the passive kittens performed normally on the tests. The major point raised by this experiment is that movement per se, in the presence of a stable optical input, is inadequate for normal visual-motor development; rather, variation in visual stimulation concurrent with and systematically dependent on self-produced movement is essential for the normal development of visual-motor coordination and visually guided spatial activity.

Hein and Held (1967) extended their research on perceptual-motor development focusing on the accuracy of the visual-placing response. They contended that there are two aspects of the placing response: the mere extensions of the forelimbs on approach to a surface and precise guidance of these limbs toward particular objects. From earlier research, they reasoned that although elicitation of the visual-placing response will usually occur to the presence of an approaching surface, the accuracy of the animal's placing response requires prior experience with sight of

Table 19.1
RATIO OF DESCENTS TO SHALLOW AND DEEP SIDES
OF VISUAL CLIFF[a, b]

Age in weeks[c]	Exposure in apparatus (in hr.)		Ratio of descents shallow/deep	
	A	P	A	P
8	33	33	12/0	6/6
8	33	33	12/0	4/8
8	30	30	12/0	7/5
9	63	63	12/0	6/6
10	33	33	12/0	7/5
10	21	21	12/0	7/5
12	9	9	12/0	5/7
12	15	15	12/0	8/4

[a] Source: Held & Hein, 1963, *56*, p. 875.
[b] A = active kitten; P = passive kitten.
[c] At the beginning of exposure in the experimental apparatus.

the actively moving limbs. It follows that a kitten reared without sight of its limbs may show the placing response to an approaching surface but not with accuracy. To test this proposition Hein and Held reared six kittens in the dark until they reached four weeks of age. They were then allowed six hours of free movement daily in an illuminated and patterned environment. However, during this time they wore lightweight opaque collars (see Figure 19.2) that prevented sight of their limbs and torso but that had little effect on their locomotion. For the remainder of the day, the collars were removed and the kittens were restricted to a lightless room. After 12 days of this treatment, all animals were tested for the visual-placing response with two different surfaces. One surface afforded a gross test for the visual-placing response. In this condition the kittens were carried toward a continuous surface, one without any interstices or interruptions. All kittens appropriately extended their paws—in short, they showed the visual-placing response. The second surface was a discontinuous surface interrupted by a series of cut-outs or prongs (see Figure 19.3). Use of this surface afforded a test of

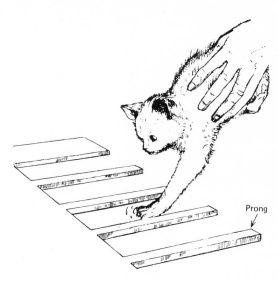

Fig. 19.3 *Kitten tested on discontinuous surface. (Source: Hein & Held, Science, 1967, 158, p. 391, October 1967. Copyright © 1967 by the American Association for the Advancement of Science.)*

the accuracy of the visual-placing response in that it provided a measure of the animal's capacity to guide its limbs toward specific portions of a surface. Notice that if the animal's response is accurately guided by its vision, then its paws should fall on the solid parts rather than the cut-out spaces. On a chance basis a prong should be contacted on half the number of placements. This, of course, would indicate poor accuracy. Of 72 limb extensions (12 trials each kitten on the interrupted surface) performed by the six experimental kittens, only half hit the prongs with their paws, whereas normally reared kittens hit the prongs on 95% of the trials. The effects of the experimental restriction on the visual-placing response were rescinded after an average of 18 hours of free movement without the collar in a normally illuminated environment.

Similar results on visually guided reaching, with monkeys reared from birth without sight of their limbs in the apparatus shown in Figure 19.4, have been reported (Held & Bauer, 1967). After 35 days of nonvisual control of limb move-

Fig. 19.2 *Kitten wearing a collar that prevents sight of limbs and torso. (Source: Hein & Held, 1967, Science, 158, p. 391, October 1967. Copyright © 1967 by the American Association for the Advancement of Science.)*

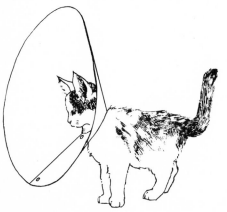

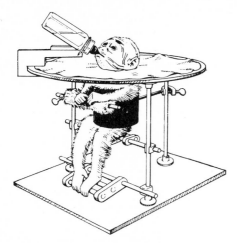

Fig. 19.4 *Apparatus for rearing an infant monkey without sight of its limbs. (Source: Held and Bauer, Science, 1967, 155, p. 719, February 1967. Copyright © 1967 by the American Association for the Advancement of Science.)*

ment, one hand was exposed to view. Visual fixation of the limb was extremely persistent and prolonged; visually guided reaching was poor but improved with experience. It appears that early experience of viewing a moving limb provides the information necessary for the animal to match the locus of its paw to target position. If movement and perception are not properly integrated, and if they do develop independently, as in the experimental arrangements described above, deficiencies in perceptual-motor development result. Extensions of this research to the human infant, particularly to perceptual-motor exploration exemplified in prehensile activity (reaching and grasping), has similarly stressed the role of proper forms of experience (e.g., White, Castle, and Held, 1964; White & Held, 1966; White, 1969; Zelazo, Zelazo, & Kolb, 1972).

We can reasonably conclude that the sight of actively moving parts of the body is essential to the development of visually coordinated movements of those parts. Moreover, depending on species, such perceptual-motor experience must likely occur over a relatively extended period of

time. This point for the human infant is stressed in the following argument by Bower (1966):

> The fact that infants will initially misreach has often been taken to show that they cannot perceive depth. If they can in fact perceive depth, the misreaching remains to be explained. A clue to an explanation is given by the fact that the most obvious change in an infant as he develops is a change in size. It seems likely that an infant who misreaches does so not because of poor depth perception but because he simply does not know how long his arm is. Since arm length is going to change drastically during development, it would be uneconomical— indeed, positively maladaptive—if the perceptual-motor system were geared at birth for a particular arm length. (P. 92)

This point is shared by others (e.g., Harris, 1965).

PERCEPTUAL ADAPTATION TO DISTORTED OPTICAL STIMULATION

A topic that is closely related to perceptual development is the modifiability of perception to systematically distorted optical stimulation. The concern here is with the consistent rearrangement or alteration in the relationship between the external environment and an organism's normal optical stimulation. A familiar example of this occurs to the novice wearer of corrective spectacles. The first day or two may be marked by visual distortion, perhaps motor disturbances such as inaccurately reaching or placing, or in general poorly executed visually guided motor activities. However, these problems soon disappear. It is likely that what follows is that the total visual system adjusts, compensates, or adapts to the initial distortion, and the world as viewed through the lenses appears normal again (indeed, there should be an overall gain in that the spectacles should aid the viewer's acuity). This general process of readjustment is referred to as adaptation, and in this context it concerns a form of learning or relearning.

There are several important reasons for studying the modifiability of the perceptual system. It is of obvious importance to examine the manner in which directional information given to the senses serves to guide spatial responses. However, some researchers have made note of the factors common to adaptation in the adult and the development of spatial coordination in the neonate. The point has been made (e.g., Kohler, 1964; Held & Hein, 1967; Held, 1968; Epstein & Shontz, 1971) that the manner in which the mature organism adapts to consistent spatial distortions basically recreates the ways in which perception normally develops in infancy. That is, the strategies that the adult employs to impose meaning on the experimentally distorted world match those processes that normally occur in infancy. If this argument is acceptable, then the study of adaptation to visual distortion provides an empirical means for studying certain features of perceptual development. Although it is an appealing comparison, it must be qualified in view of the fact that the perceptual capabilities of the adult are far more rich and complex than those of the infant. Any number of compensatory mechanisms and preestablished relationships that normally are available to the adult may be used for the adaptation process. This suggests that with optical distortions we may not be directly studying an original developmental process. However, with some reservations as to their generalizability, the findings that bear on perceptual adaptation do suggest a good deal about the organization of the visual system and may suggest some developmental trends.

An extensive and significant body of research has been performed using lens systems that impose between the eyes and the world. Generally, optical devices composed of inverting and displacing prisms that produce precisely controlled transformations of optical stimulation are used to observe changes in the viewer's response over time on specific activities. Although there are numerous precursors (e.g., Helmholtz, 1866) to this problem, we will begin with the widely cited experiments of Stratton (see Rock, 1966; Epstein, 1967; or Smith & Smith, 1962 for a general history). In 1896 George Stratton wore a specially designed optical system in front of one eye that produced an up-down inversion and a left-right reversal of the visual image. The subject, who in this case was also the experimenter, saw all objects transposed and upside down, as if the physical scene were rotated 180°. From a reading of his reports, there seems to have been initial marked disruption and disorientation of visual-motor coordination, but after several days he reported fleeting impressions of his visual world as normally oriented, and the tendency to deliberate and intentionally correct for movements decreased. With still longer experience with the displacing optical system, a greater degree of normalcy was reported (Stratton, 1897a,b). In general, there was a strong suggestion that he was making some sort of adaptation or adjustment to his new visual world although it is not clear from his account whether he began to "see" the world right side up or whether he only learned to adjust his behavior to a world that appeared upside-down. The conclusion that some adjustment was made, despite the maintenance of a retinally distorted image, is strengthened by the fact that removal of the system produced an aftereffect, in that the world appeared slightly distorted. In a general way these reports have been substantiated (Ewert, 1930; Snyder & Pronko, 1952). For example, Ivo Kohler (1962, 1964) reported from his study that adaptation to spatial inversion was good enough for the performance of complicated visual-motor activities such as skiing and bicycling. Although it is not clear whether a real change in perception occurs (i.e., the world appears reinverted or upright), an inverting optical system does offer a consistent and essentially intact source of information about the environment to the visual system, although in an altered form. On the basis of the foregoing, human observers, with sufficient experience, appear to perform the translation necessary to effect adjustment. The important question here is: What are the necessary conditions and variables that produce the translation? Before turning to some of the research performed with these optical systems, consider first a brief and relevant theoretical account of perceptual-motor integration. Many researchers have stressed the importance of active movements for effecting adaptation to optical distortions. Among the first to formulate a clear and firm hypothesis was Holst (1954). Basically Holst argued, on the basis of his observations and experiments with invertebrates and lower vertebrates, that a crucial component in gaining proper visual-motor coordination is the relation of self-produced movements of parts of the body to changes in the pattern of stimulation of the sense organs that these movements produce. He termed the changes in sensory stimulation consequent on self-produced movement *reafference* (afference refers to sensory input). That is, the sensory feedback stimulation that is dependent on self-produced movements—in which the organism makes and observes the results of his movements—is reafference. In distinction, stimulation of the sense organs produced only by changes in the external world were termed *exafference*. Exafferent and reafferent visual stimulation have different perceptual consequences even when they are optically equivalent. For an example of the distinction between exafference and reafference, consider the optically equivalent movements of the retinal image that results (if done with precision) by voluntarily moving the eye versus having the eye moved involuntarily, as in the case of applying pressure to the eye with the finger. In the former case the world appears stationary; in the latter, the world appears to move. A self-orienting animal must be capable of distinguishing between reafferent and exafferent

stimulation. This is accomplished by utilizing the information from the neural centers that control the movements of the parts of the body. (This distinction was also pointed out in Chapter 15.)

More to the point, in order to account for the organism's ability to distinguish exafference from reafference, Holst proposed that *efferent* impulses, which initiate movements, leave behind a centrally stored image or copy of the efference. The image, stored in the central nervous system, is called the *efference copy*. Thus, when the eye moves, an efference copy of the movement is available for comparison with reafference. Normally the reafference returns to the central nervous system and cancels the efference copy, with the result that the world does not appear to move as the eyes move. The critical distinction between the normal condition of reafference and the condition of exafference is that with exafference an efference copy is not available. That is, the exafference is unmatched by an efference copy. Accordingly, the ability of an organism to distinguish between stationary and moving objects when both produce identical optical stimulation is due to this difference.

Held (1961) extended Holst's hypothesis to explain adaptation phenomena and to include any motor system that can be the source of reafferent stimulation. The schematized process, shown in Figure 19.5, basically follows Holst with the addition of a *correlation storage* or memory component to take into account changes over time. The correlation storage may be thought of as a kind of memory in which traces of previous combinations of concurrent efferent and reafferent signals are retained. According to Held, the reafferent visual signal is compared (in the comparator) with a signal selected from the correlation storage by the monitored efferent signal. The currently monitored efferent signal is presumed to select from the correlation storage unit the trace combination containing the identical efferent part and to activate the corresponding reafferent trace combined with it. The resulting revived reafferent

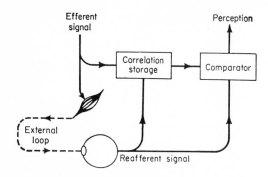

Fig. 19.5 *Schematized process assumed by Held to underlie the process of adaptation. (Source: Hein & Held, 1962. Reprinted by permission of Plenum Press.)*

signal is sent to the comparator for comparison with the current reafferent signal. The outcome of this determines perception and guides further performance.

Richard Held and his colleagues have persuasively applied this hypothesis to visual-motor adaptation in their laboratories and have designed a series of experiments that compare the effectiveness of self-produced movement with that of passive movement to a displaced visual input in adult humans (similar in many ways to the Held & Hein, 1963, carousel experiments with young kittens described earlier). Figure 19.6 shows a sketch of the apparatus that was used in several experiments on limb movements (Held & Hein, 1958; Held & Gottleib, 1958; Held & Schlank, 1959). In the apparatus the subject viewed the image of a square target reflected by a mirror. His pre- and postexposure tasks were to mark on a sheet of paper placed under the mirror the apparent position of the four corners of a square. Because of the interposition of the mirror the subject could see neither his marks nor his hand. After preexposure marking, the mirror and marking sheet were removed and substituted with a prism for the exposure task. The prism displaced the image of the hand by about 2.2 in (5.6 cm) to the right. The subjects were then assigned to one of three conditions: (*a*) no movement—the subject saw his stationary hand through the prism; (*b*)

passive movement (exafference)—the subject's arm was moved by the experimenter; and (*c*) active movement (reafference)—the subject saw his hand through the prism and also moved it from side to side. The results of the experimental manipula-

Fig. 19.6 *The apparatus, shown in A, was used to test subject's ability to guide his unseen hand to a visible target (T). The subject first marks the apparent location of the corners of the square as he sees them in the mirror (M). Notice that the subject's hand is under the mirror, and it is not visible during target markings. When the mirror is replaced by a prism (P), the subject sees his hand but not the target. The prism produces an apparent displacement of the hand as shown in B. (Source: Held & Gottlieb, 1958, p. 84.)*

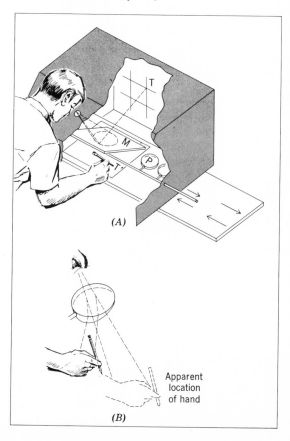

tions are best seen by comparing the target corner marking made before and after the prism exposure for the three conditions. As Figure 19.7 indicates, active movement only produced substantial compensatory shifts. These results mean that even though the eye receives the same visual input from active and passive conditions, the movement alone, without the connection between motor output and sensory input (i.e., the lack of self-produced movement with contingent reafferent stimulation), is not sufficient to produce adaptation. The active exposure had led to a change in the relationship between the visual location of the targets and the localizing movements made to touch them.

For movements of the entire body, a different experimental procedure was employed (Held & Bossom, 1961; see also Mikaelian & Held, 1964). The subject sat in a rotating chair in a darkened room and was required to position himself so that a luminous slit target was directly in front of him. After initial trials with *egocentric localization* (localization with regard to the position of one's own body rather than other objects), prism goggles were placed on the subject that produced an apparent displacement in the optical input of 11° to the left. The logic of the experiment was as

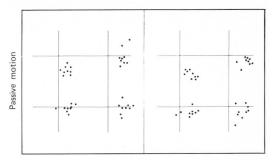

Fig. 19.7b *These marks were produced by subject whose hand was passively moved as he viewed it through the prism. The marks indicate no adaptation to the horizontal displacement of images produced by the prism viewing.*

follows: With proper experience and adaptation the subject should perceive the displaced retinal location as being straight ahead. It follows, then, that when tested after prism exposure on the egocentric localization task the adapted subject will shift his position 11° to the right of his original preexposure position. That is, the subject will perceive himself to be lined up with the

Fig. 19.7c *These marks were produced by a subject who performed active movements of his hand as he viewed it through the prism. The marks show a clear adaptation to the displacement of the images produced by prism viewing. (Reprinted with permission of publisher from Held, R., & Hein, A. V. "Adaptation of disarranged hand-eye coordination contingent upon re-afferent stimulation," Perceptual and Motor Skills, 1958, 8, 87–90.)*

Fig. 19.7 *The pre- and post-prism-exposure results on a corner marking task are given for three conditions of prism viewing shown in a, b, and c.*
Fig. 19.7a *Markings made by subject before and after looking through a prism as described in text. The subject kept his hand still while viewing it through the prism. Under this condition, no adaptation results.*

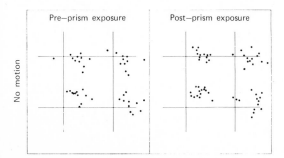

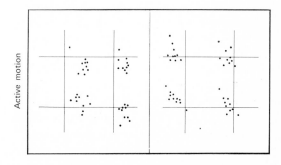

target when he is actually located 11° to its right. Two conditions of movement were employed during the exposure periods (which occurred on each of four days). Subjects in an active movement condition walked for an hour along an outdoor path; subjects in the passive condition sat in a wheelchair that was moved along the same path for the same duration. The results coincide with the previous experiments: Adaptation was significantly greater for the active subjects.

A related experiment indicated that adaptation can occur with a random scene, one that appears to be the same with or without prisms (Held & Rekosh, 1963). The apparatus consisted of a large drum that had an irregular array of small spots on its inside surface. The prisms used were wedge prisms, which result in the apparent curvature of normal surroundings. Before and after experimental exposure, each subject was tested for his perception of the straightness of a vertical line. During experimental exposure, each subject wore goggles that occluded the left eye and held a prism to the right one. Since the subject was instructed not to view any part of his body, his visual field contained only an array of spots. The active condition consisted of a half hour of walking inside the drum while viewing its surface. In the passive condition the subject viewed the surface while being wheeled around a similar path to the active condition for the same duration in a specially designed cart. Without exception the active subjects adapted to the displaced input whereas the passive subjects did not. What the active subjects then saw as a straight line was in fact a convex line. It appears that the presence of curved patterning in the visual field is not a necessary condition for generating adaptation. "Visual space can be warped solely as a result of transforming the relation between self-produced movement and its concurrent sensory feedback" (Held & Rekosh, 1963, p. 723).

Although the quality of the patterning may not be crucial, the distortion must be systematic. In other words, the causal link between actual movement and visual feedback, however

perturbed, must not be broken. If an arrangement is provided whereby signals from the motor system are made wholly independent of visual feedback, that is, *decorrelated* feedback, adaptation does not occur (Held & Freedman, 1963). Generally these are signs of environmental instability—for example, where muscular movements do not produce corresponding bodily movement (the astronaut in free flight on zero-gravity maneuvers), or passive bodily movements, produced entirely by external forces. Fortunately, under normal conditions of terrestrial life these events are rare.

Comparative studies

Adaptation to the rearrangements produced by optical displacement techniques has been shown for animals other than man. Foley (1940) reported that monkeys can adjust some of their movements after wearing an inverting lens for eight days. Similarly, Bossom and Hamilton (1963) found that monkeys could adapt to a 13° lateral visual displacement after two days. Cats have also been shown to adapt to optically displaced vision (Bishop: cited in Howard & Templeton, 1966). In contrast, negative results have been found with submammalian species. Hess (1956) fitted newly hatched experimental chicks with hoods containing prisms that displaced the visual field 7° laterally, right or left. In contrast to control animals (who viewed through a plain glass), the general course of pecking of the experimental animals remained inaccurately displaced—approximately 7° from the target. Moreover, there was little improvement in accuracy over four days of practice. The point stressed is that the chicks were not capable of adapting to a laterally displaced optical input. Similarly, Pfister (cited in Smith & Smith, 1962), using adult chickens fitted with left-right reversing prisms, reported that they also showed initial inaccuracy in pecking at grain and a subsequent lack of improvement with practice. Although not in complete agreement, other researchers (e.g.,

Moray & Jordan, 1967) have also indicated that chickens do not successfully adapt to a displaced optical input.

Of relevance to our discussion are studies that introduced spatial rearrangements by surgical modifications of the visual system. Sperry (1951), in one of a series of studies, inverted the eye of a frog. In one case, the eyeball was rotated through 180° and healed in this new position, producing a combined up-down inversion and front-back reversal. When tested for object localization, the frog reacted in the same manner as did humans with inverting lenses. As illustrated in Figure 19.8A, object movement in one direction was responded to with a head movement in the diametrically opposite direction, showing displacement in both the up-down and front-back dimensions. In other cases, the eyes were removed, interchanged, and then grafted into position on the opposite side of the head, producing either an up-down inversion or a front-back reversal. The frog's responses to these anatomical displacements are shown in Figure 19.8B and C. These inappropriate and obviously maladaptive responses (inappropriate to the physical environment, not to the visual image) persisted, uncorrected by experience.

These results suggest that there may be phylogenetic differences in adaptation in that not all species appear to benefit from systematic motor-sensory feedback. (See Taub, 1968, for a general discussion of the phylogenetic trends in adaptation to optical rearrangements.) Taub (1968) has argued that since a form of learning appears to be central to adaptation, then phylogenetic differences in the ability to adapt to optic displacements reflect phylogenetic differences in the ability to learn the necessary components for adaptation. In short, the phylogenetic locus for the possession of the kinds of learning abilities necessary for adaptation to systematic optical displacements are at or near the mammalian level.

There remain many open questions and general reservations about the direct role of active movement and reafference for adaptation. For example, what is learned when adaptations to optical distortions occur? Is the locus of adaptation visual or positional, central or peripheral (see Hardt, Held, & Steinback, 1971)? We must also note the report of studies in which passive subjects adapted to displacement (e.g., Pick & Hay, 1965; Kravitz & Wallach, 1966; Mack, 1967; Singer & Day, 1966; Templeton, Howard, & Lowman, 1966; Baily, 1972). Active movement may not, in all cases, be a necessary condition to effect adaptation. It may be that the adaptation that follows active movement is a matter of the total increased stimulation afforded to the active over the passive subject. Perhaps the passively moved subject has less motivation to engage in visual exploration; hence, he samples less of the full range of stimulation available to the active subject.

Although our main intention was to introduce the topic of adaptation as an issue pertinent to perceptual development, we must note that an issue as complex as this yields numerous alternative, though not necessarily incompatible, explanations (e.g., Taylor, 1962; Smith & Smith, 1962; Harris, 1965; Howard & Templeton, 1966; Day & Singer, 1967, and Ebenholtz, 1969). Rock (1966) offers the stimulating empiricist view that the relevant question to ask about adaptation to optically displaced vision is why the world appears distorted at all when first viewing through the distorting optical system:

> . . . there is good reason why the world ought not to appear distorted on first looking through the optical device, since the essential information conveyed by the retinal image would seem to remain intact (namely, relationships of components of the image to one another and to the self as object in the field). The explanation suggested as to why the world does appear distorted was that memories of the specific character of the normal retinal image have been established in the past and these memories influence

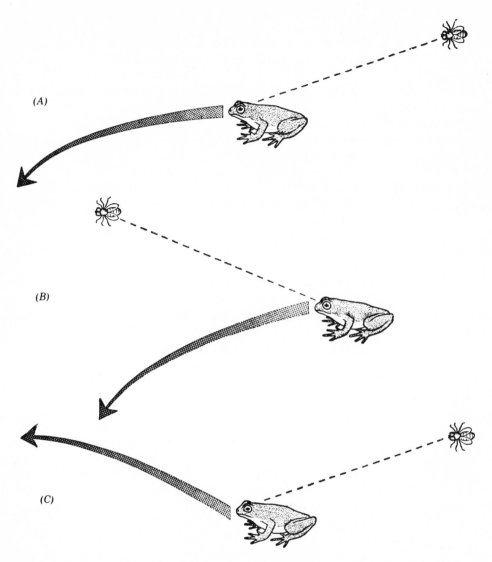

Fig. 19.8 *Errors in spatial localization of small objects following rotation and inversion of the eye. A: With eye rotated 180°, frog strikes at a point in the visual field diametrically opposite that at which the lure is actually located. B: After up–down inversion of the visual field frog strikes correctly with reference to the front–back dimensions of the visual field but inversely with reference to the up–down dimensions. C: After front–back inversion of the visual field, frog strikes correctly with reference to the up–down dimensions of the visual field, but inversely with reference to the front–back dimensions. (From R. W. Sperry, in Handbook of Experimental Psychology, edited by S. S. Stevens, Wiley, New York, 1951, p. 244. Reprinted by permission of the publisher.)*

what is now seen . . . the specific character of the retinal image becomes associated with information about spatial properties of the objects, and, thus, the former becomes a sign of the latter. (Pp. 268–269)

In this chapter we continued a discussion of perceptual development with the focus on the acquisition of perceptual-motor coordination and the development of accurate visually guided spatial locomotion. The studies reviewed on this matter employed a biased sensory input such as rearing animals lacking experience with visual stimulation concurrent with self-produced movement. It was noted that without such experience there is a deficiency in the development of visual-motor coordination and precise visually guided locomotor activity. The findings from a number of studies, employing various species including primates, suggest that if self-produced movement and visual stimulation are not properly integrated, deficiencies in perceptual-motor development result.

The topic of adaptation to systematically distorted optical stimulation was discussed. It was noted that the manner in which the adult organism adapts to consistent spatial distortions (e.g., as from viewing through distorting lens systems) may simulate the way in which perception normally develop in infancy. Research on this problem with humans indicates that so long as there is self-produced, active movement on the part of the organism there is a form of adaptation to the distorted optical input. However, this is not the case for all species, in that animals below the mammal do not appear to adapt to consistent optical displacements. Some reservations about the necessary role of active movement in adaptation was presented. There is controversy on this matter, and in general, the nature of adaptation to optical distortions is not fully understood.

The nature of time pervades many areas of intellectual thought, particularly literature, philosophy, physics, and biology. It follows that the perception of the duration of time as a subjective experience is of special interest to psychology. Of course, our main interest is not with the physicist's notion of time, but rather, with the duration of which one is aware. This subjective experience has been termed *protensity* (Woodrow, 1951) to distinguish it from physical duration. From the outset it should be clear that time perception is an oddity in that its variables are mental. There are no obvious sensory organs subserving it, nor any direct, observable source of cues that signify the subjective experience of time. Indeed, experienced time does not have the thing-like quality possessed by most experienced physical stimuli. Unlike space perception, time perception appears to be less directly dependent on sense experiences as such. Albert Einstein's query to Jean Piaget is appropriate here. Einstein had asked, "Is time immediate or derived? Is it integral with speed from the very outset?" Piaget's answer suggests that the notion of time is derived from the notions of speed and distance. He replied that ". . . the fundamental intuitions are those of distance and speed; time is gradually distinguished from these, but only insofar as the

two movements can be related to each other. . . ." (Piaget: cited in Fraisse, 1963). Although it is not fully clear whether the perception of time is a direct and immediate attribute of sensations emanating from the perception of (as yet, undefined) temporal stimuli or whether time is judged indirectly by means of some mental process, a number of authorities on time perception have stressed the latter concept (e.g., Gilliland, Hofeld, & Eckstrand, 1946; Woodrow, 1951; Fraisse, 1963; Ornstein, 1969). If it is not an immediately given property then ". . . time is a concept, somewhat like the value of pieces of money, that attaches to perception only through a judgmental process" (Woodrow, 1951, p. 1235).

Two main classes of explanations will be examined—the biological basis of time perception, and time perception as a function of cognitive processing. Of course, these classes are neither mutually exclusive nor exhaustive.

BIOLOGICAL BASIS OF TIME PERCEPTION

The cyclical nature of many bodily functions is well known. A clear-cut example in man is body temperature variation. There is about a 1.8° F difference in human temperature between the minimum at night and the maximum in the afternoon. In addition, for most animals many forms of behavior in some way reflect the cycle of day and night. The influence of the time of the day is obvious in many gross kinds of behavior such as general locomotor activity, the pattern of feeding and drinking, and in many other recurrent activities. Such activity patterns that regularly recur on a daily basis are termed *circadian rhythms* (from *circa*: about and *diem*: day, because the cycles approximate 24 hours) (for a general discussion of circadian rhythms for animal behavior, see Marler & Hamilton, 1966, Chapter 2; for human circadian rhythms, see Siegel, Gerathewohl, & Mohler, 1969). Many biological cycles show a direct dependence on natural physical events, especially daily and seasonal changes. The possession of a biological mechanism that varies bodily functions to certain temporally related environmental events offers a biological advantage to the organism, in that the internal rhythms react adaptively (e.g., bird roosting, hibernation) to periodic change (e.g., photic, thermal) in the environment (see Brown, 1972).

Understandably, a number of researchers have sought to find a chemical, neurological, or physiological mechanism in the nervous system that might serve as the workings of an internal biological clock or chronometer (Hoagland, 1933, 1935; Treisman, 1963; Holubář, 1969). According to this idea, biological time, as a matter of bodily functioning, determines experienced time. The concept of an internally directed time sense assumes that there exists some sort of automatic rhythm, occurring continuously in the body, and not easily or directly affected by environmental stimulation, with which the organism can compare the duration of stimuli or events. As noted there is evidence of the existence of biological rhythms in a number of species of animals. These rhythms may serve as the candidates for a time-measuring mechanism. For example, periodic phenomena with measurable frequencies are found in the electrical activity of the brain, pulse and heart beat, respiration, metabolic and endocrine function and general activity cycles (although many of these would not be good reference rhythms because they are markedly affected by external stimulation and hence can vary over wide ranges). Some of the internal processes have been the subject of research in time perception. In particular, the effect of temperature and metabolic processes have led to a theoretical account of time perception.

Hoagland's Hypothesis: the Biological Clock

An attempt at a theory based on an internal biological clock or chronometer was made by Hoagland (1933, 1935). It is reported that he began his work when his wife became ill and developed a fever. After she made a temporal misjudgment, he explored the possibility that her high temperature had affected her sense of time. Hoagland had her count to 60 at what she felt was a rate of one count per second. Relating this measure of her subjective minute to her oral temperature, he found the relationship between speed of counting and temperature shown in Figure 20.1. Specifically, he found that a subjective or judged minute

Fig. 20.1 *Representation of the dependence on body temperature of the estimated number of seconds in a timed minute. As temperature increases, fewer seconds are required for a subjective minute. (Based on data given in Hoagland, 1933.)*

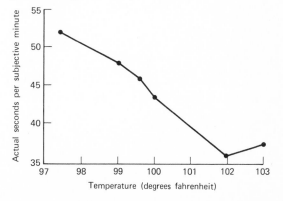

seemed shorter at the higher temperatures than at the lower ones. This suggested the existence of an inner clock, chemical chronometer, or pacemaker in the brain that controls the speed of the brain's metabolism and the rhythm of subjective time.

Hoagland was neither the only nor the first one to stress the effects of temperature on time perception. Pieron (see Cohen, 1964) suggested that if physiological processes are increased, subjective time will pass more rapidly. His pupil, M. Francois, put this to test by having some subjects tap a key at the rate of three times per second. When he raised their temperature, he found that they tapped faster. A number of studies have been performed since then in an attempt to explore the relationship between time perception and body temperature. Taken as a whole, the evidence is mixed and the results are difficult to interpret. Some researchers reported no clear-cut relationship between time perception and body temperature (Bell, C. R. & Provins, 1963; Bell, C. R., 1965; Lockhart, 1967). On the other hand, Thor (1962), Kleber, Lhamon, & Goldstone (1963), and Pfaff (1968), in basic agreement with Hoagland's notion that the internal clock accelerates when body temperature is raised, found that subjects overestimated the passage of physical time when body temperature was highest. As an interesting variation in the usual artificial employment of increased temperature (e.g., diathermy), Pfaff made use of the normal daily variations in body temperature during a 24-hour period.

Of course, it follows that time perception at reduced body temperature should have an opposite effect. Baddeley (1966) tested this with scuba divers in cold water (4° C) off the coast of Wales during cold March weather. In the test the subjects were asked to count (to themselves) to 60 at what they felt was a rate of 1 per sec (as did Hoagland with his wife). The results pertinent to our discussion are shown in Table 20.1. Clearly, the subjects were colder after the dive and, in agreement with Hoagland's notion, counted more slowly. (Notice that after diving the subjects required 70.44 sec in order to count to 60; hence, after their cold dive they underestimated the passage of physical time.)

Time Perception and the EEG

A different attempt to establish the existence of an internal measuring mechanism based on a biological rhythm is given by Holubář (1969). He argued that for the intervals of time most studied in the laboratory (seconds to minutes), the rhythmic activity of the brain could serve as the time-measuring pacemaker. Brain rhythms are autonomous, are not directly based on external stimulation, are of a comparatively consistent frequency, and do not affect metabolism or temperature. In particular, the alpha rhythm of the

Table 20.1

MEAN TEMPERATURE AND TIME-JUDGMENT BEFORE AND AFTER DIVING IN VERY COLD WATER[a]

	Oral temp. (°F)	Time judged as 1 min. (sec.)
Before diving	97.39	64.48
After diving	95.03	70.44[b]
Difference	2.36	−5.96

[a] Source: Baddeley, *American Journal of Psychology*, 1966, *79*, 475–479.
[b] Notice that after diving the subjects required 70.44 sec in order to count to 60, that is, they judged the passage of 70.44 sec to be equal to a minute. Thus, the lowered temperature produced an underestimation of time.

electroencephalogram (EEG), which assesses the electrical activity of the brain, is a sort of personal constant, not under external influences, and unchanging with age in adulthood.

An empirically interesting feature of brain rhythms is that although they are relatively immune from external influences, they can be substantially and quantitatively altered by optical stimulation of the eyes with interrupted or flickering light sources. This allowed for a test of Holubář's hypothesis that the sense of time varies with brain rhythms. The method of testing relied on Pavlovian conditioning techniques using a temporally conditioned reflex, the galvanic skin reflex (GSR), which is a measure of the change in the electrical resistance of the skin. The unconditioned stimulus was shock or loud sound (which produced a measurable GSR) that was repeatedly presented at regular intervals (30 sec). Following termination of the unconditioned stimulus, the GSR then appeared very accurately at the interval without any kind of external stimulus. A flickering light was introduced and simultaneous with GSR recordings electroencephalographic records were made. This permitted the determination of the specific effect of brain rhythms on the duration of GSR intervals. In brief, by introducing a flickering light of specified frequency the brain rhythm can be predictably altered. If the brain rhythms affect the time sense, it would show up by the manifestation of corresponding changes in the temporally conditioned interval. That is, the intervals between GSR occurrences would be altered. This would result in a psychobiological estimation of time perception.

The results from a series of experiments were that the specific effect on the temporally conditioned intervals is decisively dependent on the frequency of the flicker employed (hence dependent on the brain rhythm, since flicker alters the brain rhythm). Flicker of the frequency of the alpha rhythm (10 per second) did not affect the intervals of the GSR, nor did flicker frequencies of half (5 per second) and double (20 per second) the alpha frequency (see Table 20.2). However,

Table 20.2
EFFECT OF FLICKER ON THE INTERVALS BETWEEN TEMPORALLY CONDITIONED REFLEXES[a]

Frequency of flicker (c/sec)	Average interval (sec)
without flicker	29
5	26
7	14
10	27.5
14–15	15.5
20	23
continuous light	27

[a] Averages of the results for 4 subjects. Reprinted from the *Sense of Time* by J. Holubář, by permission of the MIT Press, Cambridge, Mass.

under the influence of frequencies that did not coincide with that of the alpha frequency, 7 and 14 to 15 per second, a decrease of the GSR intervals to about one half occurred. Holubář denotes these phenomena as the "rule of the octaves."

These findings led Holubář to conclude that "... rhythmic activity of the brain or a part of it could represent a fundamental reference rhythm which serves the organism in the measurement of time. Specifically, in man for times of the order of minutes it is the alpha rhythm, i.e., the most prominent human electroencephalographic rhythm of a frequency of about 10 per sec" (p. 83). Other sources have also implicated the alpha rhythm of the EEG to serve in some form as the basic unit of time experience. An interval of 0.1 sec, which is the phase length of the alpha rhythm (i.e., one cycle of the alpha is 0.1 sec)—referred to as the "perceptual instant" or "moment"—has been hypothesized as the basic interval unit in which all input information is integrated and processed (Stroud, 1956; White, C. T., 1963). It must be inserted, however, that the results from studies relating EEG activity to time perception are not clear-cut (see Ornstein, 1969, p. 28). For example, using very different techniques from those employed by Holubář, changes in time judgments were not matched by consistent changes in alpha frequency (Adam, Rosner, Hosick, & Clark, 1971).

As to neural correlates, Holubar is not specific on what part of the brain controls the timing of events. According to Dimond (1964), who reviewed the structural basis of time perception, including studies relevant to alpha activity, the prefrontal area of the cortex is the locus of the timing mechanism, that is, the comparison of temporally relevant information from the environment with the internal standard is performed in this area of the brain.

Drugs

There is evidence that a number of drugs influence the experience of time. Frankenhauser (1959) and Goldstone, Boardman, and Lhamon (1958) found that the administration of amphetamine lengthens time experience. In addition, Frankenhauser reported that caffein was similarly effective in lengthening time experience whereas pentobarbital, a sedative, was not. The latter effect of the shortening of time experience has also been observed with nitrous oxide (Steinberg, 1955) and other anesthetic gases (cyclopropane, ether, penthrane and ethrane) (Adam, Rosner, Hosick, & Clark, 1971). A general rule, according to Fraisse (1963) is that drugs that accelerate vital functions lead to an overestimation of time and those that slow them down have the reverse effect.

Among the most striking effects on time perception are those that occur with the administration of "psychedelic" drugs (marihuana, mescaline, psilocybin, LSD, etc.). Generally, these drugs produce a dramatic lengthening of perceived time duration relative to ordinary experience (e.g., Fisher, R., 1967; Weil, Zinberg, & Nelson, 1968). In the case of marihuana, this has also been demonstrated with the chimpanzee (Conrad, Elsmore, & Sodetz, 1972). However,

whether the psychedelics produce their effect directly by influencing an endogenous biological clock or indirectly by altering various bodily processes is not clear. Moreover, these drugs are assumed to increase awareness and alertness, which could also influence temporal experience. We will consider the implications of this point below.

COGNITIVE ASPECTS OF TIME PERCEPTION

A very different perspective of temporal experience has been taken by Ornstein (1969). He argues that the notion of an internal biological clock, whatever its locus, is of limited utility in encompassing the very diverse findings that exist on time perception. His view is that it is more economical and integrative to assume that the reported effects of psychedelic drugs on time perception are owing to their influence on cognitive rather than metabolic processes. Because they increase awareness and general mental activity, their administration could result in more information from the environment reaching consciousness. According to Ornstein, the reception of more information results in a greater perceived duration, which is in accord with the findings. However, Ornstein's notion extends beyond explaining the effects of drugs on time perception. In general, his fundamental concern lies with cognitive manipulations as opposed to endogenous bodily ones (e.g., temperature, EEG activity, etc.). To Ornstein, duration is considered as a dimension of experience. Indeed, he plausibly argues that it is difficult to maintain that an increase in the number of elements that fill an interval—which lengthens time experience—also speeds up some vaguely defined internal mechanism. In contrast, an increase in temperature, which produces the same lengthening effect on time perception, can reasonably be viewed as affecting cognitive processes.

Ornstein's basic premise is that the amount of information registered in consciousness and stored in memory determines the duration experience of a particular interval. Conceptually, he adopts an information-storage or memory approach to time perception, assuming that the perceived duration is constructed from the contents of mental storage. Relating his central theme to a computer metaphor with regard to the storage space of information, Ornstein comments:

> If information is input to a computer and instructions are given to store that information in a certain way, we can check the size of the array or the number of spaces or number of words necessary to store the input information. A more complex input would require a larger storage space than a simpler. An input composed of many varied items would similarly require more space than more homogeneous input. . . . In the storage of a given interval, either increasing the number of stored events or the complexity of those events will increase the size of storage, and as storage size increases the experience of duration lengthens. (P. 41)

Time perception described in this manner is quite amenable to an empirical examination. According to Ornstein, one would expect that an increase in the number of events occurring within a given interval, or an increase in the complexity of these events, or a reduction in efficiency in the way events are coded and stored would each lengthen the experience of duration of that interval. Ornstein has performed a series of experiments directed toward an examination of these expectations. He substantiated the findings that duration experience is a function of the number of occurrences in a given interval. He presented the subjects with three tape recordings, each of the same physical time (9 min, 20 sec), that had sounds (500 Hz tones) that occurred at the rate of 40, 80, or 120 per minute. As expected, increasing the number of stimuli within an interval produced the perception of lengthened duration. The 40 tones

per minute tape was judged shorter than the 80 tones per minute tape, and both were judged shorter than the 120 tones per minute tape. These results also have been confirmed within the visual (Mescavage, Heimer, Tatz, & Runyon, 1971; Mo, 1971) and tactual modalities (Buffardi, 1971). That is, durations with more elements were judged longer than durations with fewer elements.

In an offhanded way the results of these experiments apply to the situation where one is anxiously waiting for an event to occur, e.g., the receipt of a letter, a person's arrival, or the results of one's test performance. The lengthening of time experience is attributed to the effects of anticipation or expectation. Expectancy reasonably leads to an increased vigilance with the effect that there is a greater amount of "awareness of input" and consequently a lengthening of perceived duration (Ornstein, 1969): "A watched pot never boils." Consistent with this is the finding that anxiety induced by the expectation of electric shock also produces an increase in perceived duration (Falk & Bindra, 1954).

To test the effects of varying the complexity of a stimulus on time perception, Ornstein graded a series of stimulus figures on a complexity scale based on the number of interior angles (see Figure 20.2). Each stimulus was shown for 30 sec and the task was to judge the duration of the exposure interval. A magnitude estimation task was used in which the standard stimulus (shown in bottom right of Figure 20.2) was always shown first and the subject judged the duration intervals of the other stimulus figures relative to the perceived duration of the standard. The results are summarized in Table 20.3, which gives the ratio of the duration of each stimulus figure divided by the duration of the standard. In general, the less complex stimuli, stimuli 1 and 2, were judged shorter in duration than the standard, but stimuli 3, 4, and 5 were judged about equal in duration to the standard. It appears that as the complexity of a stimulus increased up to a

Stimulus 1   Stimulus 2

Stimulus 3

Stimulus 4

Stimulus 5

Standard

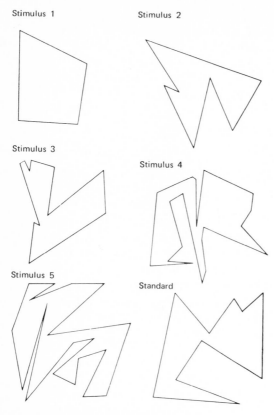

Fig. 20.2 *Stimuli of various complexity used in experiment by Ornstein. (Source: Ornstein, 1969, p. 60. Reprinted by permission of Penguin Books, Ltd.)*

limiting point, duration experience lengthened, and that further increases in complexity above that point no longer produced increases in perceived duration.

Further experiments examined the effect of

Table 20.3
RESULTS OF COMPLEXITY EXPERIMENT[a]

Stimulus	1	2	3	4	5
Duration ratio	0.81	0.92	0.99	0.96	0.97

[a] The values given are ratios of the duration for each stimulus figure divided by the duration of the standard. Source: Ornstein, 1969, p. 61. Reprinted by permission of Penguin Books, Ltd.

varying the complexity of a series of stimuli in order to manipulate the facility of coding the information. Two tapes, an "easily codible" and a "random" one, each of 5 min total duration were used. Each tape had the same total stimulus information, a series of 10 different sounds (e.g., a typewriter key striking the roller, tearing paper) presented 20 times each. On the easily codible tape the sounds were presented in an orderly fashion; each sound was played and repeated for 20 times. In contrast, the different sounds were randomly distributed on the random tape. Each subject heard the two tapes and then compared the perceived duration of one tape with the other. The overall result was that the duration of the random tape was judged on the average to be 1.33 times as long as the duration of the easily codible tape. Similar results were obtained, from essentially the same procedures, with visual stimuli (see Schiffman & Bobko, 1974). These results, according to Ornstein, suggest that an increase in complexity of the stimulus input produces an increase in perceived duration. Consistent with this is the report that time estimations are longer for more complex melodies than for simpler ones (Yeager, 1969).

Ornstein also explored the effect of some procedures that affect the processing and coding of information on duration experience. According to his notion, the perceived duration of an interval that involves the performance of a task will be shortened when the task is well practiced or familiar. In his words, ". . . a person who could respond 'automatically' to the situation would be aware of less of the stimulus array and should then experience less duration than one who could not respond in the same way" (p. 74). In one experiment he had subjects work on a simple motor task (pursuit rotor), one on which a subject could easily achieve a high degree of proficiency. All subjects worked on the motor task for 2 min after which they judged its duration. In addition there were three conditions which manipulated the experience immediately prior to the 2 minute task. In one condition the 2-min task was preceded by an additional 7 min of prior practice on the same task; a second condition allowed no other prior practice; and in a third condition the 2-min task was preceded by 7 min on an irrelevant motor task (mirror drawing). According to expectation, the subjects in the first condition, who had a good deal of practice on a simple motor task, should be aware of less of the stimulus array on that task, and thereby perceive an interval of less duration. The findings supported this: The interval of the well-practiced task was perceived as shorter than either an interval preceded by no practice or one with irrelevant practice.

In order to explore the possibility that modification of the experience of duration depends not only on the amount of input information registered but on aspects of its storage (the way the information is coded and stored) as well, a series of experiments was employed that altered the contents of storage *after* the input was registered. The following is an example. A learning task was used in which words were paired with either harsh or neutral sounds. The subject's learning task was to learn which sound went with which word. First he would hear the sounds paired with the words. Then he would hear a sound from a tape recorder, and he would have to say the appropriate word before it was also sounded. The task required seven trials that took 6 min. The temporal response utilized for assessing time perception was the estimate of the duration of the learning task. Preliminary testing indicated that words paired with harsh sounds are forgotten more quickly than words paired with neutral sounds, but neither affects initial learning time. Thus, in this experiment duration experience was investigated as a function of the amount of the information retained with the amount of input information held constant. Four groups in all were used. Half of the subjects initially heard words preceded by harsh sounds and half heard words preceded by neutral sounds. In addition, half of each of these groups estimated the duration of the learning interval immediately

after learning the task, and the other half did this two weeks later. The results were that there was no difference in the time perception of the duration of the learning interval for harsh or neutral words when assessed immediately after performance of the task. However, after two weeks elapsed the number of harsh words retained and the perceived duration of the original learning task for the harsh word group was less than for the neutral word group. According to Ornstein, during the two-week interval items dropped out of storage and as they did, the experience of duration correspondingly decreased. This experiment, along with further research, confirmed that a crucial determinant of perceived duration is the way in which information is coded and stored. These experiments could be extended to explain the common experience that pleasant or interesting events are likely to be regarded in retrospect as being longer than they were in passing. Following the previous experiment, the reason is that these sorts of events are better retained than ordinary events; hence, compared to ordinary events, they will seem longer.

Before turning from Ornstein's information-storage approach to time perception, we should note that although his is not the first to deal with temporal experience as a cognitive phenomenon (e.g., see Gilliland, Hofeld, & Eckstrand, 1946; Michon, 1966; Kristofferson, 1967), and although this approach does not explain all the phenomena of time perception, it does serve rather well to integrate a broad spectrum of findings into a very useful and general scheme (see also Allan & Kristofferson, 1974; Eisler, 1975).

Biological Versus Cognitive Basis of Time Perception

To review, there appears to be some kind of relationship between bodily activity and a time sense. Similarly, the time perception of complex events has been shown to be under cognitive influences. How are we to resolve the obvious discrepancy between the two classes of explanations?

It should be pointed out that the sorts of temporal experiences and responses assessed by experiments that support an internal biological clock basis of time perception are of a very different nature from those employed in experiments supporting an explanation of time perception based on cognitive processes. The biological clock type of experiment often employs relatively brief intervals and utilizes response measures such as the rate of tapping. Perhaps the perception of short intervals makes use of a very different psychological process from that employed in the perception of longer intervals of time. It may be that with brief intervals attention can be focused primarily on the interval itself and can reflect physiological rhythms, whereas for longer durations judgments must rely on indirect cues such as the number and kind of activities. If this is the case, then two classes of explanations may be drawn upon: The internal biological explanation of time perception can most usefully be applied to the perception of short intervals, whereas longer intervals, necessarily perceived less directly and with greater reference to external events, fall under a cognitive explanation.

TIME PERCEPTION AND SPATIAL EVENTS: THE *TAU-* AND *KAPPA-* EFFECT

A close interrelationship between experienced time and certain activities exists in that each can influence the other. Helson and King (1931) demonstrated that an observer's comparative perception of two tactual distances is influenced by the magnitudes of the temporal intervals associated with them: The greater the temporal intervals, the greater the experienced distance. This relationship between duration and distance is termed the *tau*-effect. Consider the following as an example of the *tau*-effect: If three equidistant points on the forearm of a subject are

stimulated (e.g., forming a tactual equilateral triangle) and the interval of time between stimulation of the first and the second point is greater than that between the first and third, the subject will perceive the distance between the first and second points as being greater than that between the first and third (see Figure 20.3). In other words, if an observer is judging two equal distances, that distance that is delimited by the longer interval of time will appear to be longer. A similar effect has been demonstrated in vision (Abbe, 1937).

A converse effect, in which time perception is influenced by the manipulation of distance, has also been identified and termed the *kappa*-effect (Cohen, J., Hansel, & Sylvester, 1953, 1955). Consider two equal temporal intervals defined by the onset of three successive stimuli (e.g., three lights arranged in a row as in Figure 20.4). If the distance between the first and second stimulus is

Fig. 20.3 *The tau effect. Three equidistant points are stimulated on the forearm. If the interval of time between stimulating points A and B is greater than that between A and C, then the distance between A and B will be perceived as greater than between A and C. Thus, relative time differences can affect the perception of distance.*

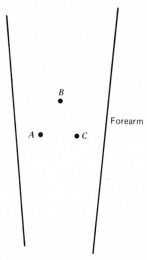

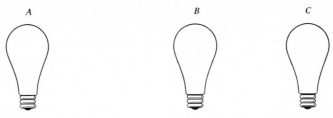

Fig. 20.4   *The kappa effect. The three lights, A, B, and C, are successively flashed at equal temporal intervals. If the distance between lights A and B is greater than between B and C, then the interval of time between the flashing of lights A and B will be perceived as longer than the interval between B and C. Thus, the relative distance between stimuli can affect the perception of time.*

greater than that between the second and third, the first interval will be perceived as being longer in duration. This has also been shown with audition (Cohen, J., Hansel & Sylvester, 1954) and with touch (Suto, 1955). It has been suggested by Suto (1955) that the influence of space or distance on time experience, when demonstrated by touch, is due to the accompaniment of touch stimulation with visual imagery. He found that subjects who had been blind since early childhood did not manifest the *kappa*-effect with touch. Since the blind do not spatialize the points of stimulation, their perception of time will not vary with the distance between stimuli.

A final point: Many matters of procedural importance have been simplified in this presentation of time perception. For example, we have not dwelled on what response features characterize underestimations or overestimations of physical duration (see Bindra & Waksberg, 1956), nor have we discussed the accuracy, reliability and implications of the various response modes used for assessing time perception (e.g., Doehring, 1961; Underwood, 1966, Chap. 2; Hornstein & Rotter, 1969; Adam, 1971). Since a thorough discussion of these matters lies beyond the province of this book it should be emphasized that manifold methodological problems complicate a clear understanding of the phenomena of time perception at this stage of knowledge.

In this chapter we have examined the perception of time or protensity. Two main classes of explanations were reviewed. A biological approach to time perception is founded on the cyclical nature of many bodily functions and processes, such as temperature variation, electrical activity of the brain, and general metabolic activities. The assumption made by its proponents is that there is some internal biological clock that controls the speed of metabolic processes and subjective time. It was noted that the findings bearing on this approach are equivocal.

A second explanation contends that time perception is a function of the kind and degree of cognitive processing. According to the general form of this notion, perceived duration is constructed from the contents of mental storage. Thus, the amount of information registered in consciousness and stored in memory determines the duration experience for a particular time interval. It was noted that for the present a cognitive approach to explaining time perception serves as a useful scheme encompassing a broad range of findings.

Finally, the relation of time perception to spatial events was outlined: The *tau*-effect refers to the effect of duration on perceived distance; the *kappa*-effect refers to the effect of physical distance on perceived duration.

Glossary

Absolute Threshold
The least amount of physical intensity of a stimulus required for its detection.

Accomodation
The variable refractive capacity of the lens that brings an image into sharp focus on the retinal surface.

Achromatic
Lacking color.

Achromatism
Total color blindness.

Acuity
The ability to detect, resolve, and perceive fine details of a visual display.

Acupuncture
An ancient Chinese medicinal practice of therapy for the general treatment of disease and control of pain. Acupuncture involves inserting needles into the body at precise loci.

Adaptation
(1) Relative loss in sensitivity or increase in threshold due to prolonged or repeated stimulation.
(2) The process of adjustment to the change in the conditions of lighting, i.e., dark or light adaptation.
In general, adaptation refers to a reversible change in the state of an organism due to the effects of environmental events.

Adaptation Level
A psychophysical concept devised by Harry Helson. It holds that judgments of certain stimulus attributes are made in terms of a subjective scale or standard value. The subjective level established by the observer as a standard is termed the adaptation level or AL.

Adaptation-Produced Potentiation
The effect of imparting a particular taste to water because of adaptation to the taste of certain chemical substances.

Additive Color Mixture
Mixtures in which the addition of the excitations produced by different wavelengths produces a specific chromatic sensation.

Aerial Perspective
A depth or distance cue in which objects whose retinal images are sharp or distinct appear closer than those whose images are blurry or otherwise indistinct.

Afferent Impulses
Neural excitations toward the brain—sensory input.

Afterimage
Sensory effect following termination of a light

stimulus. A negative afterimage is the visual sensation in which the hue and brightness of the original stimulus is reversed, e.g., yellow is the apparent hue after staring at a blue hue. Positive afterimages are rarer and are sensations of the same apparent hue and brightness as the original stimulus.

Air-Righting Reflex
The tendency of some mammals to right themselves during a fall and land upright.

Albedo
A surface property that refers to the proportion of incident light that is reflected. Also known as reflectance.

Alpha Rhythm
Brain wave frequency of 8 to 12 Hz. Alpha rhythms predominate when the body is awake but relaxed, and the eyes are closed.

Ambiguous Figures
Figures with inherent depth characteristics that may be ambiguously perceived with respect to their principle spatial orientation.

Ames Illusion
A set of demonstrations devised by Adelbert Ames and used by Transactionalists to indicate the significance of experience in organized perception.

Amplitude
The extent of displacement of vibrations in either direction from the position of rest.

Ampulla
Basal portion of the semicircular canal that contains the vestibular receptors.

Anaglyph
A form of stereo figure that is produced by printing the two patterns of the visual stereo stimuli on top of each other in different inks to produce a composite picture. When viewed through the proper filters that enable each eye to sort out a single pattern, a stereo depth effect is perceived.

Analgesic
An agent, usually chemical, for reducing the sensation of pain.

Aniseikonia
An optical anomaly in which the image in one eye is larger than that in the other, resulting in a significant disparity between the images in each eye.

Anisotropy
The change in the appearance of targets when viewed from different spatial orientations.

Anomalous Trichromatism
Defect in color vision in which a different proportion of the three primary colors than normal are needed in order to match the colors of the spectrum.

Anomaloscope
A special kind of color mixer that measures the proportions of red and green necessary to match a yellow.

Anosmia
Insensitivity to odors.

Apparent Movement
The perception of movement from a stationary stimulus.

Aqueous Humor
Gelatinous fluid between the cornea and the lens.

Astigmatism
Optic defect in which the corneal surface is not spherical.

Audio Analgesia
Certain forms and conditions of stimulation of the auditory system that reduce the sensation of pain.

Audiogram
A graph that shows hearing loss, in decibels, for pure tones as a function of frequency.

Auditory Canal
The air-filled passage from the outer ear to the ear drum or tympanic membrane.

Auditory Fatigue
The elevation in the auditory threshold after the termination of a masking tone. Also called sound-induced hearing loss and adaptation.

Auditory Masking

The rise in the threshold of one tone in the presence of a second, masking tone.

Auditory Nerve

The eighth cranial nerve. It contains the fibers from the cochlea and extends to the auditory cortex.

Autokinetic Movement

The phenomenon of apparent motion of a stationary point of light in an otherwise darkened environment.

Autonomic Nervous System

The branch of the nervous system that innervates the smooth muscles and the glands. It is divided into the sympathetic and parasympathetic systems.

Average Error, Method Of

A psychophysical technique for determining thresholds and constant errors, in which the observer manipulates a variable stimulus in relation to a standard. The mean of a number of responses is generally taken as the most representative threshold value.

Axon

Portion of the neuron or nerve cell that conducts impulses away from the cell body to adjacent neurons or to a gland or muscle.

Backward Masking

The impairment to the perception of a target stimulus by the presentation of a closely following second masking stimulus.

Basilar Membrane

A membrane upon which lies the organ of Corti.

Beat

The perception of a single throbbing tone of a single pitch, periodically varying in loudness. Beats can result from the simultaneous occurrence of two tones that are of similar intensity but slightly different in frequency.

Beta Rhythm

Brain-wave pattern of about 25 Hz, characteristic of brain waves during waking.

Bezold-Brücke Effect

The sensory effect in which the perception of long wavelength light apparently shifts toward yellow and short wavelength light shifts toward blue, with an increase in intensity.

Bilateral Symmetry

The characteristic of many organisms to have similar parts or shapes on both sides of the body.

Binaural

Involving both ears.

Binocular

Involving two eyes.

Binocular Depth Cues

Cues to the perception of depth and distance that require the use of both eyes.

Binocular Fusion

The perceptual fusion of the images presented to each eye.

Binocular Parallax or Disparity

The difference in the two retinal images that provides a strong impression of depth and three-dimensionality of space. Also termed *retinal disparity*.

Binocular Rivalry

The phenomenon that occurs when each eye is presented with different stimuli. When binocular rivalry occurs, at one moment the stimuli from one eye may be dominant with a suppression of the stimuli from the other eye.

Biological Clock

A hypothesized internal clock or chronometer in the brain that controls the speed of metabolism and the rhythm of subjective time.

Biological Motion

The perception of the pattern of movement produced by locomoting humans. These forms of motion have been labeled *biological motion* by G. Johansson.

Bipolar Cell

Cells in the intermediate retinal layer that transmit impulses from the receptors to the ganglion cells.

Blind Spot

The region of the visual field that is reflected upon the optic nerve fibers (optic disc) exiting from the eyeball. No photoreceptors lie at this region and, accordingly, the viewer cannot perceive this part of the visual field.

Bloch's Law

Stimulus intensity (I) and exposure time (T) of a stimulus bear a reciprocal relation for a constant threshold value. That is, $I \times T = $ a constant threshold value. Also known as the *Bunsen-Roscoe Law*.

Border Contrast

Subjective contrast enhancement that occurs at contours.

Bone Conduction

Process by which sound is conducted to the cochlea of the inner ear through the cranial bones, rather than by the usual conduction structures.

Brain Asymmetry

Different hemispheres of the brain predominate in the perception of certain broad characteristics of a tone.

Brightness

One of the basic psychological dimensions of light. It varies primarily with physical intensity.

Brightness Constancy

The tendency to perceive the brightness of an object as relatively unchanging despite changes in the physical energy reflected by the object to the eye.

Bunsen-Roscoe Law

Within certain limits, the threshold response to a visual stimulus is a product of its intensity (I) and exposure duration (T). That is, $T \times I = $ a constant threshold value. Also known as *Bloch's Law*.

Cataract

An opacity of the lens of the eye resulting in impaired vision.

Causalgia

A severe and prolonged burning pain produced by a lesion in peripheral nerves.

Central Tendency

The score around which most scores cluster in a frequency distribution.

Cerebellum

A brain structure that functions in bodily equilibrium and motor coordination.

Cerebral Dominance

The relative dominance of one side of the brain over the other for certain perceptual processes.

Cerebral Hemisphere

The halves of the forebrain connected by the corpus callosum.

Cerebrum

The largest part of the brain, divided into the two hemispheres connected by commissures. It serves in the activity of sensory, motor, and cognitive processes.

Chorda Tympani

Branch of the facial nerve that serves the front part of the tongue.

Choroid Coat

The middle layer of the wall of the eye that is opaque, thus preventing stray light from activating the photoreceptors. It consists of blood vessels and provides a major source of nutrition for the eye.

Chromatic Aberration

Distortion of chromatic retinal images by the lens due to greater refraction of short wavelengths than of long ones.

Ciliary Muscle

Muscle that changes the shape or curvature of the lens and effects accommodation.

Circadian Rhythms

Activity patterns that occur regularly on a daily basis.

Closure

A Gestalt principle of perceptual organization; it is a tendency to "fill in" gaps in the structure of a figure or form so that it appears complete or closed.

Cochlea

Spiral-shaped portion of the inner ear containing the receptive elements (transducers), which convert sound to neural activity.

Cochlear Canal (or Duct)

Middle canal of cochlea of inner ear. It contains the organ of Corti. Also called the *scala media*.

Cognitive Masking

An inhibitory effect on the detectability of a figure due to the presence of an emotional stimulus.

Cold Spot

Region of the skin particulary sensitive to cold stimulation.

Color Circle

An arrangement of the hues around the perimeter of a circle used to specify the relation among hues and saturations. Hues are arranged around the perimeter of the circle, and saturation extends from the center to the perimeter of the circle.

Color Memory

The effect of past experience on apparent color.

Color Solid

A three-dimensional model used to show the relation among hues, brightness, and saturation. Hues are located around the perimeter, saturation from the center to the perimeter, and brightness is arranged from top to bottom.

Commissures

The neural connections between the two hemispheres of the brain.

Complementary Colors

The hues of two colors which, when mixed in the correct proportions, yield a chromatic gray or white. Complementary colors lie opposite each other on the color circle.

Conditioned Stimulus (CS)

The initially neutral stimulus in a conditioning experiment that becomes associated with the reinforcement.

Conduction Deafness

Deficiency in hearing due to a defect in the conduction mechanism of the auditory system. Hearing loss is distributed about equally over all frequencies.

Cone

Photoreceptor cell of retina that functions in color vision and acuity. Such cells are most dense in the fovea and relatively absent in the periphery of the retina. There are approximately 6 to 8 million cones in the retina.

Congenital

Existing at or from birth.

Consonance

In audition, those combinations of tones that appear to blend well together and sound pleasant together.

Constancy, Object

The tendency of an object to be perceived as invariant regardless of changes in its retinal image produced by changes of orientation, distance, and intensity relative to a viewer.

Constant Error

A systematic error in judgment in which one stimulus tends to be either overestimated or underestimated relative to another.

Constant Stimuli, Method of

A psychophysical method employed for establishing thresholds. Each of a limited number of stimuli is presented repeatedly, and the degree to which each one elicits a sensation is used to determine the threshold value. Generally the stimulus value yielding a detection response 50% of the time is accepted as an approximation of the absolute threshold.

Contour

A dividing line separating one part of a perceptual field from adjacent parts.

Contralateral

Opposite side.

Convergence

The tendency of the eyes to turn toward each other in a coordinated action to fixate on targets located nearby. .

Cornea

The transparent outer surface of the sclerotic coat lying in front of the lens.

Corpus Callosum

The largest commissure connecting the two hemispheres of the brain.

Cortex

Neural tissue covering most of the external surface of the brain.

Crista

The base of the cupula of the semicircular canal that registers rotary movement.

Criterion

The stimulus magnitude at and above which an observer will report a stimulus present in a signal detection experiment.

Critical Fusion Frequency (CFF)

The minimum frequency of intermittent light stimulation necessary for it to be perceived as continuous.

Cross-Adaptation

The effect in which adaptation to one odorant affects the threshold or sensitivity to another odorant.

Cupula

Tongue-shaped protuberance lying within the ampulla of a semicircular canal.

Cutaneous Sensations

Sensations obtained by stimulation of the skin: such sensations are labeled pressure or touch, warmth, cold, and pain.

Cyclopean Perception

A form of stereo viewing devised by Bela Julesz based on the idea that the image on each eye is combined and synthesized in a central visual area of the brain to produce the perception of depth.

Dark Adaptation

Increase in sensitivity of the eye during the change from high to low levels of lighting.

Decibel (*db*)

One-tenth of a bel. One bel is the common logarithm of the ratio between two intensities or energies:

$$(\log_{10}\frac{p_1^{\ 2}}{p_2^{\ 2}}).$$

It is used to specify the amplitude or intensity of a sound wave.

Dendrite

Neural cellular unit that radiates from the neuron cell body and receive and transmit impulses to it.

Density

A tonal quality that refers to the compactness or tightness of a sound. Generally greater density occurs with higher frequency tones.

Dermal Optical Perception (DOP)

A form of vision in which light is assumed to be sensed through the skin.

Detection Acuity

The acuity task of detecting the presence of a target stimulus in the visual field.

Deuteranopia

Color weakness characterized by the inability to distinguish between reds and greens and a relative insensitivity to those wavelengths that appear green to normal viewers.

Dichorhinic

Stimulation with a different odorant to each nostril.

Dichotic

The condition in which each ear hears a different sound or message at the same time.

Dichromat

Color-vision defective person who matches all wavelengths of the spectrum with two rather than three colors.

Difference Tone

The sound of a difference tone has the pitch that corresponds to the frequency difference of two primary tones simultaneously sounded.

Differential Threshold

The amount of change in stimulus magnitude

of a given level of stimulation in order for a change to be detected. Also known as the *difference limen* or *just noticeable difference (jnd)*.

Diopter

The unit of refractive power of a lens. A lens with a focal length of one meter is designated as having the refractive power of one diopter. The refractive power of a lens is expressed as the reciprocal of its focal length, in meters.

Diotic

The condition in which the same tonal stimulation is applied to both ears simultaneously.

Diplopia

"Double vision" occurring when the movements of both eyes are not coordinated.

Dirhinic

Stimulation by an odorant applied to the two nostrils simultaneously.

Displacusis

An abnormality of hearing in which a simple tone is perceived as different in pitch by the two ears.

Dissonance

In audition, those combinations of tones that sound discordant or harsh when sounded together.

Doctrine of Specific Nerve Energies

Treatise of Johannes Mueller (1826) that states that the sensation elicited by a stimulus depends primarily on the nerve excited and secondarily on the stimulus itself; that is, nerves are specific to sensations.

Doppler Shift

A change in the frequency and pitch of a moving sound source relative to a stationary listener.

Dyne Per Square Centimeter (Dynes/cm^2)

Equivalent to a microbar. They are both units of pressure. Ten dynes/cm^2 equals one N/m^2 (Newtons per square meter).

Echolocation

The use of self-produced echoes to gain location information.

Efferent Impulses

Neural excitation away from the brain. Such excitations as initiating movements are examples of efferent impulse activity.

Egocentric Localization

Judging the direction of targets with reference to oneself rather than to external stimuli.

Eikonogenic Eye

Image-forming eye.

Electroencephalogram (EEG)

A measure of the electrical activity of the brain.

Elevation

A depth or distance cue in which objects appearing higher in the visual field are perceived as being farther away from the viewer than those lower in the visual field.

Emmert's Law

The apparent size of an afterimage is directly related to the apparent distance of the surface on which it is perceived.

Emmetropic Eye

Optically normal lens of the eye.

Empiricism

The view that perceptual organization is based primarily on past experience.

Environmental Orientation

The orientation of a shape with respect to gravity and to the visual frame of reference.

Equidistance Tendency

In the absence of effective distance cues there is a tendency for objects in the visual field to appear equally distant to the viewer. The strength of this tendency increases as the objects are laterally brought closer to each other in the frontal plane of the visual field.

Eustachian Tube

Tube that connects the middle ear chamber with the back of the mouth. The tube permits pressure from the outside to be equalized with air pressure in the middle ear. This is accomplished when the mouth is opened.

Exafference
Stimulation of the sense organs produced only by changes in the external world.

Extraocular Muscles
The set of muscles that control the movement of the eyeball.

Eye-Head Movement System
The system of movement perception in which the eyes track a moving stimulus.

False Alarm
Reporting the stimulus as present on a trial of a psychophysical experiment when it is not actually present. Also called *false positive*.

Feature-Specific Detectors
The presumed specific neural detectors or channels for different features of stimulation, features such as shape, movement, orientation, or color.

Fechner's Law
General law proposed by Gustav Fechner (1860) which states that the magnitude of a sensation is a logarithmic function of the stimulus.

Figural Aftereffect
Distortion effect after prolonged exposure to a given stimulus pattern or form that occurs when a new stimulus form falls on the same or nearby retinal region.

Figure-Ground
The tendency to perceive a portion of a stimulus configuration as a figure set apart from the background.

Focal Length
The distance between a lens and the sharp image it forms of a very distant object.

Foot-Candle (ft-c)
English unit of illuminance. One foot-candle is defined as the illumination received on a surface one foot square located one foot from a standard candle.

Foot-Lambert (ft-L)
English unit of luminance defined as the total amount of light emitted in all directions from a perfectly reflecting and diffusing surface receiving one foot-candle of light.

Formant
The concentration of acoustic energy that appears in spectrograms.

Forward Masking
The impairment to the perception of a target stimulus due to a preceding masking stimulus.

Fourier Analysis
The breakdown of a complex waveform into its component simple sign waves based on the mathematical theorem devised by the nineteenth century French scientist, Jean Baptiste Fourier.

Fovea
The central region of the retina. It is a small indentation about 0.3 mm across, subtending a visual angle of 1° to 2°. The fovea contains primarily cone photoreceptors.

Free Nerve Endings
Unspecialized appearing sensory neural receptors profusely distributed throughout the body.

Frequency
A characterization of sound waves by the number of cycles or pressure changes completed in a second.

Frequency Modulations
Changes in the frequency of a continuously vibrating body.

Frequency Theory
Theory that the basilar membrane vibrates as a whole to the frequency of the sound wave, thereby reproducing the vibrations of the sound. Pitch is thus determined by the frequency of impulses traveling up the auditory nerve, that is, it is directly determined by the frequency of the sound wave. Also known as the *telephone* or *periodicity theory*.

Fundamental Tone
The lowest tone of the series of tones produced by a sound-emitting instrument. It is also called the *first harmonic*.

Galvanic Skin Response (GSR)
A measure of the change in the electrical resistance of the skin.

Ganglion Cells
Intermediate layer of neurons of the retina whose axons form the optic nerve.

Ganzfeld
A completely textureless and homogeneous field of uniform brightness.

Gate Control Theory of Pain
Theory of pain that focuses on the afferent nerve impulse transmission from the skin to the spinal cord.

General Constancy Theory
Theory proposed by R. H. Day that states that if any of the traditional stimulus cues for distance normally used to preserve constancy are independently manipulated with the size of the retinal image not correspondingly changed, variations in apparent size will result.

Geniculate Bodies
Mass of cells that serve as relay stations.

Gestalt Psychology
A theoretical viewpoint of the organized nature of perception, begun by a group of German psychologists, especially Wertheimer, Köhler, and Kofka. The German word *Gestalt* means *form* or *configuration*.

Glomerulus
A relay connection in the olfactory bulb where nerve fibers connect with the brain by olfactory tracts.

Glossopharyngeal Nerve
One of the taste nerves that serves the back of the tongue.

Good Continuation
Gestalt tendency for stimulus elements to be perceptually grouped in a way so as to perceive the continuation of a line or curve in the direction that has been established.

Good Figure
The collective tendency, according to the Gestalt principles, of a certain pattern of stimuli to have the qualities of good continuation, closure, and symmetry.

Ground
The part of a total stimulus configuration that serves as the background for the apparent figure. It appears less well structured, extending behind the figure, and has less the focus of attention.

Gymnesma Sylvestre
Tasting the leaves of the Indian plant *Gymnesma sylvestre* can suppress the ability to taste sweetness without affecting the response to salty, acid, or bitter substances.

Haptic
From the Greek "to lay hold of." A sensory-perceptual channel that refers to the combined input from the skin and joints.

Harmonics
Partial tones simultaneously occurring in a complex sound. The first harmonic is the dominant frequency of the sound. Also called *overtones*.

Hemeralopia
Pathological insensitivity to dim lighting. Also called *night blindness* or *nyctalopia*.

Hertz (Hz)
The number of cycles completed within a second. Named for the nineteenth century German physicist, Heinrich Hertz.

Hit
Correctly detecting the presence of a signal in a trial of a signal detection experiment.

Homonymous Hemianopia
A form of blindness for either the left or right half of the visual field, that is, visual function is lost in the right or left halves of both retinae.

Homunculus
A topographic representation of the relative amount of brain devoted to various parts of the body.

Hue
The chromatic sensation principally produced by the wavelength of a light.

Hypermetropia
Refractive error of the lens of the eye in which the image formed of a nearby target falls on a focal plane behind the. retina. Also known as *farsightedness*.

Icon
The brief trace or fading image remaining after the presentation of a stimulus.

Illuminance
The amount of light falling on a surface.

Image-Retina Movement System
The system of movement perception in which there is a stimulation of a succession of neighboring retinal loci.

Impossible Figures
Displays containing inconsistent and contradictory sets of depth cues that cannot individually be suppressed. The graphic renderings of E. C. Escher are examples of such displays.

Incident Light
The radiant energy falling on a surface.

Incus
One of the chain of three small bones or ossicles of the middle ear. Aslo known as the *anvil*.

Induced Movement
Apparent movement of a stationary stimulus induced by movement of a nearby moving stimulus.

Intensity
A general term that refers to the magnitude of the physical energy stimulating a sense organ.

Interposition
A depth or distance cue in which the appearance of one object partially conceals or overlaps another.

Interstimulus Interval (ISI)
The duration between presentation of two stimuli.

Ipsilateral
Same side.

Iris
Circular diaphragm-type structure forming the colored portion of the eye that controls the size of the pupil opening.

Just Noticeable Difference (jnd)
The least change in the magnitude of a stimulus that is detectable.

Kappa Effect
The effect in which time perception is influenced by the distance separating two stimuli.

Kinesthesis
The reception of body-part position and movement in space of the limbs and other mobile parts of the jointed skeleton.

Kinetic Depth Effect
Moving two-dimensional patterns perceived in three-dimensions.

Krause End Bulbs
Receptors in the skin presumed to account for the sensation of coldness.

Labyrinth
Bony cavities of the inner ears of mammals.

Ladd-Franklin Theory
An evolutionary theory of color vision that holds that primitive black-white achromatic sensitivity evolved into a sensitivity to blue and yellow, and at a later stage of evolution further differentiated into a sensitivity to red and green.

Land Effect
The phenomenon, demonstrated by Edwin Land, that under certain conditions most chromatic sensations can be produced by less than three colors.

Lateral Geniculate Nucleus (LGN)
Relay center for vision located in the thalamus. Neural fibers from the LGN project to the visual area in the occipital lobe of the cortex.

Lateral Inhibition
The phenomenon in which adjacent or neighboring neural units mutually inhibit each other.

Lateral Line
A specialized sensory mechanism in fish consisting of a small fluid-filled tube that runs

under the skin and appears as a line running along the side of the body from head to tail. It contains sensory cells (neuromasts) that respond to faint vibratory stimuli.

Lens
Structure of the eye that aids in focusing light rays on the retina.

Limen
Latin term for threshold.

Limits, Method of
A psychophysical method employed for establishing thresholds. A series of stimuli of increasing or decreasing magnitude is presented until a stimulus value is reached at which the stimulus is just perceived or just fails to be perceived.

Limulus
Horseshoe crab, whose eye has been studied as a model for analyzing higher visual systems.

Linear Perspective
The geometric technique that involves systematically decreasing the size of more distant elements and the space separating them. Linear perspective is a monocular spatial cue.

Looming
The spatial and temporal information that specifies an imminent collision with an environmental object.

Loudness
The attribute of an auditory sensation in terms of which tones may be ordered from soft to loud. Loudness is primarily determined by the amplitude of a sound wave.

Luminance
The amount of light reflected from an illuminated surface.

Mach Bands
Perception of bands of brightness at borders where there are abrupt changes in luminance.

Macrosomatic
Possession of a keen sense of smell.

Macula Lutea
The yellowish retinal area that includes the fovea and adjacent regions.

Magnitude Estimation
A psychophysical method employed in scaling sensory magnitudes for Stevens' Power Law application.

Malleus
The first in the chain of three small bones or ossicles attached to the eardrum. Also know as the *hammer*.

Masking
In audition, the phenomenon in which the threshold for a tone is raised by the presence of a second tone.

McCollough Effect
The perceptual aftereffect that suggests the existence of specific feature detectors or channels for certain classes of stimulation.

Mean
A measure of central tendency (average) calculated by dividing the arithmetic sum of all scores of a set of scores by the number of scores.

Mechanoreceptors
Receptors whose excitation is dependent on mechanical stimulation.

Meissner Corpuscle
Sensory receptor in touch-sensitive hairless skin regions, presumed to be a pressure receptor.

Mel
A dimension of pitch. By definition, the pitch of a 1000 Hz tone at 40 *db* is assigned a value of 1000 mels.

Memory Color
The notion that familiarity with a chromatic stimulus influences its apparent color.

Metacontrast
Backward masking in an experimental arrangement when the target and masking stimuli fall on nonoverlapping adjacent retinal areas.

Metamers
Different lights whose mixture produces an apparent match with a third light.

Meter-Candle (m-c)
Metric unit of illuminance, defined as the illumination on a surface of one meter square

located one meter from a standard candle. One meter candle equals 0.0929 foot-candles.

Method of Limits
A procedure used to determine the threshold in which the magnitude of the stimuli are systematically increased (or reduced) until a stimulus value is obtained that is just dectectable (or just undetectable).

Microelectrode
Miniature electrode used to record neuronal activity from individual nerve cells.

Microsomatic
Relative lack of the sense of smell.

Middle Ear
It consists of a cavity containing the ossicles and the Eustachian tube.

Millilambert (mL)
Metric unit of luminance, equivalent to 0.929 foot-Lamberts. An often used alternative unit of luminance is candles-per-square-meter (c/m^2), which is equal to 0.3142 mL.

Mind-Body Relationship
A philosophical issue arising from the attempt to categorize the total organism into the two distinct categories of mind and body.

Minimum Principle
Notion that the organization that is perceived from an ambiguous configuration is the simpler one, where simplicity is specified in terms of objective physical measures.

Miraculin (*Synsepalum Dulcificum* or *Richardella Dulcifica*)
The fruit of a plant indigenous to tropical West Africa. Although the fruit is tasteless itself, exposure of the tongue to a thin layer of fruit pulp may cause any sour substance to taste sweet.

Monaural
Stimulation of one ear.

Monochromatic Light
Light of a single wavelength.

Monochromatism
A color defect in which monochromats match all wavelengths of the spectrum against any other wavelength or a white light.

Monocular
Involving one eye.

Monocular Depth Cues
Spatial cues requiring only one eye.

Monorhinic
Stimulation by an odorant to a single nostril.

Moon Illusion
The illusory perception that the moon at the horizon appears significantly larger than when it is at the zenith.

Motion Parallax
The relative apparent motion of objects in the visual field as the viewer moves his head. Motion parallax is a monocular spatial cue.

Multistable Figures
The class of figures charaterized by ambiguous and equivocal depth information.

Myopia
Refractive error of the lens of the eye in which the image of a distant target is brought to a focus in front of the retina. Also known as *nearsightedness*.

Nanometer (nm)
A billionth of a meter.

Nativism
The notion that perceptual organization is inherent in the biological structure of the organism, and therefore experience and learning play a comparatively small role.

Nature-Nurture Controversy
The controversy as to the relative contribution of innate versus learned factors in perceptual organization.

Near Point
The nearest distance from a viewer at which a target can be seen clearly.

Neonate
the period of infancy in which the infant is considered an independent individual. It begins by the cutting of the umbilical cord.

Nerve Deafness
Deficiency in hearing due to damage of the au-

ditory nerves or to the basilar membrane or other neural connection of the cochlea. Hearing loss for nerve deafness is greatest for high frequency sounds.

Neuron
The basic cellular unit of the nervous system that serves to conduct nerve impulses. It consists of a cell body, an axon, and a dendrite.

Newtons Per Square Meter (N/m^2)
A measure of sound pressure. One N/m^2 equals 10 dynes/cm^2.

Nociceptor
A receptor whose effective stimulus is harmful to the body.

Nocturnal
Pertaining to night activity.

Normal Curve
A theoretical curve having certain well-defined mathematical properties. It is a perfectly symmetrical, bell-shaped frequency curve. A distribution curve made up of many chance events approximates a normal curve.

Nyctalopia
Pathological insensitivity to dim lighting. Also called *hemeralopia* or *night blindness*.

Nystagmus
Series of reflexive, tremor-like eye movements of an oscillatory nature.

Occipital Lobe
One of the main divisions of each cerebral hemisphere that is the primary sensory area for vision.

Octave
The interval between two tones when they are separated by a frequency ratio of 2:1.

Oculogyral Illusion
An illusory perception of movement produced by stimulation of the semicircular canals when the observer experiences a period of rapid rotation in the dark while fixating on an illuminated light source that rotates with his movement.

Oculomotor System
The system of muscles that control the movements of the eyeballs in the skull sockets.

Ogive
A curve of a distribution of values whose frequencies are cumulative, that is, based on the sums of the frequencies. The cumulative frequency of any value is the sum of all frequencies of the values below plus the frequency of the value. The shape of such a distribution is sigmoidal or s-shaped.

Ohm's Acoustical Law
The ability of the ear to hear each tone separately when it is exposed to two tones simultaneously.

Olfactometer
An apparatus used for obtaining threshold measures of odorants.

Olfactory Bulb
A mass of neural tissue into which the olfactory nerve fibers enter. Nerve tracts lead from the olfactory bulb into the brain.

Olfactory Epithelium (Olfactory Mucosa)
Odor-sensitive tissue region located on both sides of the nasal cavity.

Ommatidium
Single element of a compound eye.

Operant Conditioning
A form of conditioning in which reward or reinforcement is contingent upon performance of the proper response. It is based largely on the application of B. F. Skinner's principles of reinforcement.

Opponent-Processes Theory
A theory of color perception that holds that there are three classes of neural receptors, each composed of a pair of opponent color processes: a white-black, a red-green, and a blue-yellow receptor.

Optic Chiasma
The part of the visual system at which the optic nerve fibers from the nasal part of the retina cross over to the contralateral hemispheres.

Optic Disc

Region of the retina where the optic nerve fibers leave the eye. There are no photoreceptors in this area and thus no visual response when light strikes this region. The corresponding visual field is termed the *blind spot*.

Optohapt

A system for converting printed material into touch stimulation.

Organ of Corti

Cochlear structure containing the auditory receptors. It lies between the basilar and tectorial membranes.

Osmics

The science of smell.

Ossicles

Three small bones of the middle ear that contribute to the conduction of sound to the inner ear.

Otology

The field of medicine that is concerned with the study of the ear.

Overtones

Partial tones simultaneously occurring in a complex sound that have a higher frequency and pitch than the fundamental one. Also called *harmonics*.

Pacinian Corpuscle

Bulb-like mechanoreceptor attached to nerve endings in various parts of the body, especially in the mobile portions of the jointed skeleton.

Papillae

Clusters of taste buds seen as elevations on the tongue. Four have been distinguished on the basis of shape and location: fungiform, foliate, circumvallate, and filiform.

Paracontrast

Forward masking in an experimental arrangement where the target and masking stimuli fall on nonoverlapping adjacent retinal areas.

Paradoxical Cold

A cold sensation produced when a hot stimulus is applied to a cold spot on the skin.

Perceived Causality

The perception of causality from interacting stimuli. The phenomenon has been studied most extensively by Albert Michotte.

Pheromones

Chemical substances that serve as communicants or signals secreted to the external environment and exchanged among members of the same species.

Phi Phenomenon

The phenomenon of apparent movement between two successive presentations of separate light sources. Also called *strobiscopic* or *Beta movement*.

Phon

A unit of loudness. It is a measure of the loudness level of a tone specified as the number of decibels of a standard 1000 Hz tone of equal loudness.

Phoneme

Smallest speech sound unit of a language that serves to distinguish one utterance from another.

Photon

The quantum unit of light energy.

Photopic Vision

Vision accomplished with cones.

Physiological Zero

The temperature to which a sensation of neither warmth nor cold occurs.

Pictorial Depth

Relationships between stimuli in two-dimensional material that suggest a third dimension of depth. Examples are found in photographs, movies, television.

Pinna

Part of outer ear of mammals, an earflap. Also called the *auricle*.

Piper's Law

A constant threshold response can be maintained by the reciprocal interaction of the square root of retinal area ($\sqrt{A}$) stimulated and stimulus intensity (I). That is, $\sqrt{A} \times I = $ a constant threshold value. Piper's Law holds for relatively large retinal areas; Ricco's Law applies for small areas.

Pitch

The psychological attribute of a tone that is described as high or low. Pitch is primarily mediated by the frequency of the tone.

Place Theory of Hearing

A theory that maintains that different auditory nerve fibers lying on regions of the basilar membrane are activated by different frequencies.

Point Localization

The ability to localize pressure sensations on the region of the skin where the stimulation is applied.

Point of Subjective Equality

A psychophysical measure of the estimate that the magnitude of two stimuli are perceptually equal.

Power Law

Psychophysical statement that holds that sensory magnitude grows in proportion to the physical intensity of the stimulus raised to a power.

Prägnanz, Law of

General Gestalt principle that refers to the tendency to perceive the simplest and most stable figure of all possible perceptual alternatives.

Presbyacusis

A pathological condition of the auditory system in which there is a progressive loss of sensitivity to high frequency sounds with increasing age.

Presbyopia

A refractive error of the lens of the eye in which, with increasing age, the elasticity of the lens progressively diminishes so that it becomes more difficult for the ciliary muscle to change the lens' curvature to accommodate for near objects.

Pressure Phosphenes

The subjective lights and images resulting from pressure stimulation of the eye.

Proprioception

The class of sensory information arising from vestibular and kinesthetic stimulation.

Protanopia

Color weakness characterized by the inability to distinguish between red and green and a relative insensitivity to the long wavelength end of the spectrum.

Protensity

The subjective experience of time as distinguished from clock or physical time.

Proximity

A Gestalt principle of perception that separate elements making up a configuration will be perceptually organized into wholes according to their degree of physical closeness.

Psychophysics

The study of the relation between variation in specified characteristics of the physical stimulation and the attributes and magnitude of subjective experience.

Pulfrich Effect

A perceptual distortion of physical movement produced when the two eyes are stimulated by different intensities of light.

Pupil

The opening formed by the iris of the eye through which light enters.

Pure Tone

A tone produced by sound energy emitted at a single frequency.

Purkinje Effect

The shift in relative brightness of lights from the two ends of the spectrum as illumination decreases owing to the shift from photopic (cone) to scotopic (rod) vision.

Pursuit Eye Movements

Involuntary eye movements executed in tracking moving targets.

Quantal Theory

A theory that assumes the existence of an absolute threshold, a fixed stimulus value below which a stimulus is not detectable.

Reafference
Neural excitation that is dependent on voluntary movements.

Receptive Field
An area of the visual field upon which the presentation of a stimulus of sufficient intensity and quality will produce the firing of a sensory cell.

Recognition Acuity
The acuity task of recognizing target stimuli, such as naming the letters of an eye chart (Snellen letters).

Referred Pain
Condition in which pain originating from internal organs appears to occur from another region of the body, usually the surface of the skin.

Reflectance
The proportion of illumination reflected from a surface. Also known as *albedo*.

Reflected Light
The light reaching the eye from an illuminated surface.

Reflex
A simple, involuntary, and unlearned response to a stimulus.

Relative Size
A depth or distance cue that occurs when two or more similar or identical shapes of different sizes are simultaneously viewed; the larger stimulus generally appears closer to the viewer than the smaller one.

Resolution Acuity
The acuity task of perceiving a separation between discrete elements of a pattern.

Resonance
The property of a mechanical, electrical, or biological system in which activity such as sound energy oscillating at a particular frequency, as in the case of the ear, occurs with a minimum dissipation of energy.

Retina
A photosensitive layer at the back of the eyeball consisting of interconnected nerve cells and photoreceptors that are responsive to light energy.

Reversible Figure
Stimulus patterns that give rise to oscillation between two (or more) alternative perceptual organizations. The Necker cube and Escher drawings are examples.

Rhodopsin
A light-absorbing pigment found in rods. Rhodopsin is also called *visual purple*.

Ricco's Law
A law that states that a constant threshold response can be maintained by the reciprocal interaction of retinal area (A) and stimulus intensity (I). That is, $A \times I = $ a constant threshold value. Ricco's Law holds for relatively small visual areas. For large areas Piper's Law applies.

ROC Curve
Receiver operating characteristic curves that show the relationship between the proportion of detections and false alarms in a signal detection experiment. Also called iso-sensitivity curves.

Rods
Photo-receptors of retina found principally along the periphery of the retina.

Ruffini Cylinders
Receptors of the skin presumed to mediate the sensation of warmth.

Saccade
A rapid and abrupt jump made by the eye as it moves from one fixation to another.

Sapid
Capable of being dissolved or soluble.

Satiation
Tendency for the prolonged viewing of a particular stimulus pattern to produce distortions in the continued viewing of that pattern.

Saturation
The apparent degree of concentration of the hue of a spectral light. The corresponding physical dimension of saturation is chromatic purity. In general, the narrower the band of

wavelengths comprising a light, the greater is its purity and saturation. Accordingly, white light, composed of radiant energy distributed among all wavelengths, lacks purity and appears desaturated.

Scanpath

Phenomenon of a characteristic and repeated course of eye movements toward viewing a particular stimulus configuration. The term was coined by Noton and Stark.

Sclera

Outer coat of the eye continuous with the cornea. The sclerotic coat is seen as the "white" of the eye.

Scotopic Vision

Vision accomplished with rods.

Semicircular Canals

Fluid-filled enclosures that lie above the inner ear at approximately right angles to each other and register motion of a rotary nature. The semicircular canals and the utricle comprise the vestibular organs which register gross bodily orientation.

Sensitivity

In vision, sensitivity refers to perception in conditions of low level illumination.

Set, Perceptual

A readiness to make a particular perceptual response or class of responses to particular organizations of stimuli. Sets may be established by the prior conditions of exposure.

Shading and Lighting

A depth or distance cue in which the pattern of lighting and shading affects the apparent location of objects and surfaces relative to the viewer.

Shadowing

A technique employed for studying the attention to auditory messages. Usually two messages are simultaneously presented, and the subject must attend to or "shadow" one of them.

Shape Constancy

The tendency to perceive an object as invariant in shape regardless of the orientation from which it is viewed or the shape of its image on the retina.

Sine Wave

A geometric function whose graphic depiction characterizes periodic phenomena such as air pressure changes over time as produced by a single tone.

Simultaneous Contrast

The tendency for the color of one region to affect the perception of the color of an immediately adjacent region. The adjacent region appears tinged with the complementary of the original region. Both hue and brightness are affected.

Size Constancy

The tendency to perceive the size of objects as relatively constant in spite of changes in viewing distance and changes in the size of the object's retinal images.

Size-Distance Invariance Hypothesis

If two objects project the same size retinal image but appear at different distances from the viewer, the object that appears farther from the viewer will be perceived as larger.

SL (Sensation Level)

Specification of the sound pressure for hearing in which the reference pressure for each frequency is given at its threshold value.

Smell Prism

A three-dimensional model for the representation of six primary odors and their mixtures. Henning's smell prism is an example.

Smooth Muscles

Those muscles that line the walls of all internal visceral organs including the arteries, intestines, and stomach, but not the heart.

Somesthesis

Refers to kinesthetic and cutaneous sensation.

Sone

A unit of loudness. One sone is defined as equivalent in loudness to a pure tone of 1000 Hz at 40 *db*.

Spatial Summation

The additive effect of separate stimuli spread over space.

Specific Nerve Energies

Doctrine of Johannes Mueller (1826) that states that the quality of the sensation elicited by a stimulus depends primarily on the nerve excited and secondarily on the stimulus itself. Accordingly, specific sensations are a matter of the activation of specific nerve fibers.

Spectrogram

A graphic reproduction of the frequency, spectrum, intensity, and duration of a pattern of acoustic signals.

Spherical Aberration

Distortion of the retinal image focused by a spherical lens. This is due to the fact that the light rays passing through the periphery of the lens are brought to a shorter focal plane than those passing through the center.

SPL (Sound Pressure Level)

Stimulus amplitude, utilizing the reference pressure of 0.0002 dynes/cm^2 or 0.00002 N/m^2, which approximates the least pressure necessary for the average human observer to hear a 1000 Hz tone.

Stabilized Images

A condition in which the effects of eye movements are canceled producing an invariant retinal image.

Standard Deviation (σ)

A measure of dispersion or variability of score values around the central tendency (mean) of a distribution. It is defined as the square root of the mean of the squared deviations of each score from the mean.

Stapes

The last in the chain of three small bones or ossicles that link the middle to the inner ear. The footplate of the stapes connects to the oval window of the inner ear. Also know as the *stirrup*.

Statocysts

Specialized sensory organs that serve as gravity detectors. Also know as *otocysts*.

Statoliths

Anatomical structures that lie within the statocyst cavity. They are generally free-moving and react to inertial forces and accordingly register gravity and linear movement. They are also known as *otoliths*.

Stereochemical Theory

A theory of olfaction that attempts to establish direct links between the chemical composition of substances and perceived odors. It assumes the geometric properties (size and shape) of molecules of odorants "fit" into similar size and shape receptor sites. Also known as the *steric* or *lock-and-key theory*.

Stereopsis

A perceptual experience of depth occurring as a by product of the disparity of the images projected on each eye.

Stereoscope

An optical instrument used for effecting the fusion of two images, each from a slightly different view, so as to produce an impression of depth.

Stiles-Crawford Effect

Brightness is greater for those light rays entering at the center of the pupil than light entering near the edge. This is held due to the fact that the effectiveness of a cone depends on the angle at which the light strikes it, and those rays entering at the pupil's center stimulate the cones most directly and efficiently.

Stimulation Deafness

Hearing loss due to exposure to excessive and prolonged acoustic stimulation.

Stimulus

Physical energy that activates or excites a receptor.

Stroboscopic Motion

A form of apparent movement produced by a set of flashing lights. Also referred to as *beta* movement or *phi* movement.

Subjective Colors

the productions of chromatic sensations from black and white stimulation only.

Subliminal

Stimuli whose magnitude is too weak to produce a detection response. Same as *Subthreshold*.

Subtractive Color Mixture

The apparent result of mixing two chromatic substances, such as pigments, paints, or dyes, in which there is a mutual absorption or substraction of wavelengths, canceling the reflectance of all wavelengths but those that the two substances jointly reflect.

Successive Contrast

A condition in which a chromatic stimulus is fixated producing an afterimage in the complementary color of the initial stimulus.

Summation Tones

The pitch of a summation tone corresponds to the sum of the frequencies of two simultaneously sounded primary tones.

Superior Colliculi

A pair of visual reflex centers in the roof (or tectum) of the midbrain.

Symmetry

Gestalt tendency for the perceptual grouping of stimulus elements to form symmetrical patterns rather than asymmetrical ones.

Synapse

Region where the axon of one neuron meets the dendrite of another neuron to transmit excitations.

Tabula Rasa

Term used by empiricists to describe the state of knowledge of the newborn. It refers to a "blank tablet" to which experience from the sensory inputs is gradually applied.

Tachistoscope

A projection apparatus used to show visual stimuli for very brief durations.

Talbot's Law

A generalization of the perception of intermit-

tent stimulation that states that a flashing light shown at a rate sufficient to produce fusion, that is "on" *P* percent of the time, has the same apparent brightness as the light if continuously lit but only *P* percent as intense.

Tau Effect

The relationship between distance and perceived duration. The greater the temporal interval separating the presentment of two stimuli, the greater the experienced distance.

Tectorial Membrane

Membrane extending along the top of the organ of Corti.

Texture Gradients

The gradual refinement of the size, shape, and spacing of the form of microstructure, generally seen as a texture, that is characteristic of most surfaces. Elements of the texture appear denser as distance is increased.

Thalamus

A region of the forebrain concerned with relaying nerve impulses to the cerebral cortex.

Threshold

Smallest level of stimulation (or change in stimulation) that is detectable. Also called *limen*.

Timbre

An attribute of auditory sensation corresponding to the complexity of a tone.

Tinnitus

Auditory pathological condition manifested by a "ringing" in the ears of a relatively high pitch. It is a prominent symptom of a number of ear disturbances.

Tonotopic Organization

The organization of nerve fibers of the auditory pathway and the auditory cortex in which regions along the length of the organ of Corti that react to tones of different frequency are spatially represented in an analogous way.

Transactionalism

An empiricist theory that holds that the perceptual world is, in large measure, constructed from experience. A class of demonstrations, Ames demonstrations, have been devised to demonstrate the importance of the role of learning in perception.

Transducer
A process or structure that converts one form of energy to another.

Trapezoidal Window
One of the Ames demonstrations used to show the importance of experience for perception. The window is a trapezoidal shape that projects a retinal image of a rectangular window at a slant from the viewer's gaze line.

Trichromatic Color Theory
Color theory that color sensation results from the relative stimulation of three independent receptors (cones). Also known as the *Young-Helmholtz color theory* and *trichromatic-receptor theory.*

Trigeminal Nerve
The nerve that receives its sensory input from the olfactory epithelium. It is the fifth cranial nerve.

Tritanopia
A rare form of dichromatism characterized by a deficiency in seeing blue and yellow.

Two-Point Threshold
The minimal separation in distance of two stimuli that simultaneously gives rise to two distinct impressions of touch.

Ultrasonic
Sounds above the frequency limit of human hearing.

Utricle
A membranous fluid-filled sac that registers linear acceleration and gravity.

Vagus Nerve
One of the taste nerves that serves the recesses of the throat, pharynx, and larynx.

Vascular Theory
A theory of thermal sensation in which a single mechanism for both warm and cold sensations is proposed. It holds that thermal sensations oc-

cur from the stimulation of sensory endings that occur from constriction and dilation of the smooth muscle walls of the blood vessels of the skin.

Vergence Eye Movements
Eye movements that move the eyes in opposite directions in the horizontal plane in order that both eyes focus on the same target.

Vernier Acuity (Localization Acuity)
The acuity task of detecting whether two lines, laid end to end, are continuous or whether one line is offset relative to the other.

Vestibular
Refers to the sensory structure of the labyrinth of the inner ear that reacts to head and gross bodily movement.

Vibratese
A touch "language" devised by F. A. Geldard for use on the skin surface.

Vision Substitution System
A system used for converting a visual image into a isomorphic cutaneous pattern of stimulation.

Visual Angle
The angle formed by a target on the retina. Visual angle is given in degrees, minutes, and seconds of arc and specifies the retinal area subtended by a target as a joint function of the target's size and its distance from the viewer's eye.

Visual Cliff
An apparatus used for assessing depth perception. It consists of a glass surface extending over an apparent void (deep side) and an apparent near surface (shallow side). A center-board divides the two sides and is the surface on which the experimental animal is placed.

Visual Masking
The reduction in the perception of a target stimulus when a second stimulus is present in close temporal proximity to the target stimulus.

Visual Placing Test
The automatic elicitation of a visually mediated

extension or reaching out of the paw as if to prevent collision when the animal is moved toward a surface.

Visual Purple

A photosensitive pigment found in rods that is bleached by light. Also called *rhodopsin*.

Visual Stability Center

A hypothetical center in the nervous system in which efferent signals from the brain to the eye muscles are compared with the flow of images on the retina, thereby canceling apparent movement due to the stimulation of the image-retina system.

Vitreous Humor

Gelatinous fluid filling the eyeball behind the lens.

Volatile

Characteristic of a substance to pass into a gaseous state—readily vaporizable.

Volley Principle

An assumption about neural transmission of the auditory stimulus that every nerve fiber does not fire at the same moment. Rather, the total neural activity is distributed over a series of auditory nerve fibers so that squads or volleys of fibers fire at different times. Accordingly, the neural pattern of firing corresponds to the frequency of the stimulus.

Volume

A tonal quality that refers to the size and expansiveness of a tone. Various combinations of frequency and intensity produce different volumes.

Waveform

The waveform of a tone is a graph showing the instantaneous amplitude and pressure (or intensity) changes as a function of time.

Weber's Fraction or Ratio

Psychophysical principle that holds that the greater the magnitude of a stimulus (I), the greater the change required for a difference to be detected (ΔI). It is formulated as $\dfrac{\Delta I}{I} = k,$ where k is a constant fraction that differs for different modalities.

White Noise

A complex mixture of tones of very many audible frequencies producing a "hissing" sound.

Young-Helmholtz Theory

The color theory that maintains that there are three sets of receptors (cones) that respond differentially to different wavelengths. The theory is based on the fact that three different wavelengths, when mixed appropriately, are sufficient to produce almost all the perceptible colors.

References

Abbe, M. The temporal effect upon the perception of space. *Japanese Journal of Experimental Psychology,* 1937, *4,* 83–93.

Adam, N. Mechanisms of time perception. *T.-I.-T. Journal of Life Sciences,* 1971, *1,* 41–52.

Adam, N., Rosner, B. S., Hosick, E. C., & Clark, D. L. Effect of anesthetic drugs on time production and alpha rhythm. *Perception and Psychophysics,* 1971, *10,* 133–136.

Allan, L. G. & Kristofferson, A. B. Psychophysical theories of duration discrimination. *Perception & Psychophysics,* 1974, *16,* 26–34.

Allport, G. W. & Pettigrew, T. F. Cultural influences on the perception of Movement: The trapezoid illusion among Zulus. *Journal of Abnormal and Social Psychology,* 1957, *55,* 104–120.

Alpern, M. Effector mechanisms in vision (Chap. 11). In J. W. Kling & L. A. Riggs (Eds.), *Experimental psychology* (3rd ed.). New York: Holt, Rinehart & Winston, 1971.

Alpern, M., Lawrence, M., & Wolsk, D. *Sensory processes.* Belmont, Cal.: Wordsworth Publishing Co., Inc., Brooks/Cole Publishing Co., 1967.

Altman, J. *Organic foundations of animal behavior.* New York: Holt, Rinehart & Winston, 1966.

Ames, A. Binocular vision as affected by relations between uniocular stimulus-patterns in commonplace environments. *American Journal of Psychology,* 1946, *59,* 333–357.

Ames, A. Visual perception and the rotating trapezoidal window. *Psychological Monographs,* 1951, *65* (Whole No. 324).

Amoore, J. E. Current status of the steric theory of odor. *Annals of the New York Academy of Sciences,* 1964, *116,* 457–476.

Amoore, J. E. Psychophysics of odor. *Cold Spring Harbor Symposia in Quantitative Biology,* 1965, *30,* 623–637.

Amoore, J. E., Johnston, J. W., Jr., & Rubin, M. The stereochemical theory of odor. *Scientific American,* 1964, *210,* 42–49.

Annis, R. C., & Frost, B. Human visual ecology and orientation anisotropies in acuity. *Science,* 1973, *182,* 729–731.

Anstis, S. M., & Atkinson, J. Distortions in moving figures viewed through a stationary slit. *American Journal of Psychology,* 1967, *80,* 572–586.

Anthrop, D. F. *Noise pollution.* Lexington, Massachussetts: Lexington Books (D.C. Heath), 1973.

Arlinsky, M. B. On the failure of fowl to adapt to prism induced displacement: Some theoretical analyses. *Psychonomic Science,* 1967, *7,* 237–238.

Aronson, E., & Rosenbloom, S. Space perception in early infancy: Perception within a common auditory-visual space, *Science,* 1971, *172,* 1161–1163.

Attneave, F. Multistability in perception. *Scientific American,* 1971, *225,* 63–71.

Avant, L. L. Vision in the *Ganzfeld. Psychological Bulletin,* 1965, *64,* 246–258.

Avery, G. C., & Day, R. H. Basis of the horizontal-vertical illusion. *Journal of Experimental Psychology,* 1969, *81,* 376–380.

Baddeley, A. D. Time-estimation at reduced body temperature. *American Journal of Psychology,* 1966, *79,* 475–479.

Baily, J. S. Arm-body adaptation with passive arm movements. *Perception and Psychophysics,* 1972, *12,* 39–44.

Bakan, P. Attention research in 1896 (note). *Science,* 1967, *143,* 171.

Bakan, P. The eyes have it. *Psychology Today,* 1971, April, 64–67, 96.

Baker, H. D. The instantaneous threshold and early dark adaptation. *Journal of the Optical Society of America,* 1953, *43,* 798–803.

Baker, H. D., & Rushton, W. A. H. The red-sensitive pigment in normal cones. *Journal of Physiology,* 1965, *176,* 56–72.

Ball, W., & Tronick, E. Infant responses to impending collision: Optical and real. *Science,* 1971, *171,* 818–820.

Barlow, H. B., Hill, R. M., & Levick, W. R. Retinal ganglion cells responding selectively to direction and speed of image motion in the rabbit. *Journal of Physiology,* 1964, *173,* 377–404.

Barlow, H. B., Narasimhan, R., & Rosenfeld, A. Visual pattern analysis in machine and animals. *Science,* 1972, *177,* 567–574.

Barlow, J. D. Pupillary size as an index of preference in political candidates. *Perceptual and Motor Skills,* 1969, *28,* 587–590.

Bartlett, N. R. Thresholds as dependent on some energy relations and characteristics of the sub-

ject. In C. H. Graham (Ed.), *Vision and visual perception.* New York: John Wiley, 1965.

Bartley, S. H. The psychophysiology of vision. In S. S. Stevens (Ed.), *Handbook of experimental psychology.* New York: John Wiley, 1951.

Bartoshuk, L. M. Water taste in man. *Perception and Psychophysics,* 1968, *3,* 69–72.

Bartoshuk, L. M. Water taste in man. *Perception and Psychophysics,* 1968, *3,* 69–72.

Bartoshuk, L. M. The chemical senses. I. Taste (Chap. 6). In J. W. Kling & L. A. Riggs (Eds.), *Experimental psychology* (3rd ed.). New York: Holt, Rinehart & Winston, 1971.

Bartoshuk, L. M., Dateo, G. P., Vandenbelt, D. J., Butterick, R. L., & Long, L. Effects of *Gymnema Sylvestre* and *Synsepalum Dulcificum* on taste in man. In C. Pfaffman (Ed.), *Olfaction and taste.* New York: Rockefeller University Press, 1969.

Bartoshuk, L. M., Lee, C-H., & Scarpellino, R. Sweet taste of water induced by artichoke (*Cynara Scolymus*). *Science,* 1972, *178,* 988–990.

Bartoshuk, L. M., McBurney, D. H., & Pfaffman, C. Taste of sodium chloride solutions after adaptations to sodium chloride: Implications for the "water taste." *Science,* 1964, *143,* 967–968.

Bartz, W. H., Satz, P., Fennell, E., & Lally, J. R. Meaningfulness and laterality in dichotic listening. *Journal of Experimental Psychology,* 1967, *73,* 204–210.

Batteau, D. W. Listening with the naked ear. In S. J. Freedman (Ed.), *The neuropsychology of spatially oriented behavior.* Homewood, Illinois: Dorsey Press, 1968.

Bauer, J. H. Development of visual cliff discrimination by infant hooded rats. *Journal of Comparative and Physiological Psychology,* 1973, *84,* 380–385.

Beck, J. Effect of orientation and of shape similarity on perceptual grouping. *Perception and Psychophysics,* 1966, *1,* 300–302.

Beck, J., & Gibson, J. J. The relation of apparent shape to apparent slant in the perception of objects. *Journal of Experimental Psychology,* 1955, *50,* 125–133.

Becker, H. E., & Cone, R. A. Light-stimulated electrical responses from the skin. *Science,* 1966, *154,* 1051–1053.

Beebe-Center, J. G., & Waddell, D. A general psychological scale of taste. *Journal of Psychology,* 1948, *26,* 517–524.

Beidler, L. M. Dynamics of taste cells. In Y. Zotterman (Ed.), *Olfaction and taste.* Vol. I. New York: Macmillan, 1963.

Beidler, L. M., & Gross G. W. The nature of taste receptor sites. In W. D. Neff (Ed.), *Contributions to sensory physiology.* Vol. 5. New york: Academic Press, 1971.

Békésy, G. von. On the resonance curve and the decay period at various points on the cochlear partition. *Journal of the Acoustical Society of America,* 1949, *21,* 245–249.

Békésy, G. von. Description of some mechanical properties of the organ of Corti. *Journal of Acoustical Society of America,* 1953, *25,* 770–785.

Békésy, G. von. Human skin perception of traveling waves similar to those on the cochlea. *Journal of the Acoustical Society of America,* 1955, *27,* 830–841.

Békésy, G. von. Current status of theories of hearing. *Science,* 1956, *123,* 779–783.

Békésy, G. von. The ear. *Scientific American,* 1957, *197,* 66–78. (*a*)

Békésy, G. von. Neural volleys and the similarity between some sensations produced by tones and by skin vibrations. *Journal of the Acoustical Society of America,* 1957, *29,* 1059–1069. (*b*)

Békésy, G. von. Funneling in the nervous system. *Journal of the Acoustical Society of America,* 1958, *30,* 399–412.

Békésy, G. von. Vibratory pattern of the basilar membrane. In E. G. Wever (Trans., Ed.), *Experiments in hearing.* New York: McGraw-Hill, 1960, 404–429. (*a*)

Békésy, G. von. Frequency in the cochleas of various animals. In E. G. Wever (Trans., Ed.), *Experiments in hearing.* New York: McGraw-Hill, 1960, 500–534. (*b*)

Békésy, G. von. Experimental models of the cochlea with and without nerve supply. In G. L. Rasmussen, & W. F. Windle (Eds.), *Neural mechanisms of the auditory and vestibular systems.* Springfield, Ill.: Charles C. Thomas, 1960, 3–20. (*c*)

Békésy, G. von. Hearing theories and complex sounds. *Journal of the Acoustical Society of America,* 1963, *35,* 588–601.

Békésy, G. von. Sweetness produced electrically on the tongue and its relation to taste theories. *Journal of Applied Physiology,* 1964, *19,* 1105–1113. (*a*)

Békésy, G. von. Duplexity theory of taste. *Science,* 1964, *145,* 834–835. (*b*)

Békésy, G. von. Taste theories and the chemical stimulation of single papillae. *Journal of Applied Physiology,* 1966, *21,* 1–9.

Békésy, G. von. *Sensory inhibition.* Princeton, N. J.: Princeton University Press, 1967.

Békésy, G. von. Localization of visceral pain and other sensations before and after anesthesia. *Perception and Psychophysics,* 1971, *9,* 1–4.

Békésy, G. von, & Rosenblith, W. A. The mechanical properties of the ear. In S. S. Stevens (Ed.), *Handbook of experimental psychology.* New York: John Wiley, 1951, 1075–1115.

Bell, C. R. Time estimation and increases in body temperature. *Journal of Experimental Psychology,* 1965, *70,* 232–234.

Bell, C. R., & Provins, K. A. Relation between physiological responses to environmental heat and time judgments. *Journal of Experimental Psychology,* 1963, *66,* 572–579.

Bell, F. R. The variation in taste thresholds of ruminants associated with sodium depletion. In Y. Zotterman (Ed.), *Olfaction and taste.* New York: Macmillan, 1963.

Bennett, M. V. L. Electrolocation in fish. In Orientation: sensory basis, *Annals of the New York Academy of Sciences,* 1971, *188,* 242–269.

Benson, C., & Yonas, A. Development of sensitivity to static pictorial depth information. *Perception and Psychophysics,* 1973, *13,* 361–366.

Bergeijk, W. A. van. The evolution of vertebrate hearing. In W. D. Neff (Ed.), *Contributions to sensory physiology.* Vol. 2. New York: Academic Press, 1967.

Bergeijk, W. A. van, Pierce, J. R., & David, E. E., Jr. *Waves and the ear.* Garden City, N.Y.: Anchor Books, Doubleday, 1960.

Beroza, M., & Knipling, E. F. Gypsy moth control with the sex attractant pheromone. *Science,* 1972, *177,* 19–27.

Berrien, F. K. The effects of noise. *Psychological Bulletin,* 1946, *43,* 141–161.

Bever, T. G., & Chiarello, R. J. Cerebral dominance in musicians and nonmusicians. *Science,* 1974, *185,* 537–539.

Billmeyer, F. W., & Saltzman, M. *Principles of color technology.* New York: Interscience Publishers (John Wiley), 1966.

Bindra, D., & Waksberg, H. Methods and terminology in studies of time estimation. *Psychological Bulletin,* 1956, *53,* 155–159.

Bingham, H. C. Visual perception of the chick. *Behavior Monographs,* 1922, *4* (No. 4).

Blakemore, C., & Sutton, P. Size adaptation: A new aftereffect. *Science,* 1969, *166,* 245–247.

Bliss, J. A reading machine with tactile display. In T. D. Sterling, E. A. Bering, S. V. Pollack, & H. G. Vaughan (Eds.), *Visual prosthesis.* New York: Academic Press, 1971.

Blough, D. S. Method for tracing dark adaptation in the pigeon, *Science,* 1955, *121,* 703–704.

Blough, D. S. Experiments in animal psychophysics. *Scientific American,* 1961, *205,* 113–122.

Bolles, R. C., & Bailey, D. E. Importance of object recognition in size constancy. *Journal of Experimental Psychology,* 1956, *51,* 222–225.

Borg, G., Diamant, H., Oakley, B., Ström, L., & Zotterman, Y. A. A comparative study of neural and psychophysical responses to gustatory stimuli. In T. Hayashi (Ed.), *Olfaction and taste.* Vol. II. New York: Pergamon Press, 1967.

Boring, E. G. A new ambiguous figure. *American Journal of Psychology,* 1930, *42,* 444–445.

Boring, E. G. *Sensation and perception in the history of experimental psychology.* New York: Appleton-Century-Crofts, 1942, 263–311.

Boring, E. G. The moon illusion. *American Journal of Physics,* 1943, *11,* 55–60.

Boring, E. G. *A history of experimental psychology* (2nd ed.). New York: Appleton-Century-Crofts, 1950.

Boring, E. G. Size constancy in a picture. *The American Journal of Psychology,* 1964, *77,* 494–498.

Boring, E. G., Langfeld, H. S., & Weld, H. P. *Foundations of psychology.* New York: John Wiley, 1948.

Bossom, J., & Hamilton, C. R. Interocular transfer of prism-altered coordinations in split-brain monkeys. *Journal of Comparative and Physiological Psychology,* 1963, *56,* 769–774.

Bough, E. W. Stereoscopic vision in the macaque monkey: A behavioural demonstration. *Nature,* 1970, *225,* 42–44.

Bower, T. G. R. Stimulus variables determining space perception in infants. *Science,* 1965, *149,* 88–89.

Bower, T. G. R. The visual world of infants. *Scientific American,* 1966, *215,* 80–92. (a)

Bower, T. G. R. Slant perception and shape constancy in infants. *Science,* 1966, *151,* 832–834. (b)

Bower, T. G. R. The object in the world of the infant. *Scientific American,* 1971, *225,* 30–38.

Bower, T. G. R. *Development in infancy.* San Francisco: W. H. Freeman, 1974.

Bower, T. G. R., Broughton, J. M., & Moore, M. K. The coordination of visual and tactual input in infants. *Perception and Psychophysics,* 1970, *8,* 51–53.

Bower, T. G. R., Broughton, J. M., & Moore, M. K. Infant responses to approaching objects: An indicator of response to distal variables.

Perception and Psychophysics, 1971, *9,* 193–196.

Brennan, W. M., Ames, E. W., & Moore, R. W. Age differences in infant's attention to patterns of different complexities. *Science,* 1966, *151,* 354–356.

Bridgeman, B. Visual receptive fields sensitive to absolute and relative motion during tracking. *Science,* 1972, *178,* 1106–1108.

Brindley, G. S., & Lewin, W. S. The sensations produced by electrical stimulation of the visual cortex. *Journal of Physiology,* 1968, *196,* 479–493.

Bronson, F. H. Rodent pheromones. *Biology of Reproduction,* 1971,*4,* 344–357.

Brown, J. F. The visual perception of velocity. *Psychologische Forschung,* 1931, *14,* 199–232. Reproduced in I. M. Spigel (Ed.), *Readings in the study of visually perceived movement.* New York: Harper & Row, 1965. (*a*)

Brown, J. F. The thresholds for visual movement. *Psychologische Forschung,* 1931, *14,* 249–268. Reproduced in I. M. Spigel (Ed.), *Readings in the study of visually perceived movement.* New York: Harper & Row, 1965. (*b*)

Brown, J. L. The structure of the visual system. In C. H. Graham (Ed.), *Vision and visual perception.* New York: John Wiley, 1965.

Brown, J. L., & Mueller, C. G. Brightness discrimination and brightness contrast. In C. H. Graham (Ed.), *Vision and visual perception.* New York: John Wiley, 1965.

Brown, J. L., Shively, F. D., LaMotte, R. H., & Sechzer, J. A. Color discrimination in the cat. *Journal of Comparative and Physiological Psychology,* 1973, *84,* 534–544.

Brown, P. E. Use of acupuncture in major surgery. *Lancet,* 1972, *1,* 1328–1330.

Brown, P. K., & Wald, G. Visual pigments in single rods and cones of the human retina. *Science,* 1964, *144,* 45–52.

Bruner, J. S. On perceptual readiness. *Psychological Review,* 1957, *64,* 123–152.

Bruner, J. S., & Minturn, A. L. Perceptual identification and perceptual organization. *Journal of General Psychology,* 1955, *53,* 21–28.

Bruner, J. S., & Postman, L. On the perception of incongruity. *Journal of Personality,* 1949, *18,* 206–223.

Brunswick, E. Distal focusing of perception. Size-constancy in a representative sample of situations. *Psychological Monographs,* 1944 (No. 254).

Buchsbaum, R. *Animals without backbones.* Chicago: University of Chicago Press, 1948.

Buffardi, L. Factors affecting the filled-duration illusion in the auditory, tactual, and visual modalities. *Perception and Psychophysics,* 1971, *10,* 292–294.

Burnham, R. W., Hanes, R. M., & Bartleson, C. J. *Color: A guide to basic facts and concepts.* New York: John Wiley, 1963.

Burns, W. *Noise and man* (2nd ed.). Philadelphia: J. B. Lippincott, 1973.

Buss, A. H. *Psychology: Man in perspective.* New York: John Wiley, 1973.

Butler, R. A. The monaural localization of tonal stimuli. *Perception and Psychophysics,* 1971, *9,* 99–101.

Cagan, R. H. Chemostimulatory protein: A new type of taste stimulus. *Science,* 1973, *181,* 32–35.

Camp, W., Martin, R., & Chapman, L. F. Pain threshold and discrimination of pain intensity during brief exposure to intense noise. *Science,* 1962, *135,* 788–789.

Candland, D. K. *Psychology: the experimental approach.* New York: McGraw-Hill, 1968.

Carlin, S., Ward, W. D., Gershon, A., & Ingraham, R. Sound stimulation and its effect on dental sensation threshold. *Science,* 1962, *138,* 1258–1259.

Carpenter, J. A. Species difference in taste preferences. *Journal of Comparative and Physiological Psychology,* 1956, *49,* 139–144.

Carr, W. J., & McGuigan, D. I. The stimulus basis and modification of visual cliff performance in the rat. *Animal Behavior,* 1965, *13,* 25–29.

Carraher, R. G., & Thurston, J. B. *Optical illusions and the visual arts.* New York: Reinhold, 1966.

Casey, K. L. Pain: A current view of neural mechanisms. *American Scientist,* 1973, *61,* 194–200.

Chaikin, J. D., Corbin, H. H., & Volkmann, J. Mapping a field of short-time visual search. *Science,* 1962, *138,* 1327–1328.

Chapanis, A. How we see: A summary of basic principles. In *Human factors in undersea warfare.* Washington, D.C.: National Research Council, 1949.

Chapanis, A., Garner, W. R., & Morgan, C. T. *Applied experimental psychology.* New York: John Wiley, 1949.

Chapanis, A., & Mankin, D. A. The vertical-horizontal illusion in a visually-rich environment. *Perception and Psychophysics,* 1967, *2,* 249–255.

Cheng, T. O. Accupuncture anesthesia (Letter). *Science,* 1973, *179,* 521.

Cherry, E. C. Some experiments upon the recognition of speech, with one and with two ears. *Journal of the Acoustical Society of America,* 1953, *25,* 975–979.

Christman, R. J. *Sensory experience.* Scranton, Pa.: Intext Educational Publishers, 1971.

Churchill, A. V. Effect of mode of response on judgment of size. *Journal of Experimental Psychology,* 1962, *64,* 198–199.

Clark, W. C., & Yang, J. C. Acupunctural analgesia? Evaluation by signal detection theory. *Science,* 1974, *184,* 1096–1098.

Clatworthy, J. L., & Frisby, J. P. Real and apparent visual movement: Evidence for a unitary mechanism. *Perception,* 1973,*2* 161–164.

Cohen, J. Psychological time. *Scientific American,* 1964, *211,* 116–124.

Cohen, J., Hansel, C. E. M. & Sylvester, J. D. A new phenomenon in time judgment. *Nature,* 1953, *172,* 901–903.

Cohen, J., Hansel, C. E. M., & Sylvester, J. D. Interdependence of temporal and auditory judgments. *Nature,* 1954, *174,* 642.

Cohen, J., Hansel, C. E. M., & Sylvester, J. D., Interdependence in judgments of space, time and movement. *Acta Psychologica,* 1955, *11,* 360–372.

Cohen, L. A. Analysis of position sense in human shoulder. *Journal of Neurophysiology,* 1958, *21,* 550–562.

Cohen, L. D., Kipnes, D., Kunkle, E. G., & Kubzansky, P. E. Observations of a person with congenital insensitivity to pain. *Journal of Abnormal and Social Psychology,* 1955, *51,* 333–338.

Cohen, W. Spatial and textural characteristics of the *Ganzfeld. American Journal of Psychology,* 1957, *70,* 403–410.

Cohen, W. Color-perception in the chromatic *Ganzfeld. American Journal of Psychology,* 1958, *71,* 390–394.

Cohn, R. Differential cerebral processing of noise and verbal stimuli. *Science,* 1971, *172,* 599–601.

Collins, C. C. Tactile vision synthesis. In T. D. Sterling, E. A. Bering, S. V. Pollack, & H. G. Vaughan (Eds.), *Visual prosthesis.* New York: Academic Press, 1971. (*a*)

Collins, C. C. A portable seeing aid prototype. *Journal of Biomedical Systems,* 1971, *5,* 3–10. (*b*)

Coltheart, M. Visual feature-analyzers and aftereffects of tilt and curvature. *Psychological Review,* 1971, *78,* 114–121.

Comfort, A. Communications may be odorous. *New Scientist and Science Journal,* 1971 (February 25), 412–414.

Conrad, D. G., Elsmore, T. F., & Sodetz, F. J. Δ^9-Tetrahydrocannabinol: Dose-related effects on timing behavior in chimpanzee. *Science,* 1972, *175,* 547–550.

Coren, S. Brightness contrast as a function of figure-ground relations. *Journal of Experimental Psychology,* 1969, *80,* 517–524.

Coren, S. Subjective contours and apparent depth. *Psychological Review,* 1972, *79,* 359–367.

Coren, S., & Girgus, J. S. Visual spatial illusions: Many explanations. *Science,* 1973, *179,* 503–504.

Cornsweet, T. N. *Visual Perception.* New York: Academic Press, 1970.

Corso, J. F. *The experimental psychology of sensory behavior.* New York: Holt, Rinehart & Winston, 1967.

Cotzin, M., & Dallenbach, K. M. "Facial vision:" The role of pitch and loudness in the perception of obstacles by the blind. *American Journal of Psychology,* 1950, *63,* 483–515.

Crampton, G. H., & Schwam, W. J. Turtle vestibular responses to angular acceleration with comparative data from cat and man. *Journal of Comparative and Physiological Psychology,* 1962, *55,* 3, 315–321.

Crescitelli, F., & Pollack, J. D. Color vision in the antelope ground squirrel. *Science,* 1965, *150,* 1336–1338.

Crouch, J. E. & McClintic, J. R. *Human anatomy and physiology.* New York: John Wiley, 1971.

Crovitz, H. F., & Daves, W. Tendencies to eye movement and perceptual accuracy. *Journal of Experimental Psychology,* 1962, *63,* 5, 495–498.

Crovitz, H. F., & Schiffman, H. Visual perception and xerography. *Science,* 1968, *160,* 1251–1252.

Cruikshank, R. M. The development of visual size constancy in early infancy. *Journal of Genetic Psychology,* 1941, *58,* 327–351.

Cruze, W. W. Maturation and learning in chicks. *Journal of Comparative Psychology,* 1935, *19,* 371–409.

Curry, F. K. A comparison of left-handed and right-handed subjects on verbal and nonverbal dichotic listening tasks. *Cortex,* 1967, *3,* 343–352.

Dalland, J. I. Hearing sensitivity in bats. *Science,* 1965, *150,* 1185–1187.

Dallenbach, K. M. The temperature spots and end-organs. *American Journal of Psychology,* 1927, *39,* 402–427.

Dallos, P., Billone, M. C., Durrant, J. D.,

Wang, C. Y., & Raynor, S. Cochlear inner and outer hair cells: Functional differences. *Science,* 1972, *177,* 356–358.

D'Amato, M. R. *Experimental psychology: methodology, psychophysics and learning.* New York: McGraw-Hill, 1970.

Davidson, P. W., & Whitson, T. T. Some effects of the texture density on visual cliff behavior of the domestic chick. *Journal of Comparative and Physiological Psychology,* 1973, *84,* 522–526.

Davis, C. M. & Carlson, J. A. A cross-cultural study of the strength of the Müller-Lyer illusion as a function of attentional factors. *Journal of Personality and Social Psychology,* 1970, *16,* 403–410.

Davis, H. *Hearing and deafness: a guide for laymen.* New York: Murray Hill, 1947.

Davis, H. Psychophysiology of hearing and deafness. In S. S. Stevens (Ed.), *Handbook of experimental psychology.* New York: John Wiley, 1951.

Davis, H., Benson, R. W., Corell, W. P., Fernández, C., Goldstein, R., Katsuki, Y, Legouix, J. P., McAuliffe, D. R., and Taksaki, I. Acoustic trauma in the Guinea pig. *Journal of the Acoustical Society of America,* 1953, *25,* 1180–1189.

Davis, W. J., & Ayers, J. L. Locomotion: Control by positive feed-back optokinetic responses. *Science,* 1972, *177,* 183–185.

Daw, N. W. Goldfish retina: Organization for simultaneous color contrast. *Science,* 1967, *158,* 942–944.

Dawson, W. W. Thermal stimulation of experimentally vasoconstricted human skin. *Perceptual and Motor Skills,* 1964, *19,* 775–788.

Day, M. E. An eye-movement indicator of individual differences in the physiological organization of attentional processes and anxiety. *Journal of Psychology,* 1967, *66,* 51–62.

Day, R. H. *Human perception.* New York: John Wiley, 1969.

Day, R. H. Visual spatial illusions: a general explanation. *Science,* 1972, *175,* 1335–1340.

Day, R. H., & Singer, G. Sensory adaptation and

behavioral compensation with spatially transformed vision and hearing. *Psychological Bulletin*, 1967, *67*, 307–322.

Delk, J. L., & Fillenbaum, S. Difference in perceived color as a function of characteristic color. *American Journal of Psychology*, 1965, *78*, 290–293.

Dennis, W. *Readings in the history of psychology*. New York: Appleton-Century-Crofts, Inc., 1948.

Denes, P. B. & Pinson, E. N. *The speech chain: the physics and biology of spoken language*. Garden City, New York: Anchor Books, Doubleday, 1973.

Deregowski, J. B. Perception of the two-pronged trident by two- and three-dimensional perceivers. *Journal of Experimental Psychology*, 1969, *82*, 9–13.

Deregowski, J. B. Pictorial perception and culture. *Scientific American*, 1972, *227*, 81–88.

Desor, J. A., & Beauchamp, G. K. The human capacity to transmit olfactory information. *Perception and Psychophysics*, 1974, *16*, 551–556.

Desor, J. A., Maller, O., & Turner, R. E. Taste acceptance of sugars by human infants. *Journal of Comparative and Physiological Psychology*, 1973, *84*, 496–501.

DeValois, R. L. Analysis and coding of color vision in the primate visual system. *Cold Spring Harbor Symposia*, 1965, XXX. (*a*)

DeValois, R. L. Behavioral and electrophysiological studies of primate vision. In W. D. Neff (Ed.), *Contributions to sensory physiology*. Vol. 1. New York: Academic Press, 1965. (*b*)

DeValois, R. L., Abramov, I., & Jacobs, G. H. Analysis of response patterns of LGN cells. *Journal of the Optical Society of America*, 1966, *56*, 966–977.

DeVries, H., & Stuiver, M. The absolute sensitivity of the human sense of smell. In W. A. Rosenblith (Ed.), *Sensory communication*. Cambridge, Mass.: M.I.T. Press, 1961.

Dichgans, J., Held, R., Young, L. R., & Brandt, T. Moving visual scenes influence the apparent direction of gravity. *Science*, 1972, *178*, 1217–1218.

Dimond, S. J. The structural basis of timing. *Psychological Bulletin*, 1964, *62*, 348–350.

Dobelle, W. H., Mladejovsky, M. G., & Girvin, J. P. Artificial vision for the blind: electrical stimulation of visual cortex offers a hope for a functional prosthesis. *Science*, 1974, *183*, 440–444.

Doehring, D. G. Accuracy and consistency of time-estimation by four methods of reproduction. *American Journal of Psychology*, 1961, *74*, 27–35.

Dohlman, G. Some practical and theoretical points in labyrinthology. *Proceedings of the Royal Society of Medicine*, 1935, *28*, 1371–1380.

Dowling, J. E. Night blindness. *Scientific American*, 1966, *215*, 78–84.

Dowling, J. E. The site of visual adaptation. *Science*, 1967, *155*, 273–284.

Dowling, J. E., & Boycott, B. B. Organization of the primate retina. *Proceedings of the Royal Society* (London), 1966, *166* (Series B), 80–111.

Dowling, J. E., & Wald, G. The biological function of vitamin A acid. *Proceedings of the National Society of Sciences*, 1960, *46*, 587–616.

Duke-Elder, S. *System of ophthalmology*. (Vol. 1), *The eye in evolution*. St. Louis: C. V. Mosby, 1958.

Duncker, K. The influence of past experience upon perceptual properties. *American Journal of Psychology*, 1939, *52*, 255–265.

Dzendolet, E. Theory for the mechanism of action of "miracle fruit." *Perception and Psychophysics*, 1969, *6*, 187–188.

Dzendolet, E., & Meiselman, H. L. Gustatory quality changes as a function of solution concentration. *Perception and Psychophysics*, 1967, *2*, 29–33.

Ebenholtz, S. M. Transfer and decay functions in adaptation to optical tilt. *Journal of Experimental Psychology*, 1969, *81*, 170–173.

Eisler, H. Subjective duration and psychophysics. *Psychological Review*, 1975, *82*, 429–450.

Engel, E. Binocular fusion of dissimilar figures. *Journal of Psychology*, 1958, *46*, 53–57.

Engen, T. Man's ability to perceive odors. In J. W. Johnson, D. G. Moulton, & A. Turk (Eds.), *Advances in chemoreception.* Vol. I, *Communication by chemical signals.* New York: Appleton-Century-Crofts, 1970.

Engen, T., & Pfaffman, C. Absolute judgments of odor intensity. *Journal of Experimental Psychology*, 1959, *58*, 23–26.

Enright, J. T. Stereopsis, visual latency, and three-dimensional moving pictures. *American Scientist*, 1970, *58*, 536–545.

Epstein, W. The influence of assumed size on apparent distance. *American Journal of Psychology*, 1963, *76*, 257–265.

Epstein, W. *Varieties of perceptual learning.* New York: McGraw-Hill, 1967.

Epstein, W., & Baratz, S. S. Relative size in isolation as a stimulus for relative perceived distance. *Journal of Experimental Psychology*, 1964, *67*, 507–513.

Epstein, W., & Shontz, F. *Psychology in progress.* New York: Holt, Rinehart, & Winston, 1971.

Erdelyi, M. H., & Appelbaum, A. G. Cognitive masking: The disruptive effect of an emotional stimulus upon the perception of contiguous neutral items. *Bulletin of the Psychonomic Society*, 1973, *1*, 59–61.

Erdelyi, M. H., & Blumenthal, D. G. Cognitive masking in rapid sequential processing: The effect of an emotional picture on preceding and succeeding pictures. *Memory and Cognition*, 1973, *1*, 201–204.

Erickson, R. P. Sensory neural patterns and gustation. In Y. Zotterman (Ed.), *Olfaction and taste.* New York: Macmillan, 1963.

Eriksen, C. W., & Collins, J. F. Reinterpretation of one form of backward and forward masking in visual perception. *Journal of Experimental Psychology*, 1965, *70*, 343–351.

Eriksen, C. W., & Collins, J. F. Some temporal characteristics of visual pattern recognition.

Journal of Experimental Psychology, 1967, *74,* 476–484.

Escher, M. C. *The graphic work of M. C. Escher.* New York: Ballantine, 1971.

Evans, C. R., & Marsden, R. P. A study of the effect of perfect retinal stabilization on some well-known visual illusions, using the afterimage as a method of compensating for eye movement. *British Journal of Physiological Optics*, 1966, *23*, 242–248.

Ewert, P. H. A study of the effect of inverted retinal stimulations upon spatially coordinated behavior. *Genetic Psychology Monographs*, 1930, *7*, 177–363.

Falk, J. L., & Bindra, D. Judgment of time as a function of serial position and stress. *Journal of Experimental Psychology*, 1954, *47*, 279–282.

Fantz, R. L. Form preferences in newly hatched chicks. *Journal of Comparative and Physiological Psychology*, 1957, *50*, 422–430.

Fantz, R. L. Depth discrimination in dark-hatched chicks. *Perceptual and Motor Skills*, 1958, *8*, 47–50.

Fantz, R. L. The origin of form perception. *Scientific American*, 1961, *204*, 66–72.

Fantz, R. L. Pattern vision in newborn infants. *Science*, 1963, *140*, 296–297.

Fantz, R. L. Ontogeny of perception. In A. M. Schrier, H. F. Harlow, & F. Stollnitz (Eds.), *Behavior of nonhuman primates.* Vol. II. New York: Academic Press, 1965. (a)

Fantz, R. L. Visual perception from birth as shown by pattern selectivity. *Annals of the New York Academy of Sciences*, 1965, *118*, 793–814. (b)

Fantz, R. L. Pattern discrimination and selective attention. In A. H. Kidd, & J. L. Rivoire (Eds.), *Perceptual development in children.* New York: International Universities Press, 1966.

Fantz, R. L. Visual perception and experience in early infancy: A look at the hidden side of behavior development. In H. W. Stevenson, E. H. Hess, & H. L. Rheingold (Eds.), *Early be-*

havior: comparative and developmental approaches. New York: John Wiley, 1967.

Farquhar, M., & Leibowitz, H. W. The magnitude of the Ponzo illusion as a function of age for large and for small stimulus configurations. *Psychonomic Science*, 1971, *25*, 97–99.

Favreau, O. E., Emerson, V. F., & Corballis, M. C. Motion perception: A color-contingent aftereffect. *Science*, 1972, *176*, 78–79.

Fay, R. R. Auditory frequency discrimination in the goldfish (*Carrassius Auratus*). *Journal of Comparative and Physiological Psychology*, 1970,*73*, 175–180.

Feinberg, G. Light. *Scientific American*, 1968, *219*, 50–59.

Ferris, S. H. Motion parallax and absolute distance. *Journal of Experimental Psychology*, 1972, *95*, 258–263.

Festinger, L., Allyn, M. R., & White, C. W. The perception of color with achromatic stimulation. *Vision Research*, 1971, *11*, 591–612.

Festinger, L., Burnham, C. A., Ono, H., & Bamber, D. Efference and the conscious experience of perception. *Journal of Experimental Psychology*, 1967, Monograph Supplement 74 (*4*, Whole No. 637).

Fields, P. E. Studies in concept formation. I. The development of the concept of triangularity by the white rat. *Comparative Psychology Monographs*, 1932, *9*, 1–70.

Fieandt, K., von. *The world of perception.* Homewood, Ill.: Dorsey Press, 1966.

Fillenbaum, S. Contextual effects in judgment as a function of restrictions in response-language. *American Journal of Psychology*, 1963, *76*, 103–109.

Fillenbaum, S., Schiffman, H. R., & Butcher, J. Perception of off-size versions of a familiar object under conditions of rich information. *Journal of Experimental Psychology*, 1965, *69*, 298–303.

Fisher, G. H. A common principle relating to the Müller-Lyer and Ponzo illusions. *American Journal of Psychology*, 1967, *80*, 626–631. (*a*)

Fisher, G. H. Ambiguous figure treatments in the art of Salvador Dali. *Perception and Psychophysics*, 1967, *2*, 328–330. (*b*)

Fisher, G. H. Illusions and size-constancy. *American Journal of Psychology*, 1968, *81*, 2–20.

Fisher, G. H. An experimental and theoretical appraisal of the perspective and size-constancy theories of illusions. *Quarterly Journal of Experimental Psychology*, 1970, *22*, 631–652.

Fisher, G. L., Pfaffman, C., & Brown, E. Dulcin and saccharin taste in squirrel monkeys, rats, and men. *Science*, 1965, *150*, 506–507.

Fisher, R. The biological fabric of time. In Interdisciplinary Perspectives of Time, *Annals of the New York Academy of Sciences*, 1967, *138*, 451–465.

Fletcher, H. *Speech and hearing.* New York: Van Nostrand, 1929.

Fletcher, H. *Speech and hearing* (revised ed.). New York: D van Nostrand Co., 1952.

Flock, H. R., & Moscatelli, A. Variables of surface texture and visual space perception. *Perceptual and Motor Skills*, 1964, *19*, 327–335.

Foley, J. P. An experimental investigation of the effect of prolonged inversion of the visual field in the rhesus monkey (*Macaca mulatta*). *Journal of Genetic Psychology*, 1940, *56*, 21–51.

Forgays, D. G., & Forgays, J. W. The nature of the effect of free-environmental experience in the rat. *Journal of Comparative and Physiological Psychology*, 1952, *45*, 322–328.

Forgays, D. G., & Read, J. M. Crucial periods for free-environmental experience in the rat. *Journal of Comparative and Physiological Psychology*, 1962, *55*, 816–818.

Forgus, R. H. Early visual and motor experience as determiners of complex maze learning ability under rich and reduced stimulation. *Journal of Comparative and Physiological Psychology*, 1955, *48*, 215–220.

Forgus, R. H. Advantages of early over late perceptual experience in improving form discrimination. *Canadian Journal of Psychology*, 1956, *10*, 147–155.

Forgus, R. H. The effect of different kinds of form pre-exposure on form discrimination learning. *Journal of Comparative and Physiological Psychology*, 1958, *51*, 75–78.

Forgus, R. H. *Perception: The basic process in cognitive development.* New York: McGraw-Hill, 1966.

Foulke, E. The perception of time compressed speech. In D. L. Horton & J. J. Jenkins (Eds.), *Perception of language.* Columbus, Ohio: Charles E. Merrill, 1971.

Fox, R., & Blake, R. R. Stereopsis in the cat. Paper presented at the tenth meeting of the Psychonomic Society, San Antonio, Texas, November, 1970.

Fraenkel, G. S., & Gunn, D. L. *The orientation of animals.* New York: Dover Publications, 1961.

Fraisse, P. *The psychology of time.* New York: Harper & Row,1963.

Frankenhauser, M. *Estimation of time.* Stockholm: Almqvist & Wiksell, 1959.

Freedman, S. J., & Rekosh, J. H. The functional integrity of spatial behavior. In S. J. Freedman (Ed.), *The neuropsychology of spatially oriented behavior.* Homewood, Ill.: Dorsey Press, 1968.

Freedman, S. J. & Fisher H. G. The role of the pinna in auditory localization. In S. J. Freedman (Ed.), *The neuropsychology of spatially oriented behavior.* Homewood, Ill.: Dorsey Press, 1968.

Freeman, R. B. Perspective determinants of visual size-constancy in binocular and monocular cats. *American Journal of Psychology,* 1968, *81,* 67–73.

Freeman, R. D., Mitchell, D. E., & Millodot, M. A neural effect of partial visual deprivation in humans. *Science,* 1972, *175,* 1384–1386.

Freeman, R. D., & Thibos, L. N. Electrophysiological evidence that abnormal early visual experience can modify the human brain. *Science,* 1973, *180,* 876–878.

French, N. R., & Steinberg, J. C. Factors governing the intelligibility of speech-sounds. *Journal of the Acoustical Society of America,* 1947, *19,* 90–119.

Galambos, R., & Davis, H. The response of single auditory-nerve fibers to acoustic stimulation. *Journal of Neurophysiology,* 1943, *6,* 39–57.

Galanter, E. Contemporary psychophysics. In R. Brown, E. Galanter, E. H. Hess, & G. Mandler (Eds.), *New Directions in Psychology,* New York: Holt, Rinehart & Winston, 1962.

Galanter, E. *Textbook of elementary psychology.* San Francisco: Holden-Day, 1966.

Gandelman, R., Zarrow, M. X., Denenberg, V. H., & Myers, M. Olfactory bulb removal eliminates maternal behavior in the mouse. *Science,* 1971, *171,* 210–211.

Ganz, L. Mechanism of the figural after-effects. *Psychological Review,* 1966, *73,* 128–150.

Gardner, E. *Fundamentals of neurology.* Philadelphia: W. B. Saunders, 1947.

Gardner, M. Dermo-optical perception: a peak down the nose. *Science,* 1966, *151,* 654–657.

Gardner, W. J., Licklider, J. C. R., & Weisz, A. Z. Suppression of pain by sound. *Science,* 1960, *132,* 32–33.

Garner, W. R. Good patterns have few alternatives. *American Scientist,* 1970, *58,* 34–58.

Gazzaniga, M. S. The split brain in man. *Scientific American,* 1967, *217,* 24–29.

Gazzaniga, M. S., & Hillyard, S. A. Language and speech capacity of the right hemisphere. *Neuropsychologia,* 1971, *9,* 273–280.

Geldard, F. A. Some neglected possibilities of communication. *Science,* 1960, *131,* 1583–1588.

Geldard, F. A. *Fundamentals of psychology.* New York: John Wiley, 1962.

Geldard, F. A. Cutaneous coding of optical signals: The optohapt. *Perception and Psychophysics,* 1966, *1,* 377–381.

Geldard, F. A. Body English. *Psychology Today,* December 2, 1968, 42–47. (*a*)

Geldard, F. A. Pattern perception by the skin. Chapter 13 in D. R. Kenshalo (Ed.), *The skin senses.* Springfield, Ill.: Charles C Thomas, 1968. (*b*)

Geldard, F. A. *The human senses* (2nd ed.). New York: John Wiley, 1972.

Gesteland, R. C., Lettvin, J. Y., Pitts, W. H., & Rojas, A. Odor specificities of the frog's olfactory receptors. In Y. Zotterman (Ed.), *Olfaction and taste.* New York: Pergamon Press, 1963, 19–44.

Ghent, L. Recognition by children of realistic figures presented in various orientations. *Canadian Journal of Psychology,* 1960, *14,* 249–256.

Gibson, E. J. *Principles of perceptual learning and development.* New York: Appleton-Century-Crofts, 1969.

Gibson, E. J. The development of perception as an adaptive process. *American Scientist,* 1970, *58,* 98–107.

Gibson, E. J., & Walk, R. D. The effect of prolonged exposure to visually presented patterns on learning to discriminate them. *Journal of Comparative and Physiological Psychology,* 1956, *49,* 239–242.

Gibson, E. J., Walk, R. D., Pick, H. L., & Tighe, T. J. The effect of prolonged exposure to visual patterns on learning to discriminate similar and different patterns. *Journal of Comparative and Physiological Psychology,* 1958, *51,* 584–587.

Gibson, E. J., Walk, R. D., & Tighe, T. J. Enhancement and deprivation of visual stimulation during rearing as factors in visual discrimination learning. *Journal of Comparative and Physiological Psychology,* 1959, *52,* 74–81.

Gibson, J. J. Adaptation, after-effect, and contrast in the perception of curved lines. *Journal of Experimental Psychology,* 1933, *16,* 1–31.

Gibson, J. J. The perception of the visual world. New York: Houghton Mifflin, 1950.

Gibson, J. J. The concept of the stimulus in psychology. *American Psychologist,* 1960, *11,* 694–703.

Gibson, J. J. Observations on active touch. *Psychological Review,* 1962, *69,* 477–491.

Gibson, J. J. The useful dimensions of sensitivity. *American Psychologist,* 1963, *18,* 1–15.

Gibson, J. J. *The senses considered as perceptual systems.* New York: Houghton Mifflin, 1966.

Gibson, J. J. What gives rise to the perception of motion? *Psychological Review,* 1968, *75,* 335–346.

Gibson, J. J., & Radner, M. Adaptation, after-effect and contrast in the perception of tilted lines. I. Quantitative studies. *Journal of Experimental Psychology,* 1937, *20,* 453–467.

Gibson, J. J., & Waddell, D. Homogeneous retinal stimulation and visual perception. *American Journal of Psychology,* 1952, *65,* 263–270.

Gibson, R. H. Electrical stimulation of pain and touch. (Chap. 11). In D. R. Kenshalo (Ed.), *The skin senses.* Springfield, Ill.: Charles C Thomas, 1968.

Gillam, B. A depth processing theory of the Poggendorff illusion. *Perception and Psychophysics,* 1971, *10,* 211–216.

Gilliland, A. R., Hofeld, J., & Eckstrand, G. Studies in time perception. *Psychological Bulletin,* 1946, *43,* 162–176.

Glaser, E. M., & Haven, M. Bandpass noise stimulation of the simulated basilar membrane. *Journal of the Acoustical Society of America,* 1972, *52,* 1131–1136.

Glass, B. Foreword to M. P. Kare, & O. Haller (Eds.), *The chemical senses and nutrition.* Baltimore: John Hopkins Press, 1967.

Gleason, K. K., & Reynierse, J. H. The behavioral significance of pheromones in vertebrates. *Psychological Bulletin,* 1969, *71,* 58–73.

Gogel, W. C. Size cues to visually perceived distance. *Psychological Bulletin,* 1964, *62,* 217–235.

Gogel, W. C. Size cues and the adjacency principle. *Journal of Experimental Psychology,* 1965, *70,* 289–293.

Gogel, W. C., & Hess, E. H. A study of color

constancy in the newly hatched chick by means of an innate color preference (Abst.). *American Journal of Psychology*, 1951, *6*, 282.

Goldstone, S., Boardman, W. K., & Lhamon, W. T. Effect of quinal barbitone, dextro-amphetamine, and placebo on apparent time. *British Journal of Psychology*, 1958, *49*, 324–328.

Goldwater, B. C. Psychological significance of pupillary movements. *Psychological Bulletin*, 1972, *77*, 340–355.

Goodwin, G. M., McCloskey, D. I., & Matthews, P. B. C. Proprioceptive illusions induced by muscle vibration: Contribution by muscle spindles to perception? *Science*, 1972, *175*, 1382–1384.

Gourevitch, G., & Hack, M. H. Audibility in the rat. *Journal of Comparative and Physiological Psychology*, 1966, *62*, 289–291.

Grabowski, S. R., Pinto, L. H., & Pak, W. L. Adaptation in retinal rods of Axolotl: Intracellular recordings. *Science*, 1972, *176*, 1240–1243.

Graham, C. H. *Vision and visual perception*. New York: John Wiley, 1965.

Graham, C. H., & Brown, J. L. Color contrast and color appearances: Brightness constancy and color constancy. In C. H. Graham (Ed.), *Vision and visual perception*. New York: John Wiley, 1965.

Graham, C. H., & Hsia, Y. Luminosity curves for normal and dichromatic subjects including a case of unilateral color blindness. *Science*, 1954, *120*, 780.

Graham, C. H., & Hsia, Y. Color defect and color theory. *Science*, 1958, *127*, 675–682.

Granit, R., Holmberg, T., & Zewi, M. On the mode of action of visual purple on the rod cell. *Journal of Physiology*, 1938, *94*, 430–440.

Graybiel, A., Clark, B., MacCorquodale, K., & Hupp, D. I. Role of vestibular nystagmus in the visual perception of a moving target in the dark. *American Journal of Psychology*, 1946, *59*, 259–266.

Graybiel, A., & Hupp, D. The oculo-gyral illusion: A form of apparent motion which may be observed following stimulation of the semicircular canals. *Journal of Aviation Medicine*, 1946, *17*, 3–27.

Green, D. M., & Swets, J. A. *Signal detection theory and psychophysics*. New York: John Wiley, 1966.

Greene, L. S., Desor, J. A., and Maller, O. Heredity and experience: their relative importance in the development of taste preference in man. *Journal of Comparative and Physiological Psychology*, 1975, *89*, 279–284.

Gregory, R. L. Distortion of visual space as inappropriate constancy scaling. *Nature*, 1963, *199*, 678–680.

Gregory, R. L. *Eye and brain* (1st ed.). New York: World University Library, 1966.

Gregory, R. L. Visual illusions. *Scientific American*, 1968, *219*, 66–76.

Gregory, R. L. *The intelligent eye*. New York: McGraw-Hill, 1970.

Gregory, R. L. *Eye and brain* (2nd ed.). New York: World University Library, 1973.

Gregson, R. A. M., & Matterson, H. M. Psychophysical parameters of the perception of orally-retained liquid bulk. *Perception and Psychophysics*, 1967, *2*, 89–90.

Griffin, D. R. *Listening in the dark*. New Haven: Yale University Press, 1958, 132.

Griffin, D. R. *Echoes of bats and men*. New York: Anchor Books, Doubleday, 1959.

Grinnell, A. D. The neurophysiology of audition in bats: Intensity and frequency parameters. *Journal of Physiology*, 1963, *167*, 38–66.

Gross, C. G., Bender, D. B., & Rocha-Miranda, C. E. Visual receptive fields of neurons in inferotemporal cortex of the monkey. *Science*, 1969, *166*, 1303–1306.

Gross, C. G., Rocha-Miranda, C. E., & Bender, D. B. Visual properties of neurons in inferotemporal cortex of the Macaque. *Journal of Neurophysiology*, 1972, *35*, 96–111.

Guilford, J. P. *Psychometric methods*. New York: McGraw-Hill, 1954.

Guirao, M., & Stevens, S. S. The measurement

of auditory density. *Journal of the Acoustical Society of America,* 1964, *36,* 1176–1182.

Gulick, W. L. *Hearing: Physiology and psychophysics.* New York: Oxford University Press, 1971.

Gunter, R. Visual size constancy in the cat. *British Journal of Psychology,* 1951, *42,* 288–293.

Haagen-Smit, A. J. Smell and taste. *Scientific American,* 1952, *186,* 28–32.

Haber, R. N. Limited modification of the trapezoidal illusion with experience. *American Journal of Psychology,* 1965, *78,* 651–655.

Haber, R. N. Nature of the effect of set on perception. *Psychological Review,* 1966, *73,* 335–351.

Haber, R. N., & Hershenson, M. Effects of repeated brief exposure on the growth of a percept. *Journal of Experimental Psychology,* 1965, *69,* 40–46.

Haber, R. N., & Hershenson, M. *The psychology of visual perception.* New York: Holt, Rinehart & Winston, 1973.

Haber, R. N., & Nathanson, L. S. Post-retinal storage? Some further observations of Parks' camel as seen through the eye of a needle. *Perception and Psychophysics,* 1968, *3,* 349–355.

Hagelberg, M. P. *Physics: An introduction for students of science and engineering.* Englewood Cliffs, N.J.: Prentice-Hall, 1973.

Hahn, H. Die adaptation des Geschmacksinnes. *Z. Sinnesphysiol.,* 1934, *65,* 105–145.

Hahn, H. G., Kuckulies, G., & Taeger, H. Eine systematische Untersuchung der Geschmacks—Schwellen. I. *Z. Sinnesphysiol.,* 1938, *67,* 259–306.

Halpern, B. P. Some relationships between electrophysiology and behavior in taste. In M. R. Kare and O. Maller (Eds.), *The chemical senses and nutrition.* Baltimore: John Hopkins Press, 1967.

Hardt, M. E., Held, R., & Steinbach, M. J. Adaptation to displaced vision: A change in the central control of sensorimotor coordination. *Journal of Experimental Psychology,* 1971, *89,* 229–239.

Hardy, J. D., Stolwijk, J. A. J., & Hoffman, D. Pain following step increase in skin temperature (Chap. 21). In D. R. Kenshalo (Ed.), *The skin senses.* Springfield, Ill.: Charles C Thomas, 1968.

Harmon, L. D. The recognition of faces. *Scientific American,* 1973, *229,* 70–82.

Harmon, L. D., & Julesz, B. Masking in visual recognition: Effects of two-dimensional filtered noise. *Science,* 1973, *180,* 1194–1197.

Harper, H. W., Jay, J. R., & Erickson, R. P. Chemically evoked sensations from human taste papillae. *Physiology and Behavior,* 1966, *1,* 319–325.

Harris, C. S. Perceptual adaptation to inverted, reversed and displaced vision. *Psychological Review,* 1965, *72,* 419–444.

Harris, C., & Gibson, A. Is orientation-specific color adaptation in human vision due to edge detectors, afterimages, or "dipoles"? *Science,* 1968, *162,* 1506–1507.

Harris, J. D. Pitch discrimination. USN Bureau of Medicine and Surgery Research Report, Project NM 033 041.22.04, No. 205, June 20, 1952.

Hastorf, A. H., & Way, L. Apparent size with and without distance cues. *Journal of General Psychology,* 1952, *47,* 181–188.

Hay, J., & Pick, H. Visual and proprioceptive adaptation to optical displacement of the visual stimulus. *Journal of Experimental Psychology,* 1966, *71,* 150–158.

Hayes, W. N., & Saiff, E. I. Visual alarm reactions in turtles. *Animal Behavior,* 1967, *15,* 102–106.

Haynes, H., White, B. L., & Held, R. Visual accommodation in human infants. *Science,* 1965, *148,* 528–530.

Hebb, D. O. *The organization of behavior.* New York: John Wiley, 1949.

Hebb, D. O. *Textbook of psychology* (3rd ed.). Philadelphia: W. B. Saunders, 1972.

Hecht, S., & Shlaer, S. Intermittent stimulation by light. V. The relation between intensity and critical frequency for different parts of the spectrum. *Journal of General Physiology*, 1936, *19*, 965–977.

Hecht, S., & Shlaer, S. An adaptometer for measuring human dark adaptation. *Journal of the Optical Society of America*, 1938, *28*, 269–275.

Hecht, S., Shlaer, S., & Pirenne, M. H. Energy at the threshold of vision. *Science*, 1941, *93*, 585.

Hecht, S., Shlaer, S., & Pirenne, M. H. Energy, quanta, and vision. *Journal of General Physiology*, 1942, *25*, 819–840.

Heckenmueller, E. G. Stabilization of the retinal image: A review of method, effects, and theory. *Psychological Bulletin*, 1965, *63*, 157–169.

Hein, A., & Held, R. A neural model for labile sensorimotor coordinations. In *Biological prototypes and synthetic systems*. (Vol. I). New York: Plenum Press, 1962.

Hein, A., & Held, R. Dissociation of the visual placing response into elicited and guided components. *Science*, 1967, *158*, 390–392.

Hein, A., Held, R., & Gower, E. C. Development and segmentation of visually controlled movement by selective exposure during rearing. *Journal of Comparative and Physiological Psychology*, 1970, *73*, 181–187.

Heinemann, E. G. Simultaneous brightness induction as a function of inducing- and test-field luminance. *Journal of Experimental Psychology*, 1955, *50*, 89–96.

Held, R. Exposure-history as a factor in maintaining stability of perception and coordination. *Journal of Nervous and Mental Diseases*, 1961, *132*, 26–32.

Held, R. Plasticity in sensory-motor systems. *Scientific American*, 1965, 213, *5*, 84–94.

Held, R. Plasticity in sensorimotor coordination. In S. J. Freedman (Ed.), *The neuropsychology of spatially oriented behavior*. Homewood, Ill.: Dorsey Press, 1968.

Held, R., & Bauer, J. A. Visually guided reaching in infant monkeys after restricted rearing. *Science*, 1967, *155*, 718–720.

Held, R., & Bossom, J. Neonatal deprivation and adult rearrangement: Complementary techniques for analyzing plastic sensory-motor coordinations. *Journal of Comparative and Physiological Psychology*, 1961, *54*, 33–37.

Held, R., & Freedman, S. J. Plasticity in human sensorimotor control. *Science*, 1963, *142*, 455–462.

Held, R., & Gottlieb, N. Techniques for studying adaptation to disarranged hand-eye coordination. *Perceptual and Motor Skills*, 1958, *8*, 83–86.

Held, R., & Hein, A. Adaptation of disarranged hand-eye coordination contingent upon re-afferent stimulation. *Perceptual and Motor Skills*, 1958, *8*, 87–90.

Held, R., & Hein, A. Movement-produced stimulation in the development of visually guided behavior. *Journal of Comparative and Physiological Psychology*, 1963, 56, 872–876.

Held, R., & Hein, A. On the modifiability of form perception. In W. Wathen-Dunn (Ed.), *Models for the perception of speech and visual form*. Cambridge, Mass.: M.I.T. Press, 1967.

Held, R., & Rekosh, J. Motor sensory feedback and the geometry of visual space. *Science*, 1963, *141*, 722–723.

Held, R., & Schlank, M. Adaptation to disarranged eye-hand coordination in the distance dimension. *American Journal of Psychology*, 1959, *72*, 603–605.

Held, R., & Shattuck, S. R. Color- and edge-sensitive channels in the human visual system: Tuning for orientation. *Science*, 1971, *174*, 314–316.

Heller, D. P. Absence of size constancy in visually deprived rats. *Journal of Comparative and Physiological Psychology*, 1968, *65*, 336–339.

Helmholtz, H. von. *Treatise on physiological optics*. (original publ. 1866) Vol. 3. (J. P.

Southall, Trans., Ed.) New York: Dover Press, 1962.

Helson, H. Adaptation-level as frame of reference for prediction of psychological data. *American Journal of Psychology*, 1947, *60*, 1–29.

Helson, H. *Adaptation-level Theory*. New York: Harper & Row, 1964.

Helson, H., & King, S. M. The *tau*-effect. An example of psychological relativity. *Journal of Experimental Psychology*, 1931, *14*, 202–218.

Henney, K. *Principles of radio* (3rd ed.) New York: John Wiley, 1938.

Henning, G. J., Brouwer, J. N., Van Der Wel, H., & Francke, A. Miraculin, the sweet-inducing principle from miracle fruit. In C. Pfaffman (Ed.), *Olfaction and taste*. New York: Rockefeller University Press, 1969.

Henry, G. H., & Bishop, P. O. Simple cells of the striate cortex. In W. D. Neff (Ed.), *Contributions to sensory physiology*. (Vol. 5). New York: Academic Press, 1971.

Henzel, H., & Zotterman, Y. Action potentials of cold fibers and intracutaneous temperature gradient. *Journal of Neurophysiology*, 1951, *14*, 377–385.

Hepler, N. Color: A motion-contingent aftereffect. *Science*, 1968, *162*, 376–377.

Hershberger, W. Attached-shadow orientation perceived as depth by chickens reared in an environment illuminated from below. *Journal of Comparative and Physiological Psychology*, 1970, *73*, 407–411.

Hershenson, M. Visual discrimination in the human newborn. *Journal of Comparative and Physiological Psychology*, 1964, *58*, 270–276.

Hess, E. H. Space perception in the chick. *Scientific American*, 1956, *195*, 71–80.

Hess, E. H. Attitude and pupil size. *Scientific American*, 1965, *212*, 46–54.

Hess, E. H., & Polt, J. M. Pupil size as related to interest value of visual stimuli. *Science*, 1960, *132*, 349–350.

Hess, E. H., & Polt, J. M. Pupil size in relation to mental activity during simple problem-solving. *Science*, 1964, *140*, 1190–1192.

Hess, E. H., & Polt, J. M. Changes in pupil size as a measure of taste difference. *Perceptual and Motor Skills*, 1966, *23*, 451–455.

Hess, E. H., Seltzer, A. L., & Schlien, J. M. Pupil response of hetero- and homosexual males to pictures of men and women: A pilot study. *Journal of Abnormal Psychology*, 1965, *70*, 165–168.

Hinde, R. A. *Animal behavior* (2nd ed.). New York: McGraw-Hill, 1970.

Hirsh, H. V. B., & Spinelli, D. N. Visual experience modifies distribution of horizontally and vertically oriented receptive fields in cats. *Science*, 1970, *168*, 869–871.

Hirsh, I. J. *The measurement of hearing*. New York: McGraw-Hill, 1952.

Hoagland, H. The physiological control of judgments of duration: Evidence for a chemical clock. *Journal of General Psychology*, 1933, *9*, 267–287.

Hoagland, H. *Pacemakers in relation to aspects of behavior*. New York: Macmillan, 1935.

Hochberg, C. B., & Hochberg, J. E. Familiar size and the perception of depth. *Journal of Psychology*, 1952, *34*, 107–114.

Hochberg, C. B., & McAlister, E. Relative size vs. familiar size in the perception of represented depth. *American Journal of Psychology*, 1955, *68*, 294–296.

Hochberg, J. E. Nativism and empiricism in perception. In L. Postman (Ed.), *Psychology in the making*. New York: Knopf, 1962.

Hochberg, J. E. *Perception*. Englewood Cliffs, New Jersey: Prentice-Hall, 1964.

Hochberg, J. E. In the mind's eye. In R. N. Haber (Ed.), *Contemporary theory and research in visual perception*. New York: Holt, Rinehart & Winston, 1968.

Hochberg, J. E. Perception. In J. W. Kling & L. A. Riggs (Eds.), *Experimental psychology*. New York: Holt, Rinehart & Winston, 1971.

Hochberg, J. E., & Brooks, V. The psychophysics of form: reversible-perspective drawings of spatial objects. *American Journal of Psychology*, 1960, *73*, 337–354.

Hochberg, J. E., & McAlister, E. A quantitative approach to figural goodness. *Journal of Experimental Psychology,* 1953, *46,* 361–364.

Hochberg, J. E., Triebel, W., & Seaman, G. Color adaptation under conditions of homogeneous visual stimulation (*Ganzfeld*). *Journal of Experimental Psychology,* 1951, *41,* 153–159.

Holst, E. von. Relations between the central nervous system and the peripheral organs. *British Journal of Animal Behavior,* 1954, *2,* 89–94.

Holubář, J. *The sense of time: an electrophysiological study of its mechanism in man.* Cambridge, Mass.: M.I.T. Press, 1969.

Holway, A. H., & Boring, E. G. The moon illusion and the angle of regard. *American Journal of Psychology,* 1940, *53,* 109–116.

Holway, A. H., & Boring, E. G. Determinants of apparent visual size with distance variant. *American Journal of Psychology,* 1941, *54,* 21–37.

Hornstein, A. D., & Rotter, G. S. Research methodology in temporal perception. *Journal of Experimental Psychology,* 1969, *79,* 3, 561–564.

Hotopf, W. H. N. The size-constancy theory of visual illusions. *British Journal of Psychology,* 1966, *57,* 307–318.

Howard, I. P., & Templeton, W. B. *Human spatial orientation.* New York: John Wiley, 1966.

Hsia, Y., & Graham, C. H. Color blindness. In C. H. Graham (Ed.), *Vision and visual perception.* New York: John Wiley, 1965.

Hubel, D. H. The visual cortex of the brain. *Scientific American,* 1963, *209,* 54–62.

Hubel, D. H., & Wiesel, T. N. Receptive fields of single neurons in the cat's striate cortex. *Journal of Physiology,* 1959, *148,* 574–591.

Hubel, D. H., & Wiesel, T. N. Receptive fields, binocular interaction and functional architecture in the cat's visual cortex. *Journal of Physiology,* 1962, *160,* 106–154.

Hubel, D. H., & Wiesel, T. N. Receptive fields of cells in striate cortex of very young, visually inexperienced kittens. *Journal of Neurophysiology,* 1963, *26,* 994–1002.

Hubel, D. H., & Wiesel, T. N. Receptive fields and functional architecture of monkey striate cortex. *Journal of Physiology,* 1968, *195,* 215–243.

Hurvich, L. M., & Jameson, D. A quantitative theoretical account of color vision. *Transactions of the New York Academy of Sciences,* 1955, *18,* 33–38.

Hurvich, L. M., & Jameson, D. An opponent-process theory of color vision. *Psychological Review,* 1957, *64,* 384–404.

Hurvich, L. M., & Jameson, D. Opponent processes as a model of neural organization. *American Psychologist,* 1974, *29,* 88–102.

Hymovitch, B. The effects of experimental variations on problem solving in the rat. *Journal of Comparative and Physiological Psychology,* 1952, *45,* 313–321.

Irwin, R. J. Emmert's law as a consequence of size constancy. *Perceptual and Motor Skills,* 1969, *28,* 69–70.

Ittelson, W. H. *The Ames demonstration in perception.* Princeton: Princeton University Press, 1952.

Jacobs, G. H., & Pulliam, K. A. Vision in the prairie dog. *Journal of Comparative and Physiological Psychology,* 1973, *84,* 240–245.

Jacobs, H. L. Observations on the ontogeny of saccharine preference in the neonate rat. *Psychonomic Science,* 1964, *1,* 105–106.

Jacobs, H. L. Taste and the role of experience in the regulation of food intake. In M. R. Kare & O. Maller (Eds), *The chemical senses and nutrition.* Baltimore: Johns Hopkins Press, 1967.

James, W. *The principles of psychology.* New York: Henry Holt, 1890.

Jameson, D., & Hurvich, L. M. Complexities of perceived brightness. *Science,* 1961, *133,* 174–179.

Janson, H. W. *History of art.* Englewood Cliffs, N.J.: Prentice-Hall, 1962.

Jenks, G. F., & Brown, D. A. Three-dimensional

map construction. *Science,* 1966, *154,* 857–864.

Johansson, G. Visual perception of biological motion and a model for its analysis. *Perception and Psychophysics,* 1973, *14,* 201–211.

Johnsson, L. G., & Hawkins, J. E. Sensory and neural degeneration with aging, as seen in microdissections of the human inner ear. *Annals of Otology, Rhinology and Laryngology,* 1972, *81,* 179–193.

Jones, F. N. Scales of subjective intensity for odors of diverse chemical nature. *American Journal of Psychology,* 1958, *71,* 305–310. (*a*)

Jones, F. N. Subjective scales of intensity for three odors. *American Journal of Psychology,* 1958, *71,* 423–425. (*b*)

Judd, D. B. Basic correlates of the visual stimulus. In S. S. Stevens (Ed.), *Handbook of experimental psychology.* New York: John Wiley, 1951.

Judd, D. B. *Color in business, science, and industry.* New York: John Wiley, 1952.

Julesz, B. Binocular depth perception without familiarity cues. *Science,* 1964, *145,* 356–362.

Julesz, B. Texture and visual perception. *Scientific American,* 1965, *212,* 38–48.

Julesz, B. *Foundations of cyclopean perception.* Chicago: University of Chicago Press, 1971.

Jung, R., & Spillman, L. Receptive-field estimation and perceptual integration in human vision. In F. A. Young and D. B. Lindsley (Eds.), *Early experience and visual information processing in perceptual and reading disorders.* Washington, D.C.: National Academy of Sciences, 1970.

Kaess, D. W., & Wilson, J. P. Modification of the rat's avoidance of visual depth. *Journal of Comparative and Physiological Psychology,* 1964, *58,* 151–152.

Kagan, J. The determinants of attention in the infant. *American Scientist,* 1970, *58,* 298–306.

Kahneman, D. Method, findings and theory in studies of visual masking. *Psychological Bulletin,* 1968, *70,* 404–425.

Kahneman, D., & Beatty, J. Pupil diameter and load on memory. *Science,* 1966, *154,* 1583–1585.

Kahneman, D., Beatty, J., & Pollack, I. Perceptual deficit during a mental task. *Science,* 1967, *157,* 218–219.

Kahneman, D., Onuska, L., & Wolman, R. E. Effects of grouping on the pupillary response in a short-term memory task. *Quarterly Journal of Experimental Psychology,* 1969, *79,* 164–167.

Kare, M. R., & Ficken, M. S. Comparative studies on the sense of taste. In Y. Zotterman (Ed.), *Olfaction and taste.* New York: Macmillan, 1963.

Karplus, R. *Introductory physics: A model approach.* New York: W. A. Benjamin, 1969.

Kaufman, L. *Sight and mind.* New York: Oxford University Press, 1974.

Kaufman, L., & Rock, I. The moon illusion, I. *Science,* 1962, *136,* 953–961. (*a*)

Kaufman, L., & Rock, I. The moon illusion. *Scientific American,* 1962, *207,* 120–132. (*b*)

Kellogg, R. S. Vestibular influences on orientation in zero gravity, produced by parabolic flight. In Orientation: sensory basis, *Annals of the New York Academy of Sciences,* 1971, *188,* 217–223.

Kellogg, W. N. Sonar system of the blind. *Science,* 1962, *137,* 399–404.

Kenshalo, D. R. Psychophysical studies of temperature sensitivity. In W. D. Neff (Ed.), *Contributions to sensory physiology.* (Vol. 4). New York: Academic Press, 1970.

Kenshalo, D. R. The cutaneous senses. In J. R. Kling and L. A. Riggs (Eds.), *Experimental psychology* (3rd ed.). New York: Holt, Rinehart & Winston, 1971.

Kenshalo, D. R., & Gallegos, E. S. Multiple temperature-sensitive spots innervated by single nerve fibers. *Science,* 1967, *158,* 1064–1065.

Kenshalo, D. R., & Nafe, D. R. A quantitative theory of feeling: 1960. *Psychological Review,* **1962,** *69,* 17–33.

Kenshalo, D. R., & Scott, H. A. Temporal course

of thermal adaptation. *Science,* 1966, *151,* 1095–1096.

Kerr, J. L. Visual resolution in the periphery. *Perception and Psychophysics,* 1971, *9(3B),* 375–378.

Kessen, W. Sucking and looking: Two organized congenital patterns of behavior in the human newborn. In H. W. Stevenson, E. H. Hess, & H. L. Rheingold (Eds.), *Early behavior: Comparative and developmental approaches.* New York: John Wiley, 1967.

Kilbride, P. L., & Leibowitz, H. W. Factors affecting the magnitude of the Ponzo perspective illusion among the Baganda. *Perception & Psychophysics,* 1975, *17,* 543–548.

Kilpatrick, F. P. *Explorations in transactional psychology.* New York: New York University Press, 1961.

Kimura, D. Cerebral dominance and the perception of verbal stimuli. *Canadian Journal of Psychology,* 1961, *15,* 166–171.

Kimura, D. Left-right differences in the perception of melodies. *Quarterly Journal of Experimental Psychology,* 1964, *16,* 355–358.

Kimura, D. Functional asymmetry of the brain in dichotic listening. *Cortex,* 1967, *3,* 163–178.

Kimura, K., & Beidler, L. M. Microelectrode study of taste receptors of rat and hamster. *Journal of Cellular and Comparative Physiology,* 1961, *58,* 131–139.

Kimura, D., & Folb, S. Neural processing of backwards-speech sounds. *Science,* 1968, *161,* 395–396.

King, W. L., & Gruber, H. E. Moon illusion and Emmert's law. *Science,* 1962, *135,* 1125–1126.

Kleber, R. J., Lhamon, W. T., & Goldstone, S. Hyperthermia, hyperthyroidism, and time judgment. *Journal of Comparative and Physiological Psychology,* 1963, *56,* 362–365.

Kluver, H. *Behavior mechanisms in monkeys.* Chicago, Ill.: University of Chicago Press, 1933.

Kohler, I. Experiments with goggles. *Scientific American,* 1962, *206,* 62–86.

Kohler, I. The formation and transformation of the perceptual world. *Psychological Issues,* 1964, *3*(Whole No. 4).

Köhler, W., & Wallach, H. Figural aftereffects: an investigation of visual processes. *Proceedings of the American Philosophical Society,* 1944, *88,* 269–357.

Kolers, P. A. Some differences between real and apparent visual movement. *Vision Research,* 1963, *3,* 191–206.

Kolers, P. A. The illusion of movement. *Scientific American,* 1964, *211,* 98–106.

Konishi, M. How the owl tracks its prey. *American Scientist,* 1973, *61,* 414–424.

Köster, E. P. Intensity in mixtures of odorous substances. In C. Pfaffman (Ed.), *Olfaction and taste.* New York: Rockefeller University Press, 1969.

Kraft, A. L., & Winnick, W. A. The effect of pattern and texture gradient on slant and shape judgments. *Perception and Psychophysics,* 1967, *2,* 141–147.

Kravitz, J. H., & Wallach, H. *Adaptation to displaced vision contingent upon vibrating stimulation. Psychonomic Science,* 1966, *6,* 465–466.

Krech, D., & Crutchfield, R. S. *Elements of psychology.* New York: Knopf, 1958.

Kristofferson, A. B. Attention and psychophysical time. *Acta Psychologica,* 1967, *27,* 93–100.

Krueger, L. E. David Katz's der aufbau der tastwelt (the world of taste): a synopsis. *Perception and Psychophysics,* 1970, *7,* 337–341.

Kryter, K. D. *The effect of noise on man.* New York: Academic Press, 1970.

Kuffler, S. W. Discharge patterns and functional organization of mammalian retina. *Journal of Neurophysiology,* 1953, *16,* 37–68.

Künnapas, T. M. Influence of frame size on apparent length of a line. *Journal of Experimental Psychology,* 1955, *50,* 168–170.

Künnapas, T. M. The vertical-horizontal illusion and the visual field. *Journal of Experimental Psychology,* 1957, *53,* 405–407.

Künnapas, T. M. Influence of head inclination of

the vertical-horizontal illusion. *Journal of Psychology,* 1958, *46,* 179–185.

Künnapas, T. M. The vertical-horizontal illusion in artificial visual fields. *Journal of Psychology,* 1959, *47,* 41–48.

Kurihara, K., Kurihara, Y., & Beidler, L. M. Isolation and mechanisms of taste modifiers: Taste modifying protein and gymnemic acids. In C. Pfaffman (Ed.), *Olfaction and taste.* New York: Rockefeller University Press, 1969.

Ladd-Franklin, C. *Colour and colour theories.* New York: Harcourt, Brace, 1929.

Land, E. H. Experiments in color vision. *Scientific American,* 1959, *200,* 84–99.

Land, E. H. The retinex. *American Scientist,* 1964, *52,* 247–264.

Land. E. H., & McCann, J. J. Lightness and retinex theory. *Journal of the Optical Society of America,* 1971, *61,* 1–11.

Langdon, J. The perception of changing shape. *Quarterly Journal of Experimental Psychology,* 1951, *3,* 157–165.

Langdon, J. Further studies in the perception of changing shape. *Quarterly Journal of Experimental Psychology,* 1953, *3,* 89–107.

Lashley, K. S., & Russell, J. T. The mechanism of vision: XI. A preliminary test of innate organization. *Journal of Genetic Psychology,* 1934, *45,* 136–144.

Lasko, W. J., & Lindauer, M. J. Experience with congruity in the perception of incongruity. *Psychonomic Science,* 1968, *12,* 59.

Lavallee, R. J. Effects of visual form and distance experience before maturity on adult problem-solving ability in the rat. *Developmental Psychology,* 1970, *2,* 257–263.

Lawrence, M. *Studies in human behavior.* Princeton: Princeton University Press, 1949.

Lefton, L. A. Metacontrast: a review. *Perception and Psychophysics,* 1973, *13,* 161–171.

Leibowitz, H. W. *Visual perception.* New York: Macmillan, 1965.

Leibowitz, H. W. Sensory, learned, and cognitive mechanisms of size perception. *Annals of the New York Academy of Sciences,* 1971, *188,* 47–62.

Leibowitz, H. W., Brislin, R., Perlmutter, L., & Hennessy, R. Ponzo perspective illusion as a manifestation of space perception. *Science,* 1969, *166,* 1174–1176.

Leibowitz, H. W., & Judisch, J. M. The relation between age and the magnitude of the Ponzo illusion. *American Journal of Psychology,* 1967, *80,* 105–109.

Leibowitz, H. W., & Pick, H. A. Cross-cultural and educational aspects of the Ponzo perspective illusion. *Perception and Psychophysics,* 1972, *12,* 430–432.

Leibowitz, H. W., Shiina, K., & Hennessy, R. T. Oculomotor adjustments and size constancy. *Perception and Psychophysics,* 1972, *12,* 497–500.

Leibowitz, H., Waskow, I., Loeffler, N., & Glaser, F. Intelligence level as a variable in the perception of shape. *Quarterly Journal of Experimental Psychology,* 1959, *11,* 108–112.

Lele, P. P., & Weddell, G. The relationship between neurohistology and corneal sensibility. *Brain,* 1956, *79,* 119–154.

Lenneberg, E. H. *Biological foundations of language.* New York: John Wiley, 1967.

Lettvin, J. Y., Maturana, H. R., McCulloch, W. S., & Pitts, W. H. What the frog's eye tells the frog's brain. *Proceedings of the Institute of Radio Engineers,* 1959, *47,* 1940–1951.

Leukel, F. *Introduction to physiological psychology.* St. Louis: C. V. Mosby, 1972.

Levitsky, D. A., & Barnes, R. H. Nutritional and environmental interactions in the behavioral development of the rat: Long-term effects. *Science,* 1972, *176,* 68–71.

Lewis, D. J. *Scientific principles of psychology.* Englewood Cliffs, New Jersey: Prentice-Hall, 1963.

Lewis, M. Infant's responses to facial stimuli during the first year of life. *Developmental Psychology,* 1969, *1,* 75–86.

Liberman, A. M., Cooper, F. S., Harris, K. S., MacNeilage, P. F., & Studdert-Kennedy, M.

Some observations on a model for speech perception. In W. Wathen-Dunn (Ed.), *Models for the perception of speech and visual form.* Cambridge, Mass.: M.I.T. Press, 1967.

Lichten, W., & Lurie, S. A new technique for the study of perceived size. *American Journal of Psychology,* 1950, *63,* 280–282.

Licklider, J. C. R., & Miller, G. A. The perception of speech. In S. S. Stevens (Ed.), *The handbook of experimental psychology.* New York: John Wiley, 1951.

Lieberman, P. *Information, perception, and language.* Research Monograph No. 38. Cambridge, Mass.: M.I.T. Press, 1968.

Lieberman, P., & Crelin, E. S. On the speech of Neanderthal man. *Linguistic Inquiry,* 1971, *2,* 203–222.

Lieberman, P., Crelin, E. S., & Klatt, D. H. Phonetic ability and related anatomy of the newborn and adult human, Neanderthal man, and the chimpanzee. *American Anthropologist,* 1972, *74,* 287–307.

Lim, R. K. S. Cutaneous and visceral pain, and somesthetic chemoreceptors (Chap. 22). In D. R. Kenshalo (Ed.), *The skin senses.* Springfield, Ill.: Charles C Thomas, 1968.

Lindgren, H. C., & Byrne, D. *Psychology,* New York: John Wiley, 1975.

Lindsay, P. H., & Norman, D. A. *Human information processing: An introduction to psychology.* New York: Academic Press, 1972.

Ling, B. C. Form discrimination as a learning cue in infants. *Comparative Psychology Monographs,* 1941, *17,* No. 2(Whole No. 86).

Lipscomb, D. M. *Noise: the unwanted sounds.* Chicago, Ill.: Nelson-Hall, 1974.

Lipsett, L. P. Learning in the human infant. In H. W. Stevenson, E. H. Hess, & H. L. Rheingold (Eds.), *Early behavior: Comparative and developmental approaches.* New York: John Wiley, 1967.

Livingston, W. K. The vicious circle in causalgia. *Annals of the New York Academy of Sciences,* 1948, *50,* 247–258.

Llewellyn Thomas, E. Movements of the eye. *Scientific American,* 1968, *219,* 88–95.

Llewellyn Thomas, E. Search behavior. *Radiological Clinics of North America,* 1969, *7,* 403–417.

Locher, P. J., & Nodine, C. F. The role of scanpaths in the recognition of random shapes. *Perception and Psychophysics,* 1974, *15,* 308–314.

Lockhart, J. M. Ambient temperature and time estimation. *Journal of Experimental Psychology,* 1967, *73,* 286–291.

London, I. D. A Russian report on the postoperative newly seeing. *American Journal of Psychology,* 1960, *73,* 478–482.

Lore, R., & Sawatski, D. Performance of binocular and monocular infant rats on the visual cliff. *Journal of Comparative and Physiological Psychology,* 1969, *67,* 177–181.

Luckiesh, M. *Visual illusions.* New York: Dover Publications, 1965.

Mack, A. The role of movement in perceptual adaptation to a tilted retinal image. *Perception and Psychophysics,* 1967, *2,* 65–69.

Mackay, D. M. Moving visual images produced by regular stationary patterns. *Nature,* 1957, *180,* 849–850.

Mackworth, N. H., & Morandi, A. J. The gaze selects informative details within pictures. *Perception and Psychophysics,* 1967, *2,* 547–552.

MacNichol, E. F. Three-pigment color vision. *Scientific American,* 1964, *211,* 48–56. (*a*)

MacNichol, E. F. Retinal mechanisms of color vision. *Vision Research,* 1964, *4,* 119–133. (*b*)

Maffei, L., Fiorentini, A., & Bisti, S. Neural correlate of perceptual adaptation to gratings. *Science,* 1973, *182,* 1036–1038.

Maller, O. Specific appetite. In M. R. Kare and O. Maller (Eds.), *The chemical senses and nutrition.* Baltimore: Johns Hopkins Press, 1967.

Malott, R. W., & Malott, M. K. Perception and stimulus generalizations. In W. C. Stebbins (Ed.), *Animal psychophysics.* New York: Appleton-Century-Crofts, 1970.

Malott, R. W., Malott, M. K., & Pokrzywinski, J. The effects of outward-pointing arrowheads on the Mueller-Lyer illusion in pigeons. *Psychonomic Science,* 1967, *9,* 55–56.

Manley, G. A. Some aspects on the evolution of hearing in vertebrates. *Nature,* 1971, *230,* 506–509.

Marks, L. E. On scales of sensation: Prolegomena to any future psychophysics that will be able to come forth as science. *Perception and psychophysics,* 1974, *16,* 358–376.

Marks, L. E., & Stevens, J. C. Individual brightness functions. *Perception and Psychophysics,* 1966, *1,* 17–24.

Marks, L. E., & Stevens, J. C. Perceived cold and skin temperature as functions of stimulation level and duration. *American Journal of Psychology,* 1972, *85,* 407–419.

Marks, W. B., Dobelle, W. H., & MacNichol, E. F. Visual pigments of single primate cones. *Science,* 1964, *143,* 1181–1183.

Marler, P. R. & Hamilton, W. J. *Mechanisms of Animal Behavior.* New York: John Wiley, 1966.

Marshall, D. A. A comparative study of neural coding in gustation. *Physiology and Behavior,* 1968, *3,* 1–15.

Massaro, D. W., & Anderson, N. H. A test of a perspective theory of geometrical illusions. *American Journal of Psychology,* 1970, *83,* 567–575.

Masterton, B., & Diamond, I. T. Hearing: Central neural mechanisms (Chap. 18). In E. C. Carterette and M. P. Friedman (Eds.), *Handbook of Perception.* Volume III. *Biology of perceptual systems.* New York: Academic Press, 1973.

Masterton, B., Heffner, H., & Ravizza, R. The evolution of human hearing. *Journal of the Acoustical Society of America,* 1968, *45,* 966–985.

Matsumiya, Y., Tagliasco, C. T., Lombroso, C. T., & Goodglass, H. Auditory evoked response: Meaningfulness of stimuli and interhemispheric asymmetry. *Science,* 1972, *175,* 790–792.

Matthews, L. H., & Knight, M. *The senses of animals.* London: Museum Press, 1963.

Mattingly, I. G. Speech cues and sign stimuli. *American Scientist,* 1972, *60,* 327–337.

McBurney, D. H. Magnitude estimation of the taste of sodium chloride after adaptation to sodium chloride. *Journal of Experimental Psychology,* 1966, *72,* 869–873.

McBurney, D. H. Effects of adaptation on human taste function. In C. Pfaffman (Ed.), *Olfaction and taste.* New York: Rockefeller University Press, 1969.

McBurney, D. H., & Pfaffman, C. Gustatory adaptation to saliva and sodium chloride. *Journal of Experimental Psychology,* 1963, *65,* 523–529.

McBurney, D. H., & Shick, T. R. Taste and water taste of twenty-six compounds for man. *Perception and Psychophysics,* 1971, *10,* 249–252.

McCann, J. J. Rod-cone interactions: Different color sensations from identical stimuli. *Science,* 1972, *176,* 1255–1257.

McClintic, J. R. *Basic anatomy and physiology of the human body.* New York: John Wiley, 1975.

McClintock, M. K. Menstrual synchrony and suppression. *Nature,* 1971, *229,* 244–245.

McCollough, C. Color adaptation of edge-detectors in the human visual system. *Science,* 1965, *149,* 1115–1116.

McCutcheon, N. B., & Saunders, J. Human taste papilla stimulation: Stability of quality judgments over time. *Science,* 1972, *175,* 214–216.

McKennell, A. C. Visual size and familiar size: Individual differences. *British Journal of Psychology,* 1960, *51,* 27–35.

Mednick, S. A., Higgins, J., & Kirschenbaum, J. *Psychology: Explorations in behavior and experience.* New York: John Wiley, 1975.

Meiselman, H. L., & Dzendolet, E. Variability in gustatory quality identification. *Perception and Psychophysics,* 1967, *2,* 496–498.

Melzack, R. Phantom limbs. *Psychology Today,* 1970, *4,* 63–68.

Melzack, R. *The puzzle of pain.* New York: Basic Books, 1973.

Melzack, R., & Casey, K. L. Sensory, motivational, and central control determinants of pain (Chap. 20). In D. R. Kenshalo (Ed.), *The skin senses*. Springfield, Ill.: Charles C Thomas, 1968.

Melzack, R., & Wall, P. D. Pain mechanisms: a new theory. *Science*, 1965, *150*, 971–979.

Menzer, G. W., & Thurmond, J. B. Form identification in peripheral vision. *Perception and Psychophysics*, 1970, *8*, 205–209.

Mescavage, A. A., Heimer, W. I., Tatz, S. J., & Runyon, R. P. Time estimation as a function of rate of stimulus change. Paper presented at the annual meeting of the Eastern Psychological Association, New York, April, 1971.

Messing, R. B., & Campbell, B. A. Summation of pain produced in different anatomical regions. *Perception and Psychophysics*, 1971, *10*, 225–228.

Michael, C. R. Receptive fields of single optic nerve fibers in a mammal with an all-cone retina. *Journal of Neurophysiology*, 1968, *31*, 257–267.

Michael, C. R. Retinal processing of visual images. *Scientific American*, 1969, *220*, 104–114.

Michael, R. P., Bonsall, R. W., & Warner, P. Human vaginal secretions: Volatile fatty acid content. *Science*, 1974, *186*, 1217–1219.

Michael, R. P., & Keverne, E. B. Pheromones in the communication of sexual status in primates. *Nature*, 1968, *218*, 746–749.

Michels, K. M., & Schumacher, A. W. Color vision in tree squirrels. *Psychonomic Science*, 1968, *10*, 7–8.

Michels, W. C. & Helson, H. A reformation of the Fechner law in terms of adaptation-level applied to rating-scale data. *American Journal of Psychology*, 1949, *62*, 355–368.

Michon, J. Tapping regularity as a measure of perceptual motor load. *Ergonomics*, 1966, *9*, 401–412.

Michotte, A. *The perception of causality*. New York: Basic Books, 1963.

Mikaelian, H., & Held, R. Two types of adaption to an optically-rotated visual field.

American Journal of Psychology, 1964, 77, 257–263.

Miller, D. C. *The science of musical sounds*. New York: Macmillian, 1926.

Miller, G. A. The masking of speech. *Psychological Bulletin*, 1947, *44*, 105–129.

Milne, L. J., & Milne. M. *The senses of animals and men*. New York: Atheneum, 1967.

Milner, B. Laterality effects in audition. In V. B. Mountcastle (Ed.), *Interhemispheric relations and cerebral dominance*. Baltimore: Johns Hopkins Press, 1962.

Milner, P. *Physiological psychology*. New York: Holt, Rinehart & Winston, 1970.

Mo, S. S. Judgment of temporal duration as a function of numerosity. *Psychonomic Science*, 1971, *24*, 71–72.

Moncrieff, R. W. *The chemical senses*. London: Leonard Hill, 1951.

Moncrieff, R. W. *Odour preferences*. New York: John Wiley, 1966.

Montagna, W. The skin. *Scientific American*, 1965, *212*, 56-66.

Moray, N. Attention in dichotic listening: Affective cues and the influence of instructions. *Quarterly Journal of Experimental Psychology*, 1959, *11*, 56–60.

Moray, N., & Jordan, A. Vision in chicks with distorted visual fields. *Psychonomic Science*, 1967, *9*, 303.

Mosel, J. N., & Kantrowitz, G. The effect of monosodium glutamate on acuity to the primary tastes. *American Journal of Psychology*, 1952, *65*, 573–579.

Mowrer, O. H. Maturation vs. learning in the development of vestibular and optokinetic nystagmus. *Journal of Genetic Psychology*, 1936, *48*, 383–404.

Mozell, M. M. Olfactory discrimination: Electrophysiological spatiotemporal basis. *Science*, 1964, *143*, 1336–1337.

Mozell, M. M. The spatiotemporal analysis of odorants at the level of the olfactory receptor sheet. *Journal of General Physiology*, 1966, *50*, 25–41.

Mozell, M. M. Olfaction. In J. W. Kling and L.

A. Riggs (Eds.), *Experimental psychology* (3rd ed.). New York: Holt, Rinehart and Winston, 1971.

Mueller, C. G. *Sensory psychology,* Englewood Cliffs: Prentice-Hall, 1965.

Mueller, C. G., & Rudolph, M. *Light and vision.* New York: Time-Life Books, 1966.

Mueller, J. The specific energies of nerves (1838). In W. Dennis (Ed.), *Readings in the history of psychology.* New York: Appleton-Century-Crofts, 1948.

Muir, D. W., & Mitchell, D. E. Visual resolution and experience: Acuity deficits in cats following early selective visual deprivation. *Science,* 1973, *180,* 420–422.

Munn, N. L., & Steining, B. R. The relative efficacy of form and background in a child's discrimination of visual patterns. *Journal of Genetic Psychology,* 1931, *39,* 73–90.

Muntz, W. R. A. The development of phototaxis in the frog (*Rana temporaria*). *Journal of Experimental Biology,* 1963, *40,* 371–379.

Muntz, W. R. A. Vision in frogs. *Scientific American,* 1964, *210,* 110–119.

Murch, G. M. Growth of a percept as a function of interstimulus interval. *Journal of Experimental Psychology,* 1969, *82,* 121–128.

Murch, G. M. *Visual and auditory perception.* Indianapolis: Bobbs–Merrill, 1973.

Murch, G. M., & Hirsch, J. The McCollough effect created by complementary afterimages. *American Journal of Psychology,* 1972, *85,* 241–247.

Murphy, M. R., & Schneider, G. E. Olfactory bulb removal eliminates mating behavior in the male golden hamster. *Science,* 1969, *167,* 302–303.

Mussen, P. & Rosenzweig, M. R. *Psychology: An introduction.* Lexington, Mass., D. C. Heath, 1973.

Nachman M. Taste preferences for sodium salts by adrenalectomized rats. *Journal of Comparative and Physiological Psychology,* 1962, *55,* 1124–1129.

Nachman, M. Learned aversion to the taste of

lithium chloride and generalization to other salts. *Journal of Comparative and Physiological Psychology,* 1963, *56,* 343–349.

Nafe, J. P. The pressure, pain, and temperature senses. In C. A. Murchison (Ed.), *A handbook of general experimental psychology* (Chap. 20). Worcester, Mass.: Clark University Press, 1934.

Nealey, S. M., & Edwards, B. J. Depth perception in rats without pattern-vision experience. *Journal of Comparative and Physiological Psychology,* 1960, *53,* 468–469.

Nealey, S. M., & Riley, D. A. Loss and recovery of visual depth in dark-reared rats. *American Journal of Psychology,* 1963, *76,* 329–332.

Neisser, U. *Cognitive psychology.* New York: Appleton-Century-Crofts, 1967.

Neisser, U. The processes of vision. *Scientific American,* 1968, *219,* 204–214.

Nelson, T. M., & Bartley, S. J. The perception of form in an unstructured field. *Journal of General Psychology,* 1956, *54,* 57–63.

Newman, E. B., Stevens, S. S., & Davis, H. Factors in the production of aural harmonics and combination tones. *Journal of the Acoustical Society of America,* 1937, *9,* 107–118.

Nissen, H. W., Chow, K. L., & Semmes, J. Effects of restricted opportunity for tactual, kinesthetic, and manipulative experience on the behavior of the chimpanzee. *American Journal of Psychology,* 1951, *64,* 485–507.

Noell, W. K., Delmelle, M. C. & Albrecht, R. Vitamin A deficiency effect on the retina: Dependence on light. *Science,* 1971, *172,* 72–76.

Nordsiek, F. W. The sweet tooth. *American Scientist,* 1972, *60,* 41–45.

Noton, D., & Stark, L. Scanpaths in eye movements during pattern perception. *Science,* 1971, *171,* 308–311. *(a)*

Noton, D., & Stark, L. Eye movements and visual perception. *Scientific American,* 1971, *224,* 34–43. *(b)*

Noton, D., & Stark, L. Scanpaths in saccadic eye movements while viewing and recognizing patterns. *Vision Research,* 1971, *11,* 929–942. *(c)*

Novick, A. Echolocation in bats: Some aspects of pulse design. *American Scientist,* 1971, *59,* 198–209.

Ogle, K. N. The optical space sense. In H. Davson (Ed.), *The eye.* New York: Academic Press, 1962.

Olson, R. K. Slant judgments from static and rotating trapezoids correspond to rules of perspective geometry. *Perception and Psychophysics,* 1974, *15,* 509–516.

O'Mahoney, M., & Wingate, P. The effect of interstimulus procedures on salt taste intensity functions. *Perception and Psychophysics,* 1974, *16,* 494–502.

Ono, H. Apparent distance as a function of familiar size. *Journal of Experimental Psychology,* 1969, *79,* 109–115.

Orbison, W. D. Shape as a function of the vector field. *American Journal of Psychology,* 1939, *52,* 31–45.

Ornstein, R. E. *On the experience of time.* Baltimore, Md.: Penguin Books, 1969.

Orr, D. B. A perspective on the perception of time compressed speech. In D. L. Horton and J. J. Jenkins (Eds.), *Perception of language.* Columbus, Ohio: Charles E. Merrill, 1971.

Osgood, C. E. *Method and theory in experimental psychology.* New York: Oxford University Press, 1953.

Oster, G. Phosphenes. *Scientific American,* 1970, *222,* 82–87.

Over, R. Explanations of geometrical illusions. *Psychological Bulletin,* 1968, *70,* 545–562.

Oyama, T. Figure-ground dominance as a function of sector angle, brightness, hue, and orientation. *Journal of Experimental Psychology,* 1960, *60,* 299–305.

Pantle, A., & Sekuler, R. Size-detecting mechanisms in human vision. *Science,* 1968, *162,* 1146–1148.

Parducci, A. Range-frequency compromise in judgment. *Psychological Monograph,* 1963, *77* (Whole No. 2).

Parducci, A. The relativism of absolute judgments. *Scientific American,* 1968, *219,* 84–90.

Parks, T. E. Post-retinal visual storage. *American Journal of Psychology,* 1965, *78,* 145–147.

Parrish, M., Lundy, R. M., & Leibowitz, H. W. Hypnotic age-regression and magnitudes of the Ponzo and Poggendorff illusions. *Science,* 1968, *161,* 1235–1236.

Pastore, N. Form perception and size constancy in the duckling. *Journal of Psychology,* 1958, *45,* 259–261.

Pastore, N. *Selective history of theories of visual perception.* New York: Oxford University Press, 1971.

Penfield, W., & Rasmussen, T. *The cerebral cortex of man.* New York: Macmillan, 1950.

Penrose, L. S., & Penrose, R. Impossible objects: A special type of visual illusion. *British Journal of Psychology,* 1958, *49,* 31–33.

Pettigrew, J. D., & Freeman, R. D. Visual experience without lines: Effect on developing cortical neurons. *Science,* 1973, 182, 599–601.

Pfaff, D. Effects of temperature and time of day on time judgments. *Journal of Experimental Psychology,* 1968, *76,* 419–422.

Pfaffman, C. Gustatory afferent impulses. *Journal of Cellular and Comparative Physiology,* 1941, *17,* 243–258.

Pfaffman, C. Taste and smell. In: S. S. Stevens (Ed.), *Handbook of Experimental Psychology.* New York: John Wiley, 1951.

Pfaffman, C. Gustatory nerve impulses in rat, cat, and rabbit. *Journal of Neurophysiology,* 1955, *18,* 429–440.

Pfaffman, C. The afferent code for sensory quality. *American Psychologist,* 1959, *14,* 226–232. (a)

Pfaffman, C. The sense of taste. In J. Field, H. W. Magoun, & V. E. Hall (Eds.), *Handbook of physiology.* (Vol. I). Washington, D. C.: American Physiological Society, 1959. (b)

Pfaffman, C. Taste stimulation and preference behavior. In Y. Zotterman (Ed.), *Olfaction and taste.* New York: Macmillan, 1963.

Pfaffman, C. Taste, its sensory and motivating properties. *American Scientist,* 1964, *52,* 187–206.

Pfaffman, C. The sensory coding of taste quality. In *Chemical senses and flavor*. Dordrecht-Holland: D. Reidel Co., 1974 (*a*)

Pfaffman, C. Specificity of the sweet receptors of the squirrel monkey. In *Chemical senses and flavor*. Dordrecht-Holland: D. Reidel Co., 1974 (*b*).

Pfaffman, C. Personal communication, September 26, 1975.

Pfister, H. See Smith, K. U., & Smith, W. M., *Perception and motion*. Philadelphia: Saunders, 1962.

Pick, H. L. Perception in Soviet psychology. *Psychological Bulletin*, 1964, *62*, 21–35.

Pick, H. L., & Hay, J. C. A passive test of the Held re-afference hypothesis. *Perceptual and Motor Skills*, 1965, *20*, 1070–1072.

Pick, H. L., & Pick, A. Sensory and perceptual development. In P. H. Mussen (Ed.), *Carmichael's manual of child psychology*. (Vol. I). New York: John Wiley, 1970.

Pirenne, M. H. *Optics, painting and photography*. Cambridge, Great Britain: Cambridge University Press, 1970.

Plomp, R. Old and new data on tone perception. In W. D. Neff (Ed.), *Contributions to sensory physiology*. (Vol. 5). New York: Academic Press, 1971.

Polyak, S. L. *The retina*. Chicago: University of Chicago Press, 1941.

Polyak, S. *The vertebrate visual system*. Chicago: University of Chicago Press, 1957.

Postman, L., & Egan, J. P. *Experimental Psychology*. New York: Harper & Row, 1949.

Pressey, A. W. An extension of assimilation theory to illusions of size, area, and direction. *Perception and Psychophysics*, 1971, *9*, 172–176.

Pritchard, R. M. Stabilized images on the retina. *Scientific American*, 1961, *204*, 72–78.

Pritchard, R. M., Heron, W., & Hebb, D. O. Visual perception approached by the method of stabilized images. *Canadian Journal of Psychology*, 1960, *14*, 67–77.

Purdy, D. M. The Bezold-Brücke phenomenon and contours for constant hue. *American Journal of Psychology*, 1937, *49*, 313–315.

Rasch, E., Swift, H., Riesen, A. H., & Chow, K. L. Altered structure and composition of retinal cells in dark-reared mammals. *Experimental Cell Research*, 1961, *25*, 348–363.

Raskin, L. M., & Walk, R. D. Depth perception in the light-reared and in the dark-reared rabbit. Paper read at the annual meeting of the Eastern Psychological Association, New York, April 1963.

Ratliff, F. *Machbands: quantitative studies on neural networks in the retina*. San Francisco: Holden-Day, 1965.

Ratliff, F. Contour and contrast. *Proceedings of the American Philosophical Society*, 1971, *115*, 150–163.

Ratliff, F. Contour and contrast. *Scientific American*, 1972, *226*, 90–101.

Ratliff, F., & Hartline, H. K. The responses of *Limulus* optic nerve fibers to patterns of illumination on the retinal mosaic. *Journal of General Physiology*, 1959, *42*, 1241–1255.

Ratoosh, P. On interposition as a cue for the perception of distance. *Proceedings of the National Academy of Sciences*, 1949, *35*, 257–259.

Reese, T. S., & Stevens, S. S. Subjective intensity of coffee odor. *American Journal of Psychology*, 1960, *73*, 424–428.

Restle, F. Moon illusion explained on the basis of relative size. *Science*, 1970, *167*, 1092–1096.

Rethlingshafer, D., & Hinckley, E. D. Influence of judge's characteristics upon the adaptation level. *American Journal of Psychology*, 1963, *76*, 116–119.

Reynolds, G. S., & Stevens, S. S. Binaural summation of loudness. *Journal of the Acoustical Society of America*, 1960, *32*, 1337–1344.

Rice, C. E. Human echo perception. *Science*, 1967, *155*, 656–664.

Richter, C. P. Salt taste thresholds of normal and adrenalectomized rats. *Endocrinology*, 1939, *24*, 367–371.

Richter, C. P. Total self-regulatory functions in animals and human beings. *Harvey Lectures*, 1942, *38*, 63–103.

Riesen, A. H. Arrested vision. *Scientific American,* 1950, *183,* 16–19.

Riesen, A. H. Stimulation as a requirement for growth and function in behavioral development. In D. W. Fiske & S. R. Maddi (Eds.), *Functions of varied experience.* Homewood, Ill.: Dorsey Press, 1961.

Riesen, A. H. Effects of early deprivation of photic stimulation. In S. F. Osler & R. E. Cooke (Eds.), *The biosocial basis of mental retardation.* Baltimore, Md.: Johns Hopkins Press, 1965.

Riesen, A. H. Effects of visual environment on the retina. In F. A. Young & D. B. Lindsley (Eds.), *Early experience and visual information processing in perceptual and reading disorders.* National Academy of Sciences, 1970.

Riesen, A. H., & Aarons, L. Visual movement and intensity discrimination in cats after early deprivation of pattern-vision. *Journal of Comparative and Physiological Psychology,* 1959, *52,* 142–149.

Riesen, A. H., Ramsey, R. L., & Wilson, P. D. The development of visual acuity in rhesus monkeys deprived of patterned light during early infancy. *Psychonomic Science,* 1964, *1,* 33–34.

Riggs, L. A. Visual acuity. In C. H. Graham (Ed.), *Vision and visual perception.* New York: John Wiley, 1965.

Riggs, L. A. The "looks" of Helmholtz. *Perception and Psychophysics,* 1967, *2,* 1–13.

Riggs, L. A. Vision. In J. W. Kling & L. A. Riggs (Eds.), *Experimental Psychology* (3rd ed.). New York: Holt, Rinehart & Winston, 1971.

Riggs, L. A. Curvature as a feature of pattern vision. *Science,* 1973, *181,* 1070–1072.

Riggs, L. A. White, K. D., & Eimas, P. D. Establishment and decay of orientation-contingent aftereffects of color. *Perception and Psychophysics,* 1974, *16,* 535–542.

Robinson, D. A. Eye movement control in primates. *Science,* 1968, *161,* 1219–1224.

Rock, I. *The nature of perceptual adaptation.* New York: Basic Books, 1966.

Rock, I. *Orientation and form.* New York: Academic Press, 1973.

Rock, I. The preception of disoriented figures. *Scientific American,* 1974, *230,* 78–85.

Rock, I. *An introduction to perception,* New York: Macmillan, 1975.

Rock, I., & Ebenholtz, S. The relational determination of perceived size. *Psychological Review,* 1959, *66,* 387–401.

Rock, I., & Halper, F. Form perception without a retinal image. *American Journal of Psychology,* 1969, *82,* 425–440.

Rock, I., & Harris, C. S. Vision and touch. *Scientific American,* 1967, *216,* 96–104.

Rock, I., & Kaufman, L. The moon illusion, II. *Science,* 1962, *136,* 1023–1031.

Rock, I., & Victor, J. Vision and touch: An experimentally created conflict between the senses. *Science,* 1964, *143,* 594–596.

Rodgers, W., & Rozin, P. Novel food preferences in thiamine-deficient rats. *Journal of Comparative and Physiological Psychology,* 1966, *61,* 1–4.

Rommel, S. A., & McCleave, J. D. Oceanic electric fields: Perception by American eels? *Science,* 1972, *176,* 1233–1235.

Rosenblum, L. A., & Cross, H. A. Performance of neonatal monkeys in the visual-cliff situation. *American Journal of Psychology,* 1963, *76,* 318–320.

Rosenthal, S. R. Histamine as the chemical mediator for referred pain (Chap. 24). In D. R. Kenshalo (Ed.), *The skin senses.* Springfield, Ill.: Charles C Thomas, 1968.

Rosenzweig, M. R. Representations of the two ears at the auditory cortex. *American Journal of Psychology,* 1951, *67,* 147–158.

Rosenzweig, M. R. Cortical correlates of auditory localization and of related perceptual phenomena. *Journal of Comparative and Physiological Psychology,* 1954, *47,* 269–276.

Rosenzweig, M. R. Auditory localization. *Scientific American,* 1961, *205,* 132–142.

Routtenberg, A., & Glickman, S. J. Visual cliff behavior in undomesticated rodents, land and aquatic turtles, and cats (*Panthera*). *Journal of Comparative and Physiological Psychology,* 1964, *58,* 143–146.

Rowell, T. E. Agonistic noises of the rhesus monkeys (*Macaca mulatta*). *Symposium of the Zoological Society of London,* 1962, *8,* 91–96.

Rubin, E. Figure and ground. In D. C. Beardslee & M. Wertheimer (Eds.), *Readings in perception.* New York: D. Van Nostrand, 1958. (Based on an abridged translation by Michael Wertheimer of pp. 35–101 of Rubin, E., *Visuell wahrgenommene Figuren* (translated by Peter Collett into German from the Danish *Synsoplevede Figurer,* Copenhagen: Gyldendalske, 1915). Copenhagen: Gyldendalske, 1921. Translated and printed by permission of the publishers.

Rubin, M. L., & Walls, G. L. *Fundamentals of visual science.* Springfield, Ill.: Charles C Thomas, 1969.

Rushton, W. A. H. Visual pigments in man. *Scientific American,* 1962, *207,* 120–132.

Rushton, W. A. H. Increment threshold and dark adaptation. *Journal of the Optical Society of America,* 1963, *3,* 104–109.

Rushton, W. A. H., & Westheimer, G. The effect upon the rod threshold of bleaching neighbouring rods. *Journal of Physiology,* 1962, *164,* 318–329.

Salapatek, P. The visual investigation of geometric pattern by one- and two-month-old infants. Paper read at the annual meeting of the American Association for the Advancement of Science, Boston, December, 1969.

Salapatek, P., & Kessen, W. Visual scanning of triangles by the human newborn. *Journal of Experimental Child Psychology,* 1966, *3,* 113–122.

Satran, R., & Goldstein, M. N. Pain perception: Modification of threshold of intolerance and cortical potentials by cutaneous stimulation. *Science,* 1973, *180,* 1201–1202.

Schiff, W. The perception of impending collision: A study of visually directed avoidant behavior.

Psychological Monographs, 1965, *79,* (Whole No. 604).

Schiff, W., Caviness, J. A., & Gibson, J. J. Persistent fear responses in rhesus monkeys to the optical stimulus of "looming." *Science,* 1962, *136,* 982–983.

Schiffman, H. R. Size-estimation of familiar objects under informative and reduced conditions of viewing. *American Journal of Psychology,* 1967, *80,* 229–235.

Schiffman, H. R. Physical support with and without optical support: Reaction to apparent depth by chicks and rats. *Science,* 1968, *159,* 892–894.

Schiffman, H. R. Evidence for sensory dominance: Reactions to apparent depth in rabbits, cats, and rodents. *Journal of Comparative and Physiological Psychology,* 1970, *71,* 1, 38–41.

Schiffman, H. R. Depth perception of the Syrian hamster as a function of age and photic conditions of rearing. *Journal of Comparative and Physiological Psychology,* 1971, *76,* 491–495.

Schiffman, H. R., & Bobko, D. J. Effects of stimulus complexity on the perception of brief temporal intervals. *Journal of Experimental Psychology,* 1974, *103,* 156–159.

Schiffman, H. R., & Thompson, J. The role of eye movements in the perception of the horizontal-vertical illusion. *Perception,* 1974, *3,* 49–52.

Schiffman, H. R., & Thompson, J. G. The role of figure orientation and apparent depth in the perception of the horizontal-vertical illusion. *Perception,* 1975, *4,* 79–83.

Schiffman, H. R., & Walk, R. D. Behavior on the visual cliff of monocular as compared to binocular chicks. *Journal of Comparative and Physiological Psychology,* 1963, *56,* 1064–1068.

Schiffman, S. S. The range of gustatory quality: Psychophysical and neural approaches. First Congress of the European Chemoreception Research Organization. Universite de Paris-Sud, Campus d'Orsay, July, 1974. (*a*)

Schiffman, S. S. Physiochemical correlates of

olfactory quality. *Science*, 1974, *185*, 112–117. (*b*)

Schiffman, S. S. Contributions to the physiochemical dimensions of odor: A psychophysical approach. *Annals of the New York Academy of Science*, 1974, *237*, 164–183. (*c*)

Schiffman, S. S. Personal communication, 1975.

Schiffman, S. S., & Dackis, C. Taste of nutrients: Amino acids, vitamins, and fatty acids. *Perception & Psychophysics*, 1975, *17*, 140–146.

Schiffman, S. S., & Erickson, R. P. A theoretical review: A psychophysical model for gustatory quality. *Physiology and Behavior*, 1971, *7*, 617–633.

Schlosberg, H. Stereoscopic depth from single pictures. *American Journal of Psychology*, 1941, *54*, 601–605.

Schouten, J. F. Subjective stroboscopy and a model of visual movement detectors. In W. Wathen-Dunn (Ed.), *Models for the perception of speech and visual form*. Cambridge, Massachusetts: M.I.T. Press, 1967.

Schwartzkopff, J. Hearing. *Annual Review of Physiology*, 1967, *29*, 485–512.

Sechzer, J. A., & Brown, J. L. Color discrimination in the cat. *Science*, 1964, *144*, 427–429.

Segall, M. H., Campbell, D. T., & Herskovits, M. J. *The influence of culture on visual perception*. Indianapolis, Ind.: Bobbs-Merrill, 1966.

Seitz, V., Seitz, T., & Kaufman, L. Loss of depth avoidance in chicks as a function of early environmental influences. *Journal of Comparative and Physiological Psychology*, 1973, *85*, 139–143.

Senden, M., von. Space and sight: *The perception of space and shape in congenitally blind patients before and after operation*. London: Methuen, 1960.

Shankweiler, D. Effects of temporal-lobe damage on perception of dichotically presented melodies. *Journal of Comparative and Physiological Psychology*, 1966, *62*, 115–119.

Shankweiler, D. An analysis of laterality effects in speech perception. In D. L. Horton and J. J. Jenkins (Eds.), *The perception of language*. Columbus, Ohio: Charles E. Merrill, 1971.

Sherif, M. *The psychology of social norms*. New York: Harper & Row, 1936.

Shinkman, P. G. Visual depth discrimination in animals. *Psychological Bulletin*, 1962, *59*, 489–501.

Shinkman, P. G. Visual depth discrimination in day-old chicks. *Journal of Comparative and Physiological Psychology*, 1963, *56*, 410–414.

Shlaer, R. Shift in binocular disparity causes compensatory change in the cortical structure of kittens. *Science*, 1971, *173*, 638–641.

Shlaer, R. An eagle's eye: Quality of the retinal image. *Science*, 1972, *176*, 920–922.

Shower, E. G., & Biddulph, R. Differential pitch sensitivity of the ear. *Journal of the Acoustical Society of America*, 1931, *3*, 275–287.

Siegel, P. V., Gerathewohl, S. J., & Mohler, S. R. Time-zone effects. *Science*, 1969, *164*, 1249–1256.

Simmons, F. B., Epley, J. M., Lummis, R. C., Guttman, N., Frishkopf, L. S., Harmon, L. D., & Zwicker, E. Auditory nerve: Electrical stimulation in man. *Science*, 1965, *148*, 104–106.

Simmons, J. A. The sonar receiver of the bat. *Annals of the New York Academy of Sciences*, 1971, *188*, 161–174.

Simon, H. A. An information-processing explanation of some perceptual phenomena. *British Journal of Psychology*, 1967, *58*, 1–12.

Singer, G., & Day, R. H. Spatial adaptation and aftereffect with optically transformed vision: Effects of active and passive responding and the relationship between test and exposure responses. *Journal of Experimental Psychology*, 1966, *71*, 725–731.

Singh, D., Johnston, R. J., & Klosterman, H. J. Effect on brain enzyme and behaviour in the rat of visual pattern restriction in early life. *Nature*, 1967, *216*, 1337–1338.

Siqueland, E. R., & DeLucia, C. A. Visual reinforcement of nonnutritive sucking in human infants. *Science*, 1969, *165*, 1144–1146.

Sivian, L. J., & White, S. D. On minimum audible sound fields. *Journal of the Acoustical Society of America,* 1933, *4,* 288–321.

Slack, C. W. Familiar size as a cue to size in the presence of conflicting cues. *Journal of Experimental Psychology,* 1956, *52,* 194–196.

Slack, C. W. Critique on the interpretation of cultural differences in the Ames trapezoid. *American Journal of Psychology,* 1959, *72,* 127–131.

Smith, D. V., & McBurney, D. H. Gustatory cross-adaptation: Does a single mechanism code the salty taste? *Journal of Experimental Psychology,* 1969, *80,* 101–105.

Smith, K. U., & Smith, W. M. *Perception and motion.* Philadelphia: W. B. Saunders, 1962.

Smith, K. U., Thompson, G. F., & Koster, H. Sweat in schizophrenic patients: Identification of the odorous substance. *Science,* 1969, *166,* 398–399.

Snyder, F. W., & Pronko, N. H. *Vision with spatial inversion.* Wichita, Kan.: University of Wichita Press, 1952.

Sperling, G. The information available in brief visual presentations. *Psychological Monographs,* 1960, *74,* (No. 11).

Sperling, H. G., & Harweth, R. S. Red-green cone interactions in the increment-threshold spectral sensitivity of primates. *Science,* 1971, *172,* 180–184.

Sperry, R. W. Mechanisms of neural maturation. In Stevens, S. S. (Ed.), *Handbook of experimental psychology.* New York: Wiley, 1951.

Spigel, I. M. *Visually perceived movement.* New York: Harper & Row, 1965.

Spreen, O., Spellacy, F. J., & Reid, J. R. The effect of interstimulus interval and intensity on ear asymmetry for nonverbal stimuli in dichotic listening. *Neuropsychologia,* 1970, *8,* 245–250.

Springer, S. P. Ear asymmetry in a dichotic detection task. *Perception & Psychophysics,* 1971, *10,* 239–241.

Standing, L., Haber, R. N., Cataldo, M., & Sales, D. Two types of short-term visual storage. *Perception & Psychophysics,* 1969, *5,* 193–196.

Stavrianos, B. K. The relation of shape perception to explicit judgments of inclination. *Archives of Psychology,* 1945, No. 296.

Stebbins, W. C. *Animal psychophysics: The design and conduct of sensory experiments.* New York: Appleton: Century-Crofts, 1970.

Stebbins, W. C., Green, S., & Miller, F. L. Auditory sensitivity of the monkey. *Science,* 1966, *153,* 1646–1647.

Steinberg, A. Changes in time perception induced by an anaesthetic drug. *British Journal of Psychology,* 1955, *46,* 273–279.

Steinberg, D. D. Light sensed through receptors in the skin. *American Journal of Psychology,* 1966, *79,* 324–328.

Steinman, R. M., Cunitz, R. J., Timberlake, G. T., & Herman, M. Voluntary control of microsaccades during maintained monocular fixation. *Science,* 1967, *155,* 1577–1579.

Steinman, R. M., Haddad, G. M., Skavenski, A. A., & Wyman, D. Miniature eye movements. *Science,* 1973, *181,* 810–819.

Stent, G. S. Cellular communication. *Scientific American,* 1972, *227,* 42–51.

Steven, D. M. The dermal light sense. *Biological Review,* 1963, *38,* 204–240.

Stevens, S. S. The attributes of tones. *Proceedings of the National Academy of Sciences,* 1934, *20,* 457–459.

Stevens, S. S. The relation of pitch to intensity. *Journal of the Acoustical Society of America,* 1935, *6,* 150–154.

Stevens, S. S. The direct estimate of sensory magnitudes-loudness. *American Journal of Psychology,* 1956, *69,* 1–25.

Stevens, S. S. Adaptation-level vs. the relativity of judgment. *American Journal of Psychology,* 1958, *71,* 633–646.

Stevens, S. S. The psychophysics of sensory function. *American Scientist,* 1960, *48,* 226–253.

Stevens, S. S. To honor Fechner and repeal his law. *Science,* 1961, *133,* 80–86. (*a*)

Stevens, S. S. Psychophysics of sensory function. In W. A. Rosenblith (Ed.), *Sensory Communication*. Cambridge, Mass.: M.I.T. Press, 1961. (*b*)

Stevens, S. S. On the operation known as judgment. *American Scientist*, 1966, *54*, 385–401.

Stevens, S. S. Neural events and the psychophysical law. *Science*, 1970, *170*, 1043–1050.

Stevens, S. S. *Psychophysics, and social scaling*. Morristown, N.J.: General Learning Press, 1972.

Stevens, S. S. *Psychophysics: Introduction to its perceptual, neural and social prospects*. New York: John Wiley, 1975.

Stevens, S. S., & Davis, H. *Hearing*. New York: John Wiley, 1938.

Stevens, S. S., & Volkmann, J. The relation of pitch to frequency. *American Journal of Psychology*, 1940, *53*, 329–356.

Stevens, S. S., & Warshofsky, F. *Sound and hearing*. New York: Life Science Library, 1965.

Stratton, G. M. Some preliminary experiments on vision without inversion of the retinal image. *Psychological Review*, 1896, *3*, 611–617.

Stratton, G. M. Upright vision and the retinal image. *Psychological Review*, 1897, *4*, 182–187. (*a*)

Stratton, G. M. Vision without inversion of the retinal image. *Psychological Review*, 1897, *4*, 341–360. (*b*)

Street, R. F. *A Gestalt completion test*. New York: Teachers College, Columbia University, 1931.

Stromeyer, C. F. Contour-contingent color aftereffects: Retinal area specificity. *American Journal of Psychology*, 1972, *85*, 227–235.

Stromeyer, C. F. & Mansfield, R. Colored aftereffects produced with moving edges. *Perception & Psychophysics*, 1970, *7*, 108–114.

Stoud, J. M. The fine structure of psychological time. In H. Quastler (Ed.), *Information theory and psychology*, Glencoe, Ill.: Free Press, 1956.

Supra, M., Cotzin, M. E., & Dallenbach, K. M. "Facial vision:" The perception of obstacles by the blind. *American Journal of Psychology*, 1944, *57*, 133–183.

Suto, Y. The effect of space on time estimation (*S* effect) in tactual space. II: The role of vision in the *S* effect upon the skin. *Japanese Journal of Psychology*, 1955, *26*, 94–99.

Swets, J. A. (Ed.), *Signal detection and recognition by human observers*. New York: John Wiley, 1964.

Swets, J. A. The relative operating characteristic in psychology. *Science*, 1973, *182*, 990–1000.

Tallarico, R. B., & Farrell, W. M. Studies of visual depth perception: An effect of early experience on chicks on a visual cliff. *Journal of Comparative and Physiological Psychology*, 1964, *57*, 94–96.

Taub, A. Acupunture (letter). *Science*, 1972, *178*, 9.

Taub, E. Prism compensation as a learning phenomenon: A phylogenetic perspective. In S. J. Freedman (Ed.), *The neuropsychology of spatially oriented behavior*. Homewood, Ill.: Dorsey Press, 1968.

Tausch, R. Optishe Täuschungen. *Psychologische Forschung*, 1954, *24*, 299–348.

Taylor, D. W., & Boring, E. G. The moon illusion as a function of binocular regard. *American Journal of Psychology*, 1942, *55*, 189–201.

Taylor, J. G. *The behavioral basis of perception*. New Haven, Conn: Yale University Press, 1962.

Tees, R. C. Effect of visual deprivation on development of depth perception in the rat. *Journal of Comparative and Physiological Psychology*, 1974, *86*, 300–308.

Teevan, R. C., & Birney, R. C. *Color Vision*. Princeton, New Jersey: D. Van Nostrand, 1961.

Teghtsoonian, R., & Teghtsoonian, M. Two varieties of perceived length. *Perception & Psychophysics*, 1970, *8*, 389–392.

Templeton, W. H., Howard, I. P., & Lowman, A. E. Passively generated adaptation to prismatic distortion. *Perceptual and Motor Skills,* 1966, *22,* 140–142.

Terrace, H. S., & Stevens, S. S. The quantification of tonal volume. *American Journal of Psychology,* 1962, *75,* 596–604.

Teuber, H. L. Perception. In J. Field, H. W. Magoun, and V. E. Hall (Eds.), *Handbook of physiology, Section 1, Neurophysiology, Vol. 3.* Washington, D.C.: American Physiological Society, 1960.

Teuber, H. L., Battersby, W. S., & Bender, M. B. *Visual field defects after penetrating missile wounds of the brain.* Cambridge, Mass.: Harvard University Press, 1960.

Teuber, M. L. Sources of ambiguity in the parts of Maurits C. Escher. *Scientific American,* 1974, *231,* 90–104.

Theberge, J. B. Wolf music. *Natural History,* 1971, *80,* 37–42.

Thiéry, A. Über geometrisch-optische Täuschungen. *Philosophische Studien,* 1896, *12,* 307–369.

Thomas, J. P. model of the function of receptive fields in human vision. *Psychological Review,* 1970, *77,* 121–134.

Thompson, J. G., & Schiffman, H. R. The influence of figure size and orientation on the magnitude of the horizontal-vertical illusion. *Acta Psychologica,* 1974, *38,* 413–420 (*a*).

Thompson, J., & Schiffman, H. R. The effect on the magnitude of the horizontal-vertical illusion of horizontal retinal eccentricity. *Vision Research,* 1974, *14,* 1463–1465 (*b*).

Thor, D. H. Diurnal variability in time estimation. *Perceptual and Motor Skills,* 1962, *15,* 451–454.

Thor, D. H., Winters, J. J., & Hoats, D. L. Vertical eye movement and space perception: A developmental study. *Journal of Experimental Psychology,* 1969, *82,* 163–167.

Thouless, R. H. Phenomenal regression to the real object. *British Journal of Psychology,* 1931, *21,* 338–359.

Tolansky, S. *Optical illusions.* Oxford, England: Pergamon Press, 1964.

Treisman, A. M. The effect of irrelevant material on the efficiency of selective listening. *American Journal of Psychology,* 1967, *77,* 533–546.

Treisman, M. Temporal discrimination and the indifference interval: Implications for a model of the "internal clock." *Psychological Monographs,* 1963, *77,* (Whole No. 576).

Trychin, S., & Walk, R. D. A study of the depth perception of monocular hooded rats on the visual cliff. *Psychonomic Science,* 1964, *1,* 53–54.

Underwood, B. J. Experimental Psychology (2nd ed.), Chap. 2. New York: Appleton-Century-Crofts, 1966.

Uttal, W. R. *The psychobiology of sensory coding.* New York: Harper & Row, 1973.

Valenta, J. G., & Rigby, M. K. Discrimination of the odor of stressed rats. *Science,* 1968, *161,* 599–601.

Vandenbergh, J. G., Whitsett, J. M., & Lombardi, J. R. Partial isolation of a pheromone accelerating puberty in female mice. *Journal of Reproduction and Fertility,* 1975, *43,* 515–523.

Vernon, M. D. *Perception through experience.* London: Methuen, 1970.

Verrillo, R. T. Cutaneous sensations. In B. Scharf (Ed.), *Experimental sensory psychology.* Glenview, Ill.: Scott, Foresman, 1975.

Vierck, C. J., & Jones, M. B. Size discrimination on the skin. *Science,* 1969, *158,* 488–489.

Vierling, J. S., & Rock, J. Variations of olfactory sensitivity to Exaltolide during the menstrual cycle. *Journal of Applied Physiology,* 1967, *22,* 311–315.

Volkmar, F. R., & Greenough, W. T. Rearing complexity affects branching of dendrites in the visual cortex of the rat. *Science,* 1972, *176,* 1445–1447.

Wagner, H. G., MacNichol, E. F., & Wolbarsht, M. L. The response properties of single ganglion cells in the goldfish retina. *Journal of General Physiology,* 1960, *43,* 45–62.

Wald, G. Eye and camera. *Scientific American,* 1950, *183,* 32–41.

Wald, G. Life and light. *Scientific American,* 1959, *201,* 92–108.

Walk, R. D. Can the duckling respond adequately to depth? Paper read at 33rd meeting of Eastern Psychological Association, Atlantic City, New Jersey, 1962.

Walk, R. D. The study of visual depth and distance perception in animals. In D. S. Lehrman, R. A. Hinde, & E. Shaw (Eds.) *Advances in the study of behavior.* New York: Academic Press, 1965.

Walk, R. D. VII. The development of depth perception in animals and human infants. *Child Development Monograph,* 1966, *31,* 82–108.

Walk, R. D. Monocular compared to binocular depth perception in human infants. *Science,* 1968, *162,* 473–475.

Walk, R. D., & Dodge, S. H. Visual depth perception of a 10-month-old monocular human infant. *Science,* 1962, *137,* 529–530.

Walk, R. D., & Gibson, E. J. A comparative and analytical study of visual depth perception. *Psychological Monographs,* 1961, *75,* (15, Whole No. 519).

Walk, R. D., Gibson, E. J., Pick, H. L., & Tighe, T. J. Further experiments on prolonged exposure to visual forms: The effect of single stimuli and prior reinforcement. *Journal of Comparative and Physiological Psychology,* 1958, *51,* 483–487.

Walk, R. D., Gibson, E. J., Pick, H. L. & Tighe, T. J. The effectiveness of prolonged exposure to cutouts vs. painted patterns for facilitation of discrimination. *Journal of Comparative and Physiological Psychology,* 1959, *52,* 519–521.

Walk, R. D., Gibson, E. J., & Tighe, T. J. Behavior of light- and dark-reared rats on a visual cliff. *Science,* 1957, *126,* 80–81.

Walk, R. D., Trychin, S., & Karmel, B. Z. Depth perception in the dark-reared rat as a function of time in the dark. *Psychonomic Science,* 1965, *3,* 9–10.

Walk, R. D., & Walters, C. P. Importance of texture-density preferences and motion parallax for visual depth discrimination by rats and chicks. *Journal of Comparative and Physiological Psychology,* 1974, *86,* 309–315.

Walker, J. T. Successive textual contrast: A tactual after-effect. *American Journal of Psychology,* 1966, *79,* 328–329.

Walker, J. T. A texture-contingent visual motion aftereffect. *Psychonomic Science,* 1972, *28,* 333–335.

Wall, P. D., & Sweet, W. H. Temporary abolition of pain in man. *Science,* 1967, *155,* 108–109.

Wallace, G. K. Visual scanning in the desert locust, *Schistocerca gregaria. Journal of Experimental Biology,* 1959, *36,* 512–525.

Wallach, H. Brightness constancy and the nature of achromatic colors. *Journal of Experimental Psychology,* 1948, *38,* 310–324.

Wallach, H. The perception of motion. *Scientific American,* 1959, *201,* 55–60.

Wallach, H. On the moon illusion. *Science,* 1962, *137,* 900–911.

Wallach, H. The perception of neutral colors. *Scientific American,* 1963, *208,* 107–116.

Wallach, H., & Floor, L. The use of size matching to demonstrate the effectiveness of accomodation and convergence as cues for distance. *Perception & Psychophysics,* 1971, *10,* 423–428.

Wallach, H., Newman, E. B., & Rosenzweig, M. R. The precedence effect in sound localization. *American Journal of Psychology,* 1949, *62,* 315–336.

Wallach, H., & O'Connell, D. N. The kinetic depth effect. *Journal of Experimental Psychology,* 1953, *45,* 205–217.

Walls, G. L. Land! Land! *Psychological Bulletin,* 1960, *57,* 29–48.

Walls, G. L. *The vertebrate eye and its adaptive radiation.* New York: Hafner, 1963.

Warden, C. J., & Baar, J. The Müller-Lyer illusion in the ring dove, *Turtur risorius. Journal of Comparative Psychology,* 1929, *9,* 275–292.

Warkentin, J., & Carmichael, L. A study of the development of the air–righting reflex in cats and rabbits. *Journal of Genetic Psychology,* 1939, *55,* 67–80.

Warren, R. M. Perceptual restoration of missing speech sounds. *Science,* 1970, *167,* 392–393.

Warren, R. M., & Pfaffman, C. Suppression of sweet sensitivity by potassium gymnemate. *Journal of Applied Physiology,* 1959, *14,* 40–42.

Warren, R. M., & Warren, R. P. A critique of S. S. Stevens' "New Psychophysics." *Perceptual and Motor Skills,* 1963, *16,* 797–810.

Warren, R. M., & Warren, R. P. Auditory illusions and confusions. *Scientific American,* 1970, *223,* 30–36.

Wasserman, E. A., & Jensen, D. D. Olfactory stimuli and the "pseudo-extinction" effect. *Science,* 1969, *166,* 1307–1309.

Wegel, R. L., & Lane, C. E. The auditory masking of one pure tone by another and its probable relations to the dynamics of the inner ear. *Physiological Review,* 1924, *23,* 266–285.

Wegmouth, F. W. The eye as an optical instrument. In T. C. Ruch, H. D. Patton, J. W. Woodbury, & A. L. Towe (Eds.), *Neurophysiology* (2nd ed.). Philadelphia: W. B. Saunders, 1965.

Weil, A. T., Zinberg, N. E., & Nelson, J. M. Clinical and psychological effects of marijuana in man. *Science,* 1968, *162,* 1234–1242.

Weinstein, S. Intensive and extensive aspects of tactile sensitivity as a function of body part, sex, and laterality. (Chap. 10). In D. R. Kenshalo (Ed.), *The skin senses.* Springfield, Ill.: Charles C. Thomas, 1968.

Weintraub, W. J., & Virsu, V. The misperception of angles: estimating the vertex of converging line segments. *Perception & Psychophysics,* 1971, *9,* 5–8.

Weismann, D. L. *The visual arts as human experience.* Englewood Cliffs, N.J.: Prentice-Hall, 1970.

Weisstein, N. What the frog's eye tells the human brain: Single cell analyzers in the human visual system. *Psychological Bulletin,* 1969, *72,* 157–176.

Weisstein, N. Neural symbolic activity: A psychophysical measure. *Science,* 1970, *168,* 1489–1491.

Wendt, G. R. Vestibular functions. (Chap. 31). In S. S. Stevens (Ed.), *Handbook of experimental psychology.* New York: Wiley, 1951.

Wenger, M. A., Jones, F. N., & Jones, M. H. *Physiological psychology.* New York: Holt, Rinehart and Winston, 1956.

Wenzel, B. M. Chemoreception. In E. C. Carterette & M. P. Friedman (Eds.), *Handbook of Perception.* (Vol. III). New York: Academic Press, 1973.

Wersäll, J., & Flock, A. Functional anatomy of the vestibular and lateral line organs. In W. D. Neff (Ed.), *Contributions to sensory physiology.* (Vol. 1). New York: Academic Press, 1965.

Wertheimer, Max. Principles of perceptual organization. In D. C. Beardslee and M. Wertheimer (Eds.), *Readings in perception.* New York: D. Van Nostrand, 1958. An abridged translation by Michael Wertheimer of Untersuchungen zur Lehre von der Gestalt, II. *Psychologische Forschung,* 1923, *4,* 301–350. Translated and printed by permission of the publisher, Springer, Berlin.

Wertheimer, Michael. Hebb and Senden on the role of learning in perception. *American Journal of Psychology,* 1951, *64,* 133–137.

Wertheimer, Michael. Constant errors in the measurement of kinesthetic figural aftereffects. *American Journal of Psychology,* 1954, *67,* 543–546.

Wertheimer, Michael. Psychometer coordination of auditory and visual space at birth. *Science,* 1961, *134,* 1692.

Wever, E. G. *Theory of hearing*. New York: John Wiley, 1949.

Wever, E. G., & Bray, C. W. Present possibilities for auditory theory. *Psychological Review,* 1930, *37,* 365–380.

Wever, E. G., & Bray, C. W. The perception of low tones and the resonance-volley theory. *Journal of Psychology,* 1937, *3,* 101–114.

White, B. L. Child development research: An edifice without a foundation. *Merrill-Palmer Quarterly of Behavior and Development,* 1969, *15,* 47–78.

White, B. L., Castle, P., & Held, R. Observations on the development of visually-directed reaching. *Child Development,* 1964, *35,* 349–364.

White, B. L., & Held, R. Plasticity of sensorimotor development in the human infant. In J. F. Rosenblith & W. Allinsmith (Eds.), *The causes of behavior: readings in child development and educational psychology.* Boston: Allyn and Bacon, 1966.

White, B. W., Saunders, F. A., Scadden, L., Bach-y-Rita, P., & Collins, C. C. Seeing with the skin. *Perception & Psychophysics,* 1970, *7,* 23–27.

White, C. T. Temporal numerosity and the psychological unit of duration. *Psychological Monographs,* 1963, *77* (12, Whole No. 575).

Wightman, F. L., & Green, D. M. The perception of pitch. *American Scientist,* 1974, *62,* 208–215.

Wilson, E. O. Pheromones. *Scientific American,* 1963, *208,* 100–114.

Wilson, P. D., & Riesen, A. H. Visual development in rhesus monkeys neonatally deprived of patterned light. *Journal of Comparative and Physiological Psychology,* 1966, *61,* 87–95.

Winnick, W. A., & Rogoff, I. Role of apparent slant in shape judgments. *Journal of Experimental Psychology,* 1965, *69,* 554–563.

Witkin, H. A. The perception of the upright. *Scientific American,* 1959, *200,* 50–70.

Wolf, G. Innate mechanisms for regulation of so-dium intake. In C. Pfaffman (Ed.), *Olfaction and taste.* New York: Rockefeller University Press, 1969.

Wood, C. C., Goff, W. R., & Day, R. S. Auditory evoked potentials during speech perception. *Science,* 1971, *173,* 1248–1251.

Wood, H. Psychophysics of active kinesthesis. *Journal of Experimental Psychology,* 1969, *79,* 480–485.

Woodrow, H. Time perception. In S. S. Stevens (Ed.) *Handbook of Experimental Psychology,* New York: John Wiley, 1951.

Woodworth, R. S. *Experimental psychology.* New York: Henry Holt, 1938.

Woodworth, R. S. *Psychology* (4th ed.). New York: Henry Holt, 1940.

Woodworth, R. S., & Schlosberg, H. *Experimental psychology.* New York: Henry Holt, 1954.

Worshel, P., & Dallenbach, K. M. "Facial vision": Perception of obstacles by the deaf-blind. *American Journal of Psychology,* 1947, *60,* 502–553.

Worshel, P., & Dallenbach, K. M. The vesibular sensitivity of deaf-blind subjects. *American Journal of Psychology,* 1948, *61,* 94–98.

Wright, W. D. A re-determination of trichromatic coefficients of the spectral colours. *Transactions of the Optical Society of London,* 1928–1929, *30,* 141–164.

Yarbus, A. L. *Eye movement and vision.* New York: Plenum Press, 1967.

Yeager, J. Absolute time estimates as a function of complexity and interruption of melodies. *Psychonomic Science,* 1969, *15,* 177–178.

Young, F. A. Development of optical characteristics for seeing. In F. A. Young & D. B. Lindsley (Eds.), *Early experience and visual information processing in perceptual and reading disorders.* National Academy of Sciences, 1970.

Youtz, R. P. Aphotic digital color sensing. *American Psychologist,* 1964, *19,* 734.

Zahorik, D. M., & Maier, S. F. Appetitive conditioning with recovery from thiamine deficiency as the unconditional stimulus. *Psychonomic Science*, 1969, *17,* 309–310.

Zeigler, H. P., & Leibowitz, H. Apparent visual size as a function of distance for children and adults. *American Journal of Psychology,* 1957, *70,* 106–109.

Zelazo, P. R., Zelazo, N. A., & Kolb, S. "Walking" in the newborn. *Science*, 1972, *176,* 314–315.

Zotterman, Y. Studies in the neural mechanism of taste. In W. A. Rosenblith (Ed.), *Sensory communication.* Cambridge, Mass.: M.I.T. Press, 1961.

Zubeck, J. P., & Bross, M. Depression and later enhancement of the critical flicker frequency during prolonged monocular deprivation. *Science,* 1972, *176,* 1045–1047.

Zusne, L. Visual perception of form. New York: Academic Press, 1970.

Zwicker, E., & Scharf, B. Model of loudness summation. *Psychological Review,* 1965, *72,* 3–26.

Author Index

Subject Index